High Dependency Nursing Care

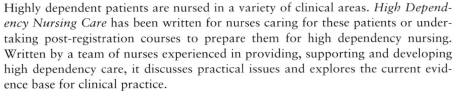

Highly dependent patients are nursed in a variety of clinical areas. *High Dependency Nursing Care* has been written for nurses caring for these patients or undertaking post-registration courses to prepare them for high dependency nursing. Written by a team of nurses experienced in providing, supporting and developing high dependency care, it discusses practical issues and explores the current evidence base for clinical practice.

Structured in four parts, the first, *Perspectives on High Dependency Care* explores the contexts of care, focusing on fundamental aspects, like sleep, nutrition, pain management and stress, demonstrating how to achieve quality nursing care. *Pathophysiology and Treatments* describes the main diseases that cause critical illness and the treatments that patients will often be given. Critically ill patients need to be monitored closely so *Monitoring and Skills* enables nurses to interpret and understand the information gained from observation and monitoring. The final part, *Professional Issues* explores topics such as Clinical Governance, Reflection, Practice Development and Managing Change to assist nurses in developing their own clinical practice and professional development.

High Dependency Nursing Care is:

- **Comprehensive** – it covers all the key areas of knowledge needed
- **User-friendly** – it includes learning outcomes, fundamental knowledge, introductions, time out exercises, implications for practice, useful websites, up-to-date references
- **Clearly written** – by a team of experienced nurses
- **Practically based** – clinical scenarios provide stimulating discussion and revision topics.

Tina Moore is a Senior Lecturer at Middlesex University, London. **Philip Woodrow** is a Practice Development Nurse in Critical Care at East Kent Hospitals NHS Trust and author of *Intensive Care Nursing* (Routledge 2000).

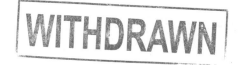

High Dependency Nursing Care

Observation, Intervention and Support

Edited by Tina Moore and Philip Woodrow

with

Sarah Coulling, Noirin Egan, Sandra Gallacher, Debbie Higgs, Vikki Howarth, Sheila O'Sullivan and Mary Tilki

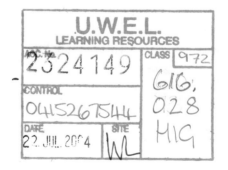
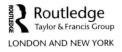

Routledge
Taylor & Francis Group

LONDON AND NEW YORK

First published 2004
by Routledge
11 New Fetter Lane, London EC4P 4EE

Simultaneously published in the USA and Canada
by Routledge
29 West 35th Street, New York, NY 10001

Routledge is an imprint of the Taylor & Francis Group

© 2004 Tina Moore and Philip Woodrow

Typeset in Sabon by Wearset Ltd, Boldon, Tyne and Wear
Printed and bound in Great Britain by The Cromwell Press, Trowbridge, Wiltshire

British Library Cataloguing in Publication Data
A catalogue record for this book is available from the British Library

Library of Congress Cataloging in Publication Data
A catalog record for this book has been requested

ISBN 0–415–26755–2 (Pb)
ISBN 0–415–26754–4 (Hb)

For my Mum, Dad and three little angels – Vincent, Charlene and Calvin

T.M.

For Laura and Michael

P.W.

Contents

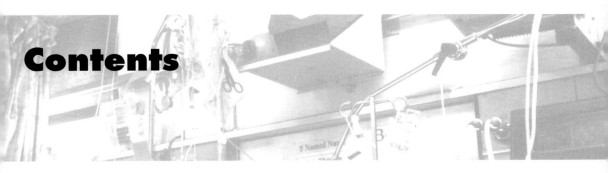

Part 2: Pathophysiology and treatments

Part 3: Monitoring and skills

Part 4: Professional issues

Figures

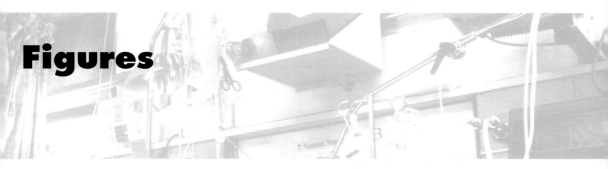

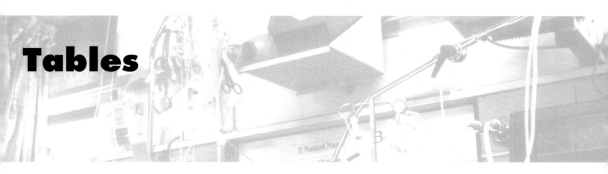

Tables

Boxes

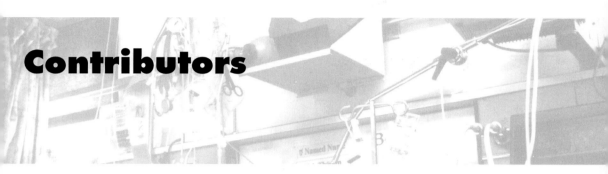

Contributors

Tina Moore is Senior Lecturer in Adult and High Dependency Nursing at Middlesex University, London. Her previous publications include journal articles relating to sensory deprivation and suctioning. She is co-writer of a chapter in a book entitled: *Managing Diversity in Nursing* (2001), published by Harcourt Brace.

Philip Woodrow is Practice Development Nurse in Critical Care at the East Kent Hospitals NHS Trust where he delivers a five-day course for ward staff caring for highly dependent (level 2) patients. His previous publications include *Intensive Care Nursing: a Framework for Practice* (Routledge 2000), *Ageing: Issues for Physiological, Psychological and Social Health* (Whurr 2002), and many articles in the nursing press.

Sarah Coulling is Clinical Nurse Specialist for Acute Pain Services at the East Kent Hospitals NHS Trust.

Noirin Egan is Senior Sister in the Coronary Care Unit at Chase Farm NHS Trust Hospital.

Sandra Gallacher is Lecturer/Practitioner in Critical Care at Middlesex University, London.

Debbie Higgs is Consultant Nurse in Critical Care at the East Kent Hospitals NHS Trust.

Vikki Howarth is Senior Nurse Manager in Intensive Care at Chase Farm Hospital NHS Trust.

Sheila O'Sullivan is Lead Nurse for Critical Care Outreach at Whittingdon Hospital NHS Trust.

Mary Tilki is Principal Lecturer and member of the Research Centre for Transcultural Studies in Health in the School of Health and Social Sciences, Middlesex University. Her publications include *Transcultural Education and Care, Older People from Minority Ethnic Groups* and *The Health of Irish People in Britain*.

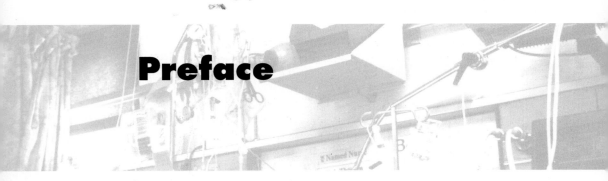

Preface

This text is adult-focused, so although pathologies and treatments may be relevant to children as well, there may be significantly different approaches to paediatric care. Readers wishing to know more about childhood conditions should seek a paediatric text.

Advances in medicine have encouraged increasing specialisation within nursing. In the second half of the twentieth century, specialised units developed to offer intensive care (ICU), coronary care (CCU), high dependency (HDU) and other critical care. However, insufficient provision resulted in some critically ill patients not being cared for in specialist critical care areas (Carr, 2002). During the 1990s, various audits, most notably by McQuillan *et al.* (1998), led the Department of Health to publish *Comprehensive Critical Care* (DOH, 2000a). This suggested radical revision of care, from being centred on geographical areas to being focused on patients' needs. It identified four levels of care:

Level 0 Patients whose needs can be met through normal ward care in an acute hospital

Level 1 Patients at risk of their condition deteriorating, or those recently relocated from higher levels of care, whose needs can be met on an acute ward with additional advice and support from the critical care team

Level 2 Patients requiring more detailed observation or intervention, including support for a single failing organ system or post-operative care and those 'stepping down' from higher levels of care

Level 3 Patients requiring advanced respiratory support alone or basic respiratory support together with support of at least two organ systems. This level includes all complex patients requiring support for multi-organ failure.

There is a continuum stretching from level 0 to level 3, with some inevitable overlap. The Intensive Care Society (2002) suggests that examples of level 2 (the focus of this book) include patients who:

- are receiving more than 50% oxygen
- are haemodynamic unstable due to hypovolaemia/haemorrhage/sepsis
- have acute impairment of renal, electrolyte or metabolic function
- have had major elective surgery
- have a tachycardia above 120 beats per minute
- are hypotensive with a systolic below 80 mmHg for more than 1 hour
- have a Glasgow Coma Scale score below 10 and are at risk of acute deterioration.

Aspects of this book are applicable to other (level 0, 1 and 3) patients, so nurses should use their professional skills to assess and plan care to meet individual needs. The book is written primarily for qualified nurses, so although the authors hope that material is useful for student nurses and other healthcare professionals, material in the text assumes that readers already have the knowledge and experience of qualified nurses. Where foreknowledge is assumed, chapters identify *Fundamental knowledge* at the start so readers can assess whether they need to revise anything before reading the chapter. *Clinical scenarios* are also included in each chapter to enable readers to relate theory to their practice. Many chapters include *Time out* exercises to help readers reflect on practice.

Throughout the text the word 'patient' includes any recipient of healthcare services, who may also be described as a 'client'.

Tina Moore and Philip Woodrow

Acknowledgements

We would like to acknowledge Edwina Welham for commissioning the book, and everyone at Routledge involved in the production and marketing and sales process. Our special thanks go to Moira Taylor, Senior Development Editor at Routledge, for developing and supporting the book throughout a long writing process, and to John Albarran at the University of the West of England and Jane Roe at St George's Hospital, London, for their exceptional input as reviewers. We thank all those who also read single chapters during this period.

Part 1

Perspectives on high dependency care

Chapter 1

The nature of high dependency nursing

Tina Moore

Contents

Learning outcomes

After reading this chapter you will be able to:

- Demonstrate knowledge of the changes occurring within critical care
- Understand the principles of high dependency nursing
- Appreciate the role of advocacy and the critically ill patient.

Fundamental knowledge

Humanism, health promotion, ethics, clinical governance (see Chapters 2, 10, 12, 36).

Introduction

The philosophy of high dependency nursing pervades this book. This particular chapter will provide a summary/overview of the nature of high dependency nursing.

Time out 1.1

1   Think back to when you first cared for critically ill patients. What do you consider to be the main aspects of care?
2   Write down the current approaches to care that you have been involved in.
3   Have you noticed any changes in the way these patients are cared for?
4   If so, why do you think these changes have occurred?

During the 1990s the adequacy of intensive care provision was questioned, mainly following media coverage and damning reports that highlighted inadequate/failing critical care services. This led to a report by the Department of Health in 1995 exploring the provision of intensive care services throughout the country (DOH, 1995). Its findings were that:

■   The number, distribution and use of intensive care beds varied around the country
■   Admission criteria varied (and were absent in some units)
■   Admissions were frequently refused because of staff shortages
■   One in six referrals to intensive care was inappropriate.

Research by Goldhill and Sumner (1998) suggested that the patient group with the highest mortality in intensive care units comprised those patients admitted from hospital wards. These reports prompted a review of adult critical care services by the Department of Health in April 1999 and an expert group was appointed to develop a framework for the future organisation and delivery of critical care. This expert group consisted largely of doctors and managers, with few nurses but no other healthcare professionals. As a result of this review, critical care has seen a number of significant changes in the approach to caring for the critically ill patient. Until recently, development has been unplanned and haphazard and has largely relied on the interest of local clinicians. Today, however, there is a more consistent approach to the organisation of critical care services, achieved through the strategic publication *Comprehensive Critical Care* (DOH, 2000a).

The strategy describes a complete process of care for the critically ill and focuses on the level of care needed by individual patients and their families at any point during their illness (DOH, 2001a). It is referred to as a 'whole systems' approach that attends to the needs of those at risk of critical illness as well as those who are critically ill, thus adopting a proactive approach. The Comprehensive Critical Care strategy is seen as a uniform standard throughout the NHS, regardless of location or speciality – i.e. it is a 'no walls' philosophy. It is viewed as a new speciality based on the severity of illness, and with a focus on the needs of the patient being central to the service provided.

This approach outlines a modernisation programme to develop consistent and comprehensive critical care services, and highlights the need for action in four areas:

Patient allocation should be based on the skill mix and competency within the nursing ratio, enabling those observations to be understood, analysed and acted upon 24 hours a day.

The traditional role of the intensive care nurse has been developed by the addition of medical tasks (RCN Critical Care Forum, 1997), creating a blurring of boundaries between contemporary nursing and medical roles. The RCN (2003:93) defines a critical care nurse as 'a registered nurse who has the right knowledge, skills and competence to meet the needs of the critically ill patient without direct supervision'. Critical care skills are not only important in providing appropriate and safe nursing care but should also aid the prevention of critical illness. Constant observation of the vulnerable critically ill is imperative. This involves the assimilation, interpretation and evaluation of a patient's physical and psychological status.

Nurses caring for critically ill patients need to have the ability to:

■ Collect data, interpret information and act appropriately
■ Based on patient cues, make decisions quickly, accurately and often independently
■ Be attentive to the minute detail of patient care for prolonged periods of time
■ Be proactive, make predictions and prevent complications, and provide prompt and skilled intervention in the event of sudden deterioration (RCN, 2003)
■ Gain a specialist body of knowledge pertinent to the care of critically ill patients, and promote competent care
■ Respond quickly and effectively in a variety of emergency situations
■ Be an effective team member
■ Work efficiently within a potentially stressful environment
■ Deliver holistic care including the family and significant others.

Advocacy

Time out 1.2

1 Write down your definition of advocacy, highlighting the key words.
2 Consider how you advocate for the patients within your care.
3 Compare your actions to the words previously highlighted. Is there any difference?

The term 'advocacy' has become a convenient 'buzzword' that is linked with concepts of morality, ethics, autonomy and patient empowerment (Snowball, 1996). The interpretation of advocacy in nursing varies from place to place. The American view is concerned with empowering clients to self-advocate through a two-fold process of informing and supporting (Teasdale, 1998), but in the UK most writers dispute this view. Baldwin (2003) has, through a concept analysis, highlighted that in most cases when nurses act as advocates for patients, they do so by attempting to influence a third party on behalf of their clients. This debate over the meaning of advocacy must be resolved. If the profession is unable to clarify the meaning of advocacy, nurses will be ill prepared to promote advocacy as part of their professional role (Mallik, 1997).

Within critical care the majority of patients are dependent, and this places a demand on the nurse to shoulder the role of advocate (Lindahl and Sandman, 1998). Reservations have been expressed regarding the suitability of nurses to act as patient advocates (Allmark and Klarzynski, 1992). Woodrow (1997) asserts that, contrary to the meaning of the law, if patients are unable to choose their nurse, it follows that they cannot choose their advocate. Oddly, as nurses are not chosen as advocates by the patients themselves, the patients may need an advocate to protect them from the nurse (Chadwick and Tadd, 1992). Woodrow (1997) suggests that such autocratic implementation militates against effective advocacy. Within critical care there is no alternative; the majority of patients are in no position to choose their advocate, although the situation may change once a patient's condition improves. Relatives may undertake advocacy, but without the patient's choice or consent.

There is a moral duty to protect patients' rights and autonomy, and it may be difficult for nurses to advocate for patients they don't know (due to severity of illness, unconsciousness, etc.). Once healthcare interventions have been adapted to meet the special needs of the patient, the nurse's role is to articulate the patient's needs within the multidisciplinary team, creating a patient-centred approach to care.

The advocacy role of the nurse has been hindered by the limited practical guidance offered on how this role should be interpreted in clinical practice. Empirical evidence is sparse and a few individuals ground theories in anecdotal accounts (Hewitt, 2002). A small-scale study conducted by Lindahl and Sandman (1998) highlighted the following themes within the role of an advocate:

■   Building a caring relationship
■   Being committed to the patient
■   Empowering the patient (shifting of appropriate power)
■   Being a moral agent
■   Creating a recovery and trusting atmosphere conducive to recovery.

Advocacy should be viewed as a temporary role. In order to promote the nurses' role as advocate, they need to be willing to hand over power and control to the patient (see Chapter 10); this can be achieved through educating nurses in theory and practice. One aim of promoting the advocacy role is that the patient's autonomy is secured. Literature addressing nursing ethics also notes that patient advocacy is supported by the principle of autonomy because the nurse is obliged to enable patients to be self-determining. A therapeutic nurse–patient relationship should secure patients' freedom and self-determination. Nurses have a role in promoting and protecting patients' rights to be involved in decision-making and informed consent.

Implications for practice

- Assessment of the patient is dependent upon his or her care needs, and not the location
- Nurses need to be willing to take on the responsibility for advocacy and for releasing control
- Nurses should actively be involved in constantly enhancing the quality of care provision
- Critical care nurses need sound generic knowledge together with critical care knowledge.

Summary

Nursing the critically ill patient is not restricted to traditional intensive care and high dependency units and therefore ward staff will need to expand their level of expertise to be able to care for these patients effectively and efficiently. Care is not just physiologically orientated, but should be holistic, acknowledging psychological, emotional and social influences.

Bibliography

Useful websites

www.doh.gov.uk/jointunit/jip.htm
www.doh.gov.uk/nhsexec.compcritcare.htm
www.lscn.co.uk (London Standing conference – Critical Care website)

Key reading

DOH documents.

Further reading

Baldwin, M. (2003) provides a comprehensive analysis of advocacy.

Chapter 2

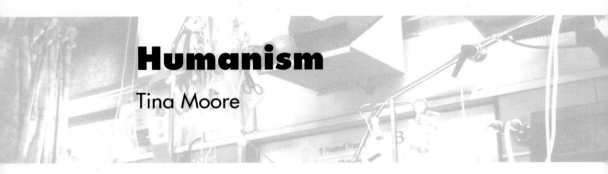

Humanism

Tina Moore

Contents

Learning outcomes

After reading this chapter you will be able to:

- Identify the characteristics of dehumanisation
- Understand the effects that technology can have on the patient
- Comprehend the importance of delivering appropriate, sensitive care to patients within high dependency units.

Introduction

In recent years the development and spread of modern technology within health care has occurred at a phenomenal rate. More highly sophisticated machines are being placed at the bedside in an attempt to provide further continuous and accurate monitoring and in some cases to assist in the diagnostic process. Consequently, technology has become one of the major determinants that shape the delivery of critical care. This is a reciprocal relationship that will not end, and therefore, nurses should try to minimise the potentially conflicting demands of technology and the needs of humanity.

This chapter identifies problems associated with the use of technology, particularly those relating to humanity. Suggestions will be offered enabling nurses to create and maintain a balance between delivering a humanistic approach to care, and the demands incurred by technology.

Time out 2.1

Write down your views about the use of technology within your area of practice. Make a list of advantages and disadvantages.

Can technology be dehumanising?

Technology can be viewed as having an intrusive and imposing presence within the critical care environment. Its dominance may cause experiences of care being invisible. In view of this, the concept of inhumanity has been linked to critical care.

Mitcham (1994) identifies two perspectives of technology – technological optimism and technological romanticism. Technological optimism views technology as being beneficial for nursing, whereas technological romanticism suggests that technology is disruptive and even dangerous to nursing. Generally, nurses share a combination of these views.

Table 2.1 highlights the tensions caused by technology.

Table 2.1 Opposing characteristics of personal and technological care (Cooper, 1993)

People	Technology
Non-invasive	Invasive
Irrational	Rational
Care	Cure
Subjective	Objective
Unpredictable	Predictable
Vulnerable	Invulnerable
Semi-obtrusive	Obtrusive
Empowerment	Helplessness

Mitcham (1994) rightly states that technology is neither inherently good nor bad (a neutral view), but rather will have good effects if used appropriately and bad effects if misused or abused. There is a need to create a balance.

Technology can create a barrier to human interactions, inducing dehumanisation. Families may be reluctant to touch loved ones who are connected to machines. This often results from the fear of upsetting equipment and causing possible malfunctions. Patients who are confined or restricted by and dependent on equipment may remind family members of the loss of control that they have, not only over their loved ones but also over their own destiny. This can lead to feelings of vulnerability and helplessness. Owing to the demands of technology, nurses may become distracted from being involved in the personal emotional care. Andrew (1998) tries to address this point, and states that amongst the technology there is a person who is a precious and significant part of the family's life.

Factors that contribute to dehumanisation in the critical setting include:

- Inconsistent philosophies about patient care delivery and decision-making (e.g. paternalism versus patient autonomy)
- Personal and professional value conflicts (e.g. prolonging life, care versus cure)
- Poor communication patterns (e.g. one-way communication, missing patient cues)
- Unresolved ethical dilemmas (e.g. withholding information, failure to respect patient autonomy)
- Increased technology (e.g. clinical information systems, extra monitoring equipment)
- Shortages of human and material resources (e.g. shortage of technical support, poor patient ratios)
- Inadequate support systems for staff delivering care (e.g. lack of clinical supervision, performance reviews and staff development plans)
- Lack of professional skill in the various dimensions of humane care (e.g. patient consent, advocacy)
- Inadequate administrative support (e.g. nurses having to answer telephones rather than deliver care)
- The physical design of the unit environment (e.g. bed-space small, difficulty in reaching the patient).

(Harvey *et al.*, 1992)

The nature of the critical illness necessitates the initial prioritisation of physical needs, but in doing so a number of human needs – psychological, social and general – may be compromised (Carnevale, 1991).

Technical optimists suggest that technology is not necessarily opposed to humanised care, but can indeed specifically and deliberately engage in the service of humanising it (Barnard and Sandelowski, 2001). Hence, technology is seen as a means to an end.

In an attempt to increase the professional status of nursing and to prove that nursing has its own body of knowledge, there has been a preoccupation to make nursing more scientifically based. As a result, nursing has become infused with a positivistic ideology that is based upon a rationalistic approach to caring. Scientific knowledge is the basis of medicine and technology, as well as being associated with the dehumanisation, depersonalisation and objectification of patients. Dehumanisation can be associated with depriving patients of their individuality, subjectivity and dignity as human beings, with overcoming the alienation between self and body, and with separating nurses from their mission to care (Barnard and Sandelowski, 2001). Historically, technology has been linked to the medicalisation (medical model based on positivism) of nursing and, as a consequence, the loss of nursing's own identity.

The philosophy of positivism includes:

■ The knowledge of factors that have developed from things that are directly observable (empiricism)
■ The belief that human experiences can be reduced to quantifiable logical data (reductionism)
■ Explanation, prediction and control
■ Observations that are objective and value-free.

Indeed, Playle (1995) warns that there is a danger in the acceptance of objectivity. He suggests that the objective attitude and positivist definitions of science will cause continuing dehumanisation of people and processes. Rushton (1991) predicts that the dehumanisation process could go beyond the patient to the caregivers and families. Hence, an important dimension of human caring could be lost.

Time out 2.2

Having read the content above, are the views cited similar to your own? Think of differences and similarities.

Humanism

Nursing's art versus science debate is an ongoing one. Humanism may be seen as being in tension and conflict with scientific values. The identification/realisation of a more humanistic approach to nursing care and the increasing emphasis on the nurse–patient relationship has had a major impact on the way in which nursing is practised and taught.

Nursing has seen a gradual shift away from the illness-cure model towards a more holistic individualised and person-centred approach. Humanism refers to any system or mode of thought or action in which human interest, value and dignity predominate (Rushton, 1991). It reflects a philosophy that emphasises an individual's uniqueness and freedom to choose a particular course of action. This is grounded in the idea that as individuals we are the only ones who can know our perceptions; we are therefore the best experts on ourselves. If patients are unable to achieve this self-knowledge (and many of them within the critical care unit are not), then the family should be involved in the delivery of care, including decision-making. As the patient's advocate, nurses still need to embark upon a sensitive approach to delivering care in accordance to their perceptions of the patient's needs.

According to Harvey *et al.* (1991) the principles of humanism suggest that:

- Each individual is unique and has specific needs, values and beliefs
- Individuals are the source of expertise and authority regarding their own unique needs
- The patient's and the patient's family's autonomy is to be preserved
- Patient and family privacy is to be respected
- The patient and loved ones participate in healthcare decisions to the extent they desire
- The quest for humane care should not compromise patient safety, and nor should it cross regulatory, legal or ethical boundaries.

The need for patient-centred care through a humanistic framework

Buus-Frank (1999) formulated eight guidelines for integrating technology within care. Although the work is written specifically for neonatal intensive care setting, its main principles can be generalised across the critical care environment, as all human needs are similar irrespective of the clinical location.

Guideline 1: Technology systems must be patient-centred

There may be situations where nurses enter the patient's bed space and attend to the machines first before looking at or acknowledging the patient. It is vital that the potential impact of any new technology on the patient and family is always considered. Nurses should be extremely careful not to create an environment or culture in which caring is diverted to machines, rather than patients and families (White, 1996).

Guideline 2: Technology must be thoughtfully applied

Technology must demonstrate a clear benefit to the patient, the family or the provider. Solid evidence is needed to support safety, efficacy and the appropriate use of new technologies. The impact on outcomes and cost (particularly risks and benefits) must also be analysed (Brans, 1991).

Guideline 3: Technology should have an invisible interface when possible

The bright lights and noxious sounds of a critical care unit are extremely frightening and intimidating to the patient and relatives. This foreign environment places them in a dependent role, and may influence the family's access to and involvement with care (Miles *et al.*, 1993).

Guideline 4: Technology should be carefully integrated

Wherever possible, physiological monitoring and therapeutic machines need to work in harmony, or 'talk to each other'.

Guideline 5: Nurses must avoid an over-reliance on technology

There is a critical need for nurses to interpret the data using other senses and experience, which means observing the patient in addition to the data output of the machine (see Chapter 28).

Guideline 6: Technology must be evaluated

Evaluation and assessment of new technology should occur in order to ensure optimum use and outcomes.

Guideline 7: Sometimes less is best!

There may be an over-reliance on technology that is perhaps not required.

Guideline 8: Technology cannot replace humanity

Cooper (1993) describes the highly technical critical care environment as an alien world to the patients and families who face it.

Time out 2.3

Technology is an essential component of critical care nursing. How could you minimise the effects of such an invasion on the patients and relatives?

Optimising patient care through a humanistic framework

The relationship between technology and care is paradoxical, holding in tension the objective values of science and the subjective values of human well-being (Cooper, 1993). Patients and their families see nurses as the interface between themselves and the technology (McConnell, 1996).

Nurses who are effective in their care delivery will know how to interact with technology and with people. They will understand the principles behind the technology they use in order to be able to recognise and respond to patient needs, particularly when a problem develops or a patient's condition changes. For example, if a patient is having arterial blood pressure monitoring and a flattened waveform occurs, there is a need to look beyond the equipment at the patient's searching for other indicators to support the technological findings. Nurses must be able to solve problems and think critically. Care has been described as a moral imperative for nurses, relying on empirical, aesthetic, ethical and personal knowledge (Carper, 1978).

Critical care nurses should continually assess the patient and the effect that technology has or may have on the patient, and take appropriate action to minimise this effect. For example, if a patient is to have non-invasive ventilation (NIV), the nurse should explain (using simple language) the equipment and enable as much movement as possible, perhaps even allowing the patient to sit out of bed. Nurses are in a unique position, as people who have special knowledge and skills about others and their responses to illness and as a result should be able to make sense of the patients' human experience (Taylor, 1994). The balance between the delivery of competent care through the use of modern technology and the humanity of care poses a challenge to nurses within the critical care environment. With each recounting of a caring experience by nurses (possibly through reflective practice), care becomes more visible and valued.

Optimising the human experience includes:

- Being there
- Sharing
- Supporting
- Involving
- Interpreting
- Advocating.

(Andrew, 1998)

The concept of 'being there', as described by Watson (1999) and Ashworth (1990) goes beyond being physically present and involves connectedness in a holistic way – i.e. being empathetic and emotionally/psychologically available. However, it is necessary to give a sense of space and time to both the patient and family members. The notion of presence requires the nurse to recognise that simply being with a patient (mentally as well as physically) can be therapeutic in itself, and therefore the nurse is seen as a therapeutic tool (Walsh, 2000). In order to achieve this, it is vital that nurses are self-aware and in touch with their own values and beliefs.

Humane care recognises the uniqueness of each patient and strives to provide a holistic approach to caring. The provision of care within a humanistic framework is dynamic, individualised, and also requires the involvement of the patient and his or her carers (where possible) (Rushton, 1991). Watson (1999) provides the links between the concepts of humanism and care. She states that caring is viewed as the moral ideal of nursing, where there is utmost concern for human dignity and preservation of humanity. Fostering humane care for patients and their families cannot occur unless the environment also treats the caregivers humanely.

Implications for practice

- Nurses should continually assess the patient and family for the effect technology has on them
- The delivery of safe, efficient and effective care needs to be balanced with sensitive, caring approaches

- The concept of humanism should be integral to the provision of care
- Nurses need to be self-aware before they can embark upon the delivery of humanistic care.

Summary

As technology continues to evolve, the challenge for critical care nurses remains clear: to function effectively within a patient-driven system in which nurses can care for patients and their families in a holistic fashion. That challenge gives a clear mandate for critical care technology: it must function efficiently and invisibly so nurses can spend less time staring at monitors and writing in charts and more time interacting directly with patients and families (McConnell, 1996). Modern technology should be utilised to allow just that, releasing more time for nurses to provide emotional, psychological and sociological care. Hence, technology should be used to help critical care nurses to care in an efficient and effective manner.

Nursing is both an art and a science, and therefore it is in nursing's best interest to be conversant with changes for its own survival but not at the expense of humane caring. Technology has to be integrated into everyday practices. For that reason, nurses must retain the caring humanistic qualities that have threaded through the profession, as well as the evidence-based practice. It is important not to lose sight of the foundations of caring, as identified by Roach (1987) when she identified the five 'C's of professional caring:

- Compassion
- Competence
- Confidence
- Commitment
- Conscience.

There is a need to integrate care and technology to the extent where technology does not impede care but enhances it. Nurses must be competent in managing the technology, even though technological competence does not necessarily have an easy relationship with the response of care.

Clinical scenario

Anna Cummings, 46 years old, is behaving in an agitated manner; she looks anxious and in pain. Cardiovascularly, she has a tachycardia of 148 bpm, her BP is 150/100 mmHg and she is sweaty. One of her ECG electrodes becomes disconnected, and the monitor alarms repeatedly. Noise from the alarm further upsets Anna. When the nurse approaches, Anna apologises profusely for setting off the monitor alarm.

1   How should the nurse respond? (Analyse the tensions between caring and technology.)

2   Formulate a plan to humanise the patient's environment.

3   Analyse why the patient felt she was the cause of the equipment alarming (consider the nurse's behaviour – non-verbal, observing and touching equipment more than the patient).

Bibliography

Key reading

Andrew (1998) provides insight into the experiences of families.

Further reading

Playle (1995) presents thought-provoking arguments relating to humanism and positivism.

Chapter 3

Stress

Tina Moore

Contents

Learning outcomes

After reading this chapter you will be able to:

- Identify the major causes of stress within the critical care unit for both the patient and the nurse
- Discuss the physiological changes that occur in response to stress
- Understand the management of stress.

Fundamental knowledge

Physiological signs of anxiety.

Introduction

It is debatable whether caring for the critically ill is more stressful than other areas of nursing. Nurses working in critical care units are exposed to different types of stressors, e.g. life-sustaining treatment, complex decision-making, continuous crisis atmosphere and complex technology. Stress is a subjective phenomenon and is dependent upon multiple variables – e.g. the nurse's level of competence and experience, the severity of the patient's illness, past experiences, perceptions of the situation, and the complexity of decision-making. Considering these variables, any clinical environment has the potential to be stressful.

There are various definitions of stress, each containing many meanings, which makes them confusing and ill-defined. Nevertheless, they all have a common attribute – the relationship between environmental influences and the individual.

Stress is a constant state of tension to which an individual is subjected whilst being incapable of controlling or finding adequate responses to it (Goldhill and Worthington, 1999). Stress can be viewed as a response to perceived demand, and is therefore a situation that is created when an individual is faced with any stimulus that causes disequilibrium in homeostatic functioning (Hudak *et al.*, 1998). This function is dependent upon the individual's ability to perceive and appraise the situation. Consequently, any situation can activate stress.

There is a tendency to concentrate on the negative components of stress and, where possible, to attempt to avoid stress-provoking situations. Stress can and does act as a motivator. This can be seen in individuals who work in critical care environments for significant periods of time, and in those who thrive on some degree of stress. A certain amount of stress is considered to be desirable for adaptation to occur. Problems arise when coping mechanisms fail and stress becomes counterproductive. Initial signs include lack of concentration, anxiety and insomnia.

This chapter aims to identify some of the sources of stress from both patient and nurse perspectives.

Stressors

The inability to cope with excess demand will possibly lead to prolonged stress and abnormal responses (physical and/or psychological), affecting the quality of life and performance. Stressors may be:

- Biological (injury or illness)
- Psychosocial (interpersonal conflicts, poor communication)
- Environmental (unfamiliarity with the surroundings, technology).

Stressors can be harmful, threatening or indeed challenging. Individuals' ability to cope will be different depending upon their perception and appraisal, and the supportive mechanisms in place, as well as their own health status. The more uncontrollable an event seems, the more likely it is to be perceived as stressful.

Coping strategies can be problem-focused and/or emotion-focused (Lookinland, 1995). Problem-focused strategies are directed towards alerting the stressor, and involve identification of the problem and the generation of ideas to solve it.

Emotion-focused strategies involve developing and regulating the accompanying distressful emotions. Strategies may involve distancing, escape avoidance, self-control, positive appraisal and acceptance of responsibility (Lookinland, 1995). Patients may view similar situations in different ways, resulting in different consequences for long-term adjustment.

Models of stress

There are various models of stress. Stimulus-based models relate to the relationship between the external causes of stress and the individuals who are exposed to it. These models may be useful in identifying external stressors, such as noise or poor air quality, but they fail to identify the individual's responses to the stressor(s).

Probably the most well-known model is Selye's (1956) General Adaptation Syndrome (GAS), an example of a response-based model involving physiological responses to stress. It recognises the individual's ability to respond and adapt to the environment. This is demonstrated in three progressive phases:

1   The alarm state – the body mobilises to confront the threat ('fight and flight')
2   Resistance, or adaptation – physical and nervous energy is used up; coping mechanisms vary
3   Exhaustion and death – response to stress is initially appropriate and useful in aiding coping; responses in the long term will be detrimental.

Time out 3.1

1   Think of a situation when you felt stressed. What were the causes? Do you think it could have been prevented?
2   List the feelings you had.
3   Now consider the patients that you have cared for. Write down the causes of their stress.

The patient's experience of stress

Causes

Causes of stress in patients include:

■   Physical or psychological discomfort
■   Staff interactions
■   Family
■   Fear of dying (Chen, 1990)
■   Difficulty in communicating fears, pain

■   Sense of isolation
■   Vulnerability, loss of control
■   The environment and an unsettled pattern of activity
■   The illness itself
■   Effects of drug therapy.

Clinical features

Stressful situations can precipitate physiological and psychological reactions. The stress response occurs when a cascade of metabolic and neurohormonal changes creates a defensive mechanism in order for coping to take place.

Stress-induced hyperglycaemia is attributed to hypersecretion of the counter-regulatory hormones: catecholamines – adrenaline (epinephrine) and noradrenaline (norepinephrine) – glucagons, cortisol and growth hormone. Release of catecholamines results in decreased insulin and increased glucagon secretion by the pancreas (Ganong, 2003). The effect is a surge in circulating glucose derived from glycogenolysis and impaired utilisation of glucose (hyperglycaemia itself impairs glucose utilisation and residual insulin secretion).

Patients who are insulinopenic (reduced insulin) and taking fixed dosages of insulin are unable to increase insulin production. Secretion is inadequate to counteract these intense catabolic effects. The sympathetic branch of the autonomic nervous system plays a key role in the stress-mediated glycaemic response. Ketoacidosis may develop in patients with the most severe insulin deficiency.

Autonomic physiological responses also occur; for example, sympathetic nervous activity is increased, affecting the cardiovascular system. This results in increased heart rate, respiratory rate and blood pressure. The patient's physiological response to stress can cause considerable added strain on failing organs.

Psychologically, responses to stress include anxiety, worry and apprehension. Major symptoms include feelings of estrangement from others, sleep disturbance (Topf and Thompson, 2001) and difficulty in concentration.

Responses to stress are useful as a coping strategy in the short term, but can have detrimental effects on recovery in the long term. The continued breakdown of protein stores will lead to muscle wasting and fatigue; suppression of the inflammatory response may lead to infection; and the increased extracellular fluid volume will produce oedema and altered fluid balance (Adam and Osbourne, 1997).

Management

Critical illness can create predictable stressors. Being able to predict the occurrence of a stressful event, even if the individual cannot control it, can usually reduce the severity of the stress. Where possible, preventative strategies should be adopted – particularly when the stressor is environmental.

The condition of critically ill patients can deteriorate very quickly, with a rapid reversal of their coping strategies. This is something that nurses often cannot control or indeed predict. Including the patient (where possible) in the decision-making processes can foster a sense of control. A holistic approach to the delivery of care should be adopted. Nurses should develop a caring, non-judgmental relationship with patients, and try and understand their perspective, allowing them to express themselves freely. Nurses should introduce themselves at the start of the shift and reinforce this information throughout. Coping can be judged only in terms of the consequences. Patients' psychological and emotional needs should also be addressed; they should be given information about their condition and other information, such as the day and time of the week. Visits should be encouraged from the family and friends, who can bring in familiar objects to help orientate the patient.

Complementary therapy, although thousands of years old, is still in its infancy as a mode of treatment within hospital settings. Aromatherapy can be administered via inhalation or massage therapy (touch can also prove to be therapeutic); lemon balm and chamomile have calming properties. Lemon balm and orange blossom can reduce depression and anxiety, while lavender promotes a peaceful mood and creates a sense of calm (Chevallier, 1996). When administering such therapies, contraindications should be noted.

Severe hyperglycaemia is best treated by the intravenous infusion of insulin via a sliding-scale regime to keep glucose levels within normal parameters. Capillary blood glucose monitoring should not be relied upon and laboratory results should therefore be obtained intermittently (see Chapter 25).

Many critically ill patients require sedation to control their stress levels. Sedation (e.g. opiates) aims to control the undesirable hypertension and tachycardia caused by anxiety and fatigue, and to reduce oxygen consumption. Sedation should be appropriately selected to enable patient comfort with minimal lowering of consciousness and few side effects.

In the event of booked admission to critical care, nurses may take advantage of planned visits, enabling the patient and family (where appropriate) to prepare psychologically for admission. However, this should be optional for patients, as their stress levels may increase when confronted with the critical care environment and the visit would therefore be counterproductive.

Transfer of patients from a critical care unit

Time out 3.2

1 Have you received patients from a critical care unit? Did the transfer go well?
2 If not, what improvements would you like to see?

Transfer can and does cause anxiety (relocation stress). Some patients and their relatives may view critical care units as being secure, safe and familiar environments. A transitional period is required, where the patient can be prepared for and psychologically adjust to the impending transfer, and should occur once the patient's condition allows. However, this is not always possible. Occasionally there is not enough time to prepare adequately for discharge; however, patients should never be in a situation when they are totally unprepared.

Studies have produced inconsistencies regarding the effects of transfer on the patient. Research has variously found that patients:

- Are not affected (Compton, 1991)
- Show great fear (Jones and O'Donnell, 1994)
- Have mixed feelings – both positive and negative (Odell, 2000)
- Have difficulty in adjusting from a one-to-one relationship to a higher nurse–patient ratio (Green, 1996)
- View transfer as a sign of improvement (McKinney and Deeny, 2002).
- Find abrupt transfers, particularly at night, problematic (Goldfrad and Rowan, 2000).

Negative experiences should be treated with caution, as there are many influencing variables. There is not enough evidence to suggest that a negative experience equates to a stressful one (McKinney and Deeny, 2002).

Preparing the patient for discharge should include:

- Planning transfer (wherever possible)
- Reducing the quantity of monitoring equipment and the frequency of monitoring
- Providing information regarding the levels of care in the new ward, the type of ward the patient is being transferred to, type of patients etc.
- A nurse from the ward visiting the patient (Adam and Osbourne, 1997)
- Highlighting the patient's psychological and physical needs to ward staff
- Communication with the outreach teams.

Stress in the nurse

Caring for the critically ill patient may be stressful. If stress remains unrecognised or unalleviated, burn-out is likely to occur. The quality of care may deteriorate (clinical errors) and staff may avoid or distance themselves from all but the absolutely necessary interactions with the patient. Staff dissatisfaction at work may become evident in the form of sickness and absenteeism.

Causes

Causal factors of stress can be interpersonal (conflicts within a multidisciplinary team, bureaucracy, inadequacies of nursing care by others) or extrapersonal (environmental). Kincey et al. (2003) identified that a combination of workload, resources and a global sense of the NHS caused stress.

Clinical features

Stress can interfere with individuals' appraisal of their situation – 'can't see the wood for the trees' syndrome. Clinical features of stress may be:

- Emotional – increasing irritability
- Behavioural – indecisiveness
- Psychological – increasing suspiciousness and distrust
- Cognitive – inability to concentrate or listen
- Physiological – stress response (discussed earlier).

(Roberts, 1986)

Long-term stress can lead to ill health, e.g. gastric ulcers, coronary heart disease and a compromised immune system (increased infection, common colds).

Management

Management comprises prevention and coping strategies. Crisis situations cannot be totally avoided, but strategies involve identifying the stress and taking ownership in working towards reducing stress to a manageable level.

Albert Einstein (cited in Davidson, 1999) suggested that the significant problems we face cannot be solved at the same level of thinking we were at when we created them. Therefore, stress challenges us to take a 'mental helicopter' to a point above the situation so that we can get a different view on it and be prepared to entertain new thoughts and ideas and develop a new focus and perspective. Strategies involve identifying the stress and taking ownership in working towards reducing stress, but in order to do this, stress needs to be of a manageable level.

Kincey *et al.* (2003) identified that junior staff are more vulnerable to the negative aspects of stress. Coping with stress needs a supportive working environment through preceptorship and effective teamwork. Keeping a diary or journal as a way of expressing oneself may be useful. The use of reflection through clinical supervision may help nurses to examine their practice critically and learn through this process, identifying areas for future development. Debriefing can be offered by a supervisor, but this requires great skill (see Chapter 38). Active teaching programmes and regular appraisals can help facilitate knowledge and skill development, and detailed induction programmes for new staff should help to reduce stress.

Nurses need to be able to prioritise the management and delivery of care. This involves breaking work down into series of tasks and placing these tasks in a logical order. Implications of those tasks should be examined.

Thinking ahead, making predictions and creating deadlines for the completion of tasks should help nurses to manage their time and efforts effectively and efficiently. This will leave time for real crises, should they arise.

As a coping mechanism, some nurses detach themselves from patients by being 'too efficient' or 'too busy', and therefore adopt a depersonalised approach to care. Balancing engagement and detachment should enable nurses to care efficiently and effectively for the patient and themselves. Carmack (1997) suggests the following strategies to aid the balancing of engagement and detachment:

- Maintain consciousness and pragmatism – be realistic about what can and cannot be achieved, and be aware of your limitations
- Set limits and boundaries
- Monitor yourself – a sense of personal control is essential
- Practise self-care – it is important not to become too immersed in care; looking after yourself is also important
- Let go of the outcomes and the need to control the outcome.

Implications for practice

- Stress can and does have detrimental effects upon the nurse and patient
- Patients are at risk of developing internal and external stressors that may compromise their health and recovery from illness
- Nurses are responsible for identifying potential stressors and adopting strategies to prevent or minimise their effects
- Appropriate strategies need to be utilised to help individuals cope with stress
- Transfer to the ward must be encouraged as a positive step forward in the patient's recovery
- Pre-transfer programmes should be implemented before transferring a patient from the critical care unit
- Involvement in reflection and clinical supervision may help to support nurses and possibly reduce stress.

Summary

Stress is an individual concept that manifests itself in different ways. Our perception of the situation or experience will determine how we react to stress. Ideally, predicting and avoiding stressful situations is the best strategy to adopt. If this is unavoidable, as in many situations, then a variety of strategies may need to be adopted.

Clinical scenario

Susan Butcher (D grade, qualified for six months) has been working in the critical care unit for two weeks. It is a busy six-bedded unit, constantly full to its bed capacity. At interview she was informed that she would have a preceptor and be well supported, but in her opinion this has failed to happen.

Colleagues have noticed that she is becoming increasingly irritable, has made errors of judgment, is constantly late for work and looks tired. She has been heard to say that she cannot cope with the demands of the job and wants to leave.

1 Identify the stressors for Susan.

2 Discuss the detrimental affects that could occur.

3 Devise a plan of action to help support Susan and increase her coping strategies.

Bibliography

Key reading

Davidson, B (1999) is a helpful book that is easily read. The content is 'light hearted' with plenty of humour, making it interesting to read. It gives a general overview of stress and coping strategies. Numerous activities are available to aid understanding and application of the content.

Further reading

McKinney, A., Deeny, P. (2002).

Chapter 4

Psychological disturbances

Tina Moore

Contents

Learning outcomes

After reading this chapter you will be able to:

- Identify causative factors of psychological disturbances
- Discuss the normal sensory process
- Analyse present practices and suggest strategies to minimise the likelihood of the patient developing psychological disturbances
- Appreciate the need for early discharge planning (to the wards) and patient preparation.

Fundamental knowledge

- Physiology of stress (see Chapter 3).

Introduction

Admission to hospital, whether planned or not, can be a highly stressful experience for the patient. This may be detrimental to their psychological as well as their physiological well-being. Such psychological disturbances can affect the patient not only on admission to critical care units, but also on discharge to the general ward setting (Leith, 1998).

Much of the literature pertaining to the psychological needs of patients originates from the intensive care environment. However, the characteristics of critical illness will be the same wherever the patient is located. This point is stressed in the Department of Health's publication *Comprehensive Critical Care* (DOH, 2000a). In effect, a great deal can be learnt from the experiences of intensive care nurses.

This chapter identifies the types of psychological disturbances that patients can acquire, and discusses appropriate preventative measures.

Psychological labels

A variety of labels is used to describe these psychological disturbances, potentially leading to confusion amongst staff. Common terminology includes:

- Intensive care psychosis
- Post-traumatic stress disorder
- Delirium
- ICU (intensive care unit) syndrome
- Sensoristrain.

Despite these multiple labels, there appears to be congruency between the contributing factors. Psychological symptoms correlate to the diagnosis of delirium as identified by *The Diagnostic and Statistical Manual of Mental Disorders* (*DSM*; American Psychiatric Association, 1994) and include: disturbance of consciousness, disorientation, confusion, hallucinations and delusions. Symptoms develop over a short period of time (usually hours). Although the *DSM* is American in origin, it is widely adopted, within the mental health setting, in Britain. The description used for delirium is pertinent to the psychological disturbances experienced by the critically ill patient.

Delirium has been referred to as 'everyman's psychosis' (Clark, 1993). This seems to be an appropriate expression, as everyone is susceptible to developing this disorder; it does not discriminate. Studies by Hafsteindóttir (1996) and Laitinen (1996) confirm that delirium within ICU is indeed a real issue, with estimates indicating a prevalence ranging from 7 per cent to a staggering 72 per cent (Armstrong *et al.*, 1997). Roberts (2001) warns that this figure is escalating as a result of increases in the number of older and more severely ill patients admitted.

There is an urgent need to take action to reduce this figure. Lessons should be learnt from the failures of the past and strategies adopted in order to heighten an awareness of the problem.

Delirium can fall into one of three categories (Liptzin and Leukoff, 1992):

1 Hyperactive (hyperalert)
2 Hypoactive (hypoalert)
3 Mixed.

Contributing factors

The cause of psychological disturbances is multifactorial, but the factors can be bracketed under three main headings:

1 *Pathophysiological*. Cerebral illness associated with advancing age, e.g. dementia and Alzheimer's disease, or a history of alcohol or substance abuse (Clark, 1993), can lead to delirium. Other contributing factors include metabolic and haemodynamic instability, particularly those aggravating an underlying chronic systemic illness; hypoxaemia; acidosis and electrolyte imbalances; severe infections; and intracerebral abnormalities.
2 *Pharmacological/medical*. Sedation (e.g. opiates) and the sudden withdrawal of narcotics can cause an acute delirious episode. Other drugs that have an influence include corticosteroids, inotropes, antibiotics and anti-arrhythmic drugs.
3 *Environmental* (sensory imbalances). Nurses can and do have a great deal of influence and control over the environmental stressors that patients are exposed to in critical care units. The situation contributes to the patient becoming dependent and so feeling helpless, and some patients may also feel isolated, both socially and environmentally. When confronted by an intensive barrage of stressors or stimuli, they are probably less emotionally resilient and less able to adapt to them.

   Sensory deprivation and sensory overload indicate that external environment stimuli are having an adverse effect upon people's ability to make sense of their surroundings. Sensory deprivation is an absolute reduction in the variety and intensity of sensory input, with or without a change in pattern. Homeostatic mechanisms create a situation where the individual strives to maintain an internal balance, a variation in stimuli to the cerebral cortex as mediated by the reticular activating system (RAS).

Time out 4.1

1 Find out how the brain processes information received from the five senses.
2 What are the normal processes that occur to enable us to control the stimulation of the environment?
3 How do you think these processes alter for a patient who is exposed to environmental stressors?

The reticular activating system

The RAS acts as a filter that removes most (99 per cent) of the information received via the senses, which prevents the cerebral cortex from being overloaded with irrelevant information and therefore helps to maintain sanity.

The RAS has an adaptation level that is stimulated through the five senses. The RAS in turn stimulates the cortex and this is necessary for normal perception, learning and emotion. When this regulating system is upset there are disturbances in sensory input, and compensatory adjustments are made. When these adjustments fail, behaviour becomes disorganised.

There are three main causes of upset to the RAS balance:

1   Reduced sensory input, in which poorly functioning receptors block adequate stimuli and this results in sensory underload
2   Relevance deprivation, which occurs with a reduction of the patterning or meaningfulness of the stimulation
3   Alteration of the RAS, which changes the mechanisms for general arousal and alerting.

Critically ill patients' responses to isolation are markedly intensified compared to those of healthy adults because of the additional stressors. The patients' condition and increased disturbance (caused by frequent monitoring) may lead to sleep deprivation. The experience of sensory imbalance may not allow the critically ill patient to derive meaning. When the deprivation barrier cannot be overcome, the unfulfilled need for sensory input leads to behaviour characterised by regression, disorganisation of sensory co-ordination and difficulty in thinking coherently. The intensity of the environment and the supportive devices create feelings of fear. This fear reduces patients' ability both to hear what is happening around them and to make appropriate interpretations of the sounds.

Time out 4.2

Find a noisy location (train station, shopping centre etc.), and close your eyes for approximately five minutes. Imagine half-a-dozen unknown pairs of hands working on you, doing different things. All you can feel is pain, and all you can hear is a confusion of sounds and voices. Write down your immediate thoughts.

Now imagine the situation intensifying and prolonging.
1   How do you feel now?
2   What strategies would you like to see implemented in order to eradicate or reduce these feelings?

Clinical features

Within a few days of critical illness, symptoms associated with delirium can begin to manifest themselves. They will resolve either during the patient's stay, or a short time afterwards (Curtis, 1999). Delirium is often a frightening experience for both patients and their relatives. Disorientation is probably the most common clinical sign, and other symptoms are variable depending on the severity of the illness. Mild delirium includes an inability to concentrate or remember complete thoughts. Patients can appear to be alert and wakeful, but the next moment are absent and drowsy.

Hypoactive delirium patients are usually quiet, sleepy, slow in responding, and have vivid hallucinations. Some patients may become withdrawn and passive, 'giving up' (Borgbom-Engberg, 1991). Some patients may refuse contact with others, they often show no expression in their faces, and sometimes look very frightened and tense (American Psychiatric Association, 1994).

Severe aggression can be seen in patients with hyperactive delirium, to the point where they may attempt to assault staff and visitors. Some patients risk unintentional self-harm (American Psychiatric Association, 1994) through dislodging essential life-support and monitoring equipment.

Disorientation and confusion regarding the identity of friends, relatives and even themselves occurs in the more serious form. Hallucinations are a result of the cortex attempting to arrange available stimuli and find meaning in the environment, thus maintaining arousal. An alert state is the result of highly co-ordinated interplay between the cortex and the reticular formation. Hallucinations are often visual, and sometimes manifest as paranoid delusions. Bizarre bodily sensations are quite usual (patients attempting to pick objects off the bedclothes or themselves) (American Psychiatric Association, 1994).

Physiological symptoms include the following:

- Adrenocorticotrophic hormone (ACTH) stimulates the secretion of catecholamines, enabling the flight or fight response; the heart rate is increased (tachycardia)
- Vasodilatation occurs, increasing blood supply to the organs, enabling coping with emergencies (hypertension)
- The bronchi dilate, allowing an increased intake of oxygen/inspired air (tachypnoea), and more oxygen is supplied to the muscles. Immunity is also suppressed, initiating the stimulation of glycogenesis and thus raising serum blood sugar.

If prolonged, haemodynamic and respiratory deterioration will occur. Agitation leading to hypermetabolism at the muscular level will contribute to metabolic acidosis, possibly resulting in worsening organ dysfunction. Physiological arousal will be such as to prompt exhaustive coping mechanisms, which may result in a fatal outcome (McCartney, 1994).

Management (medical)

Medical management involves diagnosis, removing the underlying causes, and treating the signs and symptoms (Roberts, 2001). If the patient is displaying unsafe behaviour to self and others, including insomnia, agitation and/or delusions, pharmacological intervention may be required.

Haloperidol and droperidol may be prescribed. Droperidol is a faster-acting agent with quicker results. Benzodiazepines, e.g. lorazepam, midazolam and diazepam, will enhance delirium due to their anticholinergic effects. If the patient's mental status does not improve, then referral to a psychiatrist may be indicated.

Management (nursing)

Although staff within the critical care units are aware of psychological issues, acute physical symptoms are often given higher concern and priority than psychological ones because of the life-threatening situation. There may also be uncertainty and unfamiliarity with the initial clinical signs of delirium (Granberg-Axèll et al., 2001). Care of the patient goes beyond physical care, and Dyer (1995) suggests that although the presenting illness does play a role, the key factor in the development of psychological impairment is the environment. Linkages between exposure to ICU experiences and the effects of torture have been identified (Dyer, 1995).

Assessing the patient

Objective assessment is often inaccurate, carried out by general nurses who consistently underestimate or do not notice psychological complications that are later reported by patients (Dyer, 1995). A comprehensive assessment is required. When faced with a confused, agitated patient, the nurse should first consider the possible physiological causes. When these have been ruled out, consideration should be given to the environment or treatment as the possible cause.

The assessment should also include the patient's behaviour, emotions and perceptions of the environment. The patient's ability to communicate, hear, see, move and understand should be noted, in addition to any medication that could modify the patient's perception and interpretation of information.

Reality orientation

Nurses should understand the importance of reality orientation and the need for structuring sensory input by explaining any treatment or procedure. Orientating the patient to day and night, through the use of digital clocks (patients often forget how to read normal clocks) and calendars, should help. Patients need to keep in touch with the outside world, and the use of radios, televisions and newspapers, and visits from relatives and friends, should be encouraged. For many patients, relatives are the only contact with the real world outside. Wherever possible, visual stimulation should be increased by appropriate positioning of the patient or supplying a mirror to enlarge his or her visual field.

Alterations in sensory experiences may manifest as perceptions of altered body image, which may cause patients to view their body as less perfect and withdraw from others. Nurses should provide patients with correct information about themselves in reference to the environment. As patients disclose their body image perceptions, the nurse should assist them in developing adaptive modes for dealing with this.

The use of invasive techniques and therapies can result in patients experiencing feelings of being 'tied down' (Clifford, 1985), producing further sensations of fear, anxiety and helplessness (Granberg *et al.*, 1996). There is a possibility that nurses' communication with critically ill patients may be task-focused, relatively uninformative, nurse-controlled, and associated mainly with physical procedures. However, effective communication is a key strategy in preventing delirium. Explanation of patients' condition and progress is essential. The messages received from staff regarding their illness and progress must be at the level of the patients' comprehension. Communication between nurses and patients is likely to be as vital as it is difficult.

Therapeutic use of touch

Patients should be allowed time to communicate their feelings. If they are unable to do this verbally, tactile communication should be encouraged. This helps patients to respond in whatever way they can and should make them feel active participants in the conversation and activities about them. For unconscious patients unable to open their eyes, verbal communication or touch may be an important part of their limited stimulation. Touch may help to reduce the physiological effects of stress. There is concern amongst staff and visitors that touching the critically ill patient may paradoxically produce harmful physiological effects on the patient. Some studies have found that touch has a negative/positive effect on physiological response. A study by Witcher and Fisher (1979) cited in Niven (2000:10) on pre-operative patients demonstrated that female patients who were touched reported less anxiety, greater positive feelings, and had a lower blood pressure, whilst male patients who were touched reported anxiety, more negative feelings and had a higher blood pressure.

When sensory disturbances are likely, patients need to be warned and reassured that this is common and temporary (if this is the case). By discussing the symptoms relating to psychological disturbances, patients can be reassured that they are not going mad. Patients have a need to order the stimuli in their own environment into a meaningful pattern. Without explanation of the purpose of objects and machines in their environment, they are left alone with meaningless machinery and anxiety increases.

The nurse can be an environmental cause of psychological instability, but at the same time has a certain amount of power to control the patient's environment by reducing or eliminating factors contributing to instability. Helpful strategies include: minimising unfamiliar noises; explaining a new noise; creating a familiar environment; having the patient's pictures close by; explaining and removing supportive devices as soon as possible; and encouraging family contact.

Transfer to the ward

Discharge to the ward has the potential to cause relocation stress, and major characteristics include apprehension, anxiety, depression, increased confusion and loneliness (Leith, 1998). Discharge planning processes need to be in place to reduce the stress by preparing patients for transfer. After being transferred to the ward, some patients may still have nightmares from their experiences in critical care units. Reducing non-essential monitoring and nursing care prior to discharge will help (Cutler and Garner, 1995) to reduce dependence. The aim is to empower patients to take more control in the decision-making processes and participate more in their own care.

Implications for practice

- Critically ill patients are considered to be at high risk of developing psychological disturbances
- Nurses should conduct a comprehensive assessment in an attempt to identify those patients at risk
- Patients should be isolated (side room) only when necessary
- Patients should be warned of the potential symptoms of psychological disturbances, explaining the normal processes that may be affected
- Family members should be encouraged to be involved in the patients' care.

Summary

The manifestation of psychological disturbances is a real issue because it has detrimental effects on both psychological (humanitarian) care and physiological responses (e.g. the stress response). It is also an experience that is increasing amongst patients. To minimise the occurrence of psychological disturbances, nurses should aim to identify those at risk through a comprehensive assessment. They should promote a normal sensory environment for patients and assist them with perceptual or thought disturbances.

Gelling (1999) rightly indicates that nothing has improved since the 1950s, when these problems were first identified. Too little time is spent on preventative measures (Dyer, 1995). There is an urgent need for high dependency staff to develop appropriate strategies to minimise or prevent the risk of psychological disturbances occurring. This may help to reduce the associated morbidity.

Clinical scenario

Kathleen Winsor, a 64-year-old retired schoolteacher, is admitted to the critical care unit after presenting in Accident and Emergency with severe headaches and photophobia. She is pyrexial, B/P 160/110, heart rate 98 irregular.

A provisional diagnosis of meningococcal meningitis has been made. Kathleen is nursed in isolation and requires hourly monitoring.

1 Describe your assessment of Kathleen in relation to her psychological needs.

2 What criteria would you use to determine whether Kathleen is at risk of developing symptoms related to psychological disturbances?

3 Discuss the strategies that need to be adopted in order to minimise the risk of developing psychological disturbances.

Bibliography

Key reading

Roberts, B.L. (2001) provides a detailed and useful text in relation to delirium and its management within the critical care setting.

Further reading

Whittaker and Ball (2000) offers a valuable insight from the ward perspective in relation to receiving patients from critical care areas. The article also suggests appropriate strategies for managing the psychological disturbances on transfer from critical care areas to the ward and enhancing coping mechanisms of the ward staff.

Chapter 5

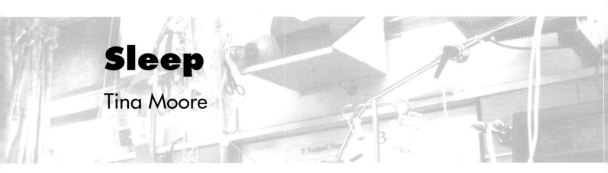

Sleep

Tina Moore

Contents

Learning outcomes

After reading this chapter you will be able to:

- Identify the stages of sleep
- Identify the factors affecting sleep
- Understand the effects of sleep deprivation on critically ill patients
- Suggest strategies to prevent/reduce the effects of sleep deprivation.

Fundamental knowledge

- Circadian rhythms.

Introduction

Sleep deprivation is not a new concept in critical care nursing. Problems with sleep deprivation date back to when the first ICUs evolved. Despite the developments over the past few decades, sleep deprivation is one problem that persists. There was a significant amount of interest in sleep deprivation during the 1970s, but this interest appears to have declined and there is a noticeable lack of recent empirical research on this topic in relation to the critically ill patient. It may be viewed as an inevitable part of critical illness but, despite the difficulties, nurses should try to promote sleep. Adequate sleep is crucial for critically ill patients, as sleep deprivation can have detrimental effects on their already compromised well-being.

This chapter will discuss the normal physiology of sleep before proceeding to sleep deprivation and the effects it has on the individual.

Purpose of sleep

Sleep has been defined as a state of unconsciousness from which individuals can be aroused by sensory stimuli (Horne, 1998). It is a natural and beneficial state, essential for the physiological and psychological well-being of human beings. Little conclusive evidence is available regarding the purpose of sleep, but it is believed that sleep has a restorative function and provides protection from fatigue in addition to compensating for the energy deficit acquired during daily activities. The amount of sleep required is variable. On average, adults who are allowed to sleep without restriction will sleep for about 8 hours a night (Merritt, 2000). Periods of enforced wakefulness result in increased sluggishness, irritability, and even psychotic behaviour (Hubbard and Mechan, 1997). The ageing process is associated with changes in the normal sleep pattern, increased nocturnal awakenings, sleep deficiency and early morning awakening. In addition, the number and length of naps may be increased for those over 75 years of age; this undoubtedly increases their total sleep time.

The sleep cycle

The reticular activating system (see Chapter 4) is associated with the level of arousal and wakefulness, and is thus a contributing factor in the sleep/wake cycle. The circadian rhythm of sleep and wakefulness represents a relationship between activity and inactivity (Gustafsson and Ek, 1992).

The mean time for one normal sleep cycle is 70–120 minutes (Hudak *et al.*, 1998), with an average of six cycles in 24 hours. The hypothalamus is responsible for the timing of these cycles.

Often, critically ill patients require hourly invasive and non-invasive monitoring. Non-invasive monitoring can still disturb the patient (e.g. Dynamaps®). An exploratory study of patients' experiences revealed that 42 per cent reported being unable to sleep. Whilst some managed to 'drift in and out of sleep', their total amount and quality of sleep was still inadequate.

Normal sleep is divided into five stages. The first four stages are non-rapid eye movement (NREM), also known as slow wave sleep (SWS), and the fifth stage is rapid eye movement (REM). NREM sleep is believed to be restorative sleep for the body, whilst REM sleep is thought to be restorative sleep for the brain's mental processes (Shapiro, 1993). Sleep is therefore a time of energy conservation and renewal.

Non-rapid eye movement sleep

Stage 1 (sleep latency) equates to a transitional state of the lightest level of sleep, lasting only 1–20 minutes. Characteristics include aimless thoughts, a drifting sensation, and frequent myoclonic jerks of the face, hands and feet. Individuals can easily be awakened.

Stage 2 (light sleep) lasts from 5–15 minutes. Individuals are more relaxed, but can still easily be awakened.

Stages 3 and 4 (deep slow wave sleep) are the deepest levels of sleep, and random stimuli do not arouse the individual. Sleep time is variable in these stages (15 to 30 minutes).

In the average young adult, NREM constitutes 50–60 per cent of the total sleep time for stages 1 and 2 (Urden, 2000), implying that younger patients can tolerate sleep disturbances better than the older person.

Rapid eye movement sleep

Stage 5 is sometimes referred to as paradoxical sleep and usually accounts for 20–25 per cent of the total night's sleep (Guyton and Hall, 2000). Here, some parts of the brain are active whilst other parts are suppressed. During REM it is more difficult to waken the individual than in any of the other stages. Sleep is more intense; as a result sleep deprivation is probably more significant when it occurs during this stage.

Within the sleep cycle there is normal progression through repetitive sequences, starting with stage 1 and moving through stages 2, 3 and 4, followed by stages 3 and 2 and then the REM stage (see Figure 5.1).

Sleep changes accompany normal ageing, and include increased fragmentation of night-time sleep due to periods of wakefulness, and less time spent in the deeper stages of sleep (i.e. stages 3 and 4).

Physiology of sleep

Although there is a deficit of research evidence, activities associated with NREM sleep are believed to include protein synthesis and tissue repair, such as of the epithelial and specialised cells of the brain, skin, bone marrow and gastric mucosa (Krachman *et al.*, 1995). In addition, growth hormones are secreted by the anterior pituitary gland and function to promote protein synthesis while sparing catabolic breakdown.

Activities from the parasympathetic nervous system predominate during

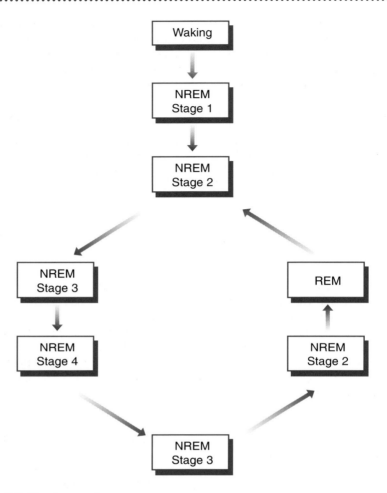

Figure 5.1 **The sleep cycle**

NREM sleep. During sleep the brain's cortical activity is depressed and reduced brain stem activity and lowering of the metabolic rate cause a reduction in respiratory rate, heart rate and blood pressure, which can sometimes be erratic (Guyton and Hall, 2000). Core body temperature is low; therefore it is important to keep the body surface well covered to avoid chills (MacPherson, 1994). Muscle tone and reflex activities are depressed, and deep tendon responses are practically absent (Fox, 1999).

Sympathetic nervous activity predominates during REM. There is sudden dilation of the pupils (Bray *et al.*, 1999), indicating caution when monitoring pupil reaction. Premature ventricular contractions and tachydysrhythmias associated with respiratory pauses may also occur during REM (Verrier and Kirby, 1988 cited in Urden, 2000).

In preparation for physical activity, the release of catecholamine peaks around 6 am (Todd, 1997); this may be responsible for episodes of ischaemia and early morning cardiac death and strokes. Secretory rates of adrenocorticotropic hormone and cortisol are higher in the early hours of the morning (between 4 am and 6 am), thus putting the body in a 'stress-like' state.

Time out 5.1

1   Reflect upon your experiences during night duty; consider the factors that can cause sleep disturbances with critically ill patients.
2   Have you personally suffered from sleep deprivation? What were the causes? How did you feel?

Sleep deprivation

A sleep disorder exists when the inability to sleep well leads to impaired daytime functioning or excessive sleepiness (Fox, 1999). An integrated review of sleep in acute care settings by Redeker (2000) concluded that few studies have shown the outcomes of sleep disturbances in these environments.

As indicated, sleep may be of great biological and psychological importance. Factors affecting sleep are many, and discussed below are a few significant reasons for sleep pattern disturbances in hospital. However, conflicting evidence exists which highlights the complex and subjective nature of sleep and possible environmental influences.

Factors that disturb sleep in hospitals include:

■   Environmental factors, such as noise (staff, machinery, other patients); lighting; store room positioning
■   The design of some coronary care units; higher noise levels were recorded in areas with more patients (Meyer *et al.*, 1994; Southwell and Wistow, 1995)
■   The delivery of patient care, which often requires frequent disruptions to the patient throughout the day and night
■   Subjective factors, such as a limited amount of personal space, limited privacy, physical restrictions (for example caused by intravenous tubes); pain; discomfort; anxiety and worry
■   Age (Southwell and Wistow, 1995), although no age difference was found by Simpson *et al.* (1996).

The relationship between hospitalisation and sleep disturbances is well documented (Southwell and Wistow, 1995; Redeker and Wykpisz, 1999; Redeker, 2000). Patients admitted to critical care units often suffer an altered sleep pattern due to the critical illness itself, frequent treatments, 24-hour intensive monitoring, anxiety, and fear of not waking up.

The combination of the physiological problems and the experiences that patients have during their period of critical illness (environment, treatment, illness itself) contribute to their feelings of fatigue. Symptoms vary between individuals, but influencing factors include age, a premorbid personality, motivation, and the environment. A single night's disturbed sleep leads to a decrease in the functioning of white blood cell activity and decreased production of T-cell cytokines, thereby compromising immunity (Dinges *et al.*, 1994). Patients are therefore more susceptible to hospital-acquired infection.

Kubitz (1999) suggests that approximately 70 per cent of growth hormone secretion takes place during deep sleep, and decreased secretion of thyroid-stimulating hormone and adrenocorticotropic hormone also occurs, thus having an effect on wound healing.

Sleep also has a psychological restorative function. Decreased REM sleep leads to impaired memory for cognitive functioning (Brown, 1999), and lack of sleep leads to memory lapses and difficulty in concentrating. This may suggest why patients sometimes have difficulty in remembering what they have been told, or events experienced.

NREM sleep deprivation symptoms include fatigue, anxiety, and increased severity of illness. REM sleep deprivation is more detrimental, with symptoms often occurring within 72 hours (Urden, 2000). These include irritability, apathy, decreased alertness and increased senility. Continued loss of REM sleep may lead to perceptual distortion and significant disturbances in mental and emotional functions ranging from disorientation and restlessness to auditory and visual hallucinations with personality changes (including paranoia).

Time out 5.2

Consider how you promote sleep for the patients within your care. What strategies do you (or should you) undertake with the critically ill?

Promoting sleep

Human beings possess a 24-hour biological clock that is resistant to change, and long-term disruption can be fatal. The provision of adequate sleep is an important but often overlooked component of critical care. The goal is to foster as much uninterrupted sleep as possible, while continuing with the safe monitoring and intervention of care.

Each patient has a right to undisturbed sleep (Fox, 1999). However, this right is often impossible to honour for the critically ill, as they also have a fundamental right to be looked after safely. Those patients who require nursing intervention at night should be nursed efficiently and quietly, with the minimum of disturbance to themselves and other patients.

Nurses within critical care should treat disturbance to the patient's sleep seriously, and take appropriate action to prevent it. Continual assessment of the patient's current sleep pattern should be undertaken and compared with the patient's normal sleep pattern, and outcomes should be reflected in communication, documentation, discussion and individual care-planning to determine whether the individual's needs are being met (Roper *et al.*, 2000). Potential threats to disturbed sleep should be identified, involving consideration of all environmental factors and subjective perceptions of the patient involving sleep.

Wherever possible, a minimum of at least 4 hours of uninterrupted sleep in every 24 hours should be achieved in order to maintain minimal performance. Frequent naps (20–90 minutes in length) should be encouraged. Accurate knowledge of sleep should assist nurses in monitoring patients safely while ensuring that they achieve optimal quality of sleep. At night, only essential monitoring should be performed. Fox (1999) further suggests that there should be a policy in place providing advice and guidance on how nurses can arrange care at night to ensure that optimum sleep is enhanced. For the safety of the patient, however, machine alarms should *not* be turned off.

Clustering of patient-care activities is vital in an attempt to maintain normal sleep cycles. This requires careful planning, and sometimes means that the nurse must act as an advocate for the patient in relation to other members of the team.

During REM sleep patients' vital signs may change, resulting in concern that their condition is worsening. Consequently, nurses may increase the frequency of monitoring, adjust intravenous fluids and measure vital signs in response. Hence, patients may not get the sleep they require. Nurses must be aware of these factors and observational data must be analysed with this in mind, as unsubstantiated actions may have detrimental effects.

At night low lighting should be used (although bright enough to enable close monitoring of patients, particularly their skin colour). Artificial light can replicate differences between day and night (with higher levels during the day and lower levels at night); this may help patients to determine day and night and thus aid the maintenance of the circadian rhythm. This is particularly useful in areas where there are no windows. Therapeutic use of light has been demonstrated as an effective treatment for circadian sleep disorders and depression (Terman *et al.*, 1995).

A study by Southwell and Wistow (1995) highlighted the differences in nurses' and patients' perceptions, with nurses reporting noise less frequently. A significant number of patients were disturbed by noise (Hofhuis and Bakker, 1998). Therefore, there must be consideration of the patient's perspective and experiences. Noise levels should be reduced to a minimum by staff wearing soft-soled shoes, speaking quietly, and avoiding unnecessary conversation during the night. Unnecessary and noisy telephone calls should be avoided (some units have a silent flashing bulb/light to alert a telephone call) and supplies and equipment planned in advance. The room temperature and ventilation should be regulated.

Sedatives and analgesia should not be withheld unless indicated. Nevertheless, critically ill patients often suffer from renal and/or liver disease, or a decrease in metabolism. This can cause the effects of sedatives continuing into the daytime, leading to confusion and sluggishness. Some hypnotic drugs have been found to promote the lighter stages of sleep, and may be the cause of night terrors, hallucinations and agitation in the older person.

Other strategies include the use of curtains or screens for privacy; this may help to promote sleep, but discretion must be used as screens cannot compromise the patient's monitoring.

Visitors should be made aware of the importance of sleep, not only for the patient but also for themselves. Indeed, some critical care units adopt a restful period of 2 hours in the afternoon, where only essential care is carried out. This allows patients to rest during the day, thus increasing their total sleep time in 24 hours. This is not an ideal situation, as patients should benefit from continuous sleep, but it is better than losing the sleep entirely.

Implications for practice

- Nurses should include sleep in the assessment and planning of care, as the majority of critically ill patients are at risk of suffering disrupted sleep patterns
- Older patients are more susceptible to sleep deprivation
- Sleep deprivation can have detrimental physiological and psychological effects on critically ill patients
- At night only essential care and monitoring should be performed, maintaining a safe level of care provision
- Nurses should ensure that the benefits of interventions outweigh those of undisturbed sleep (Southwell and Wistow, 1995)
- Care should be clustered to allow a maximum time of undisturbed sleep
- If patients are disturbed in their sleep during the night, restful periods during the day should be encouraged.

Summary

Adequate sleep is an essential component of critical care. Disturbances to sleep affects a significant amount of patients. Sleep has physiological and psychological restorative functions, and the promotion of sleep should be viewed as a natural part of care.

Clinical scenario

Jo Gibson, 72 years old, has been admitted from the ward to the critical care unit with uncontrolled type-one respiratory failure. She requires CPAP therapy, with hourly monitoring of vital signs and arterial blood gas via an arterial line.

1 State why Mrs Gibson is at risk of developing sleep deprivation.

2 What symptoms would you expect this patient to have? Provide a rationale for your answer.

3 At night her temperature is significantly lowered, her blood pressure decreases, her heart rate is labile with the occasional premature ventricu-

lar contraction (PVC), and her respiratory rate increases and is irregular. There is also a reduction in her oxygen saturation levels. Indicate why this is the case.

4 What strategies can be adopted to promote sleep?

Bibliography

Key reading

Redeker (2000) provides a comprehensive literature review of sleep and the critically/acutely ill patient.

Further reading

Southwell and Wistow (1995) presents a study highlighting sources of disturbances to sleep from the patient's perspective.

Chapter 6

Nutrition

Philip Woodrow

Contents

Learning outcomes

After reading this chapter you will be able to:

- Understand the risks and effects of malnutrition during critical illness
- Assess which types of nutrition are most appropriate for individual patients
- Plan and provide nutritional care for patients, including preventing or minimising complications caused by feeding

■ Analyse when withholding nutrition is inappropriate, and to be able to advocate for patients' nutritional needs.

Fundamental knowledge

■ Anatomy and physiology of the gastrointestinal tract.

Introduction

Nutrition is fundamental to health, providing energy for body function, repair of damaged tissue and healing. Mortality rates reflect malnutrition (Kennedy, 1997), yet up to 40 per cent of hospital patients remain malnourished (Pearce and Duncan, 2002). Some patients are malnourished on admission, but many become more, rather than less, malnourished during their hospital stay (McWhirter and Pennington, 1994). Critically ill patients may

■ Be unable to eat
■ Be nil by mouth
■ Have diets restricted by disease (e.g. renal diets)
■ Have poor appetites (e.g. from nausea or pain).

They may therefore need nutrition or supplements through an alternative route. Malnourishment frequently remains unidentified until it has progressed (Kinn and Scott, 2001), often to the extent of causing complications. Nutrition is a key target in *Essence of Care* (DOH, 2001).

Serving and clearing away meals has been largely delegated from nurses to support staff (Grieve and Finnie, 2002), so nurses seldom see what is given to, or eaten by, their patients. Many patients can report what they have eaten, but critically ill patients may forget, be confused, or have impaired communication due to their treatments.

Many critically ill patients cannot take a normal oral diet. They feel too unwell to eat (e.g. breathlessness) or their medical treatment limits or prevents them from eating (e.g. patients receiving non-invasive ventilation or following gastric surgery). These patients rely on nursing and other staff to supply nutrition enterally or parenterally.

Nutritional support is often delayed or overlooked (Kinn and Scott, 2001). Once commenced, many critically ill patients receive only 50–85 per cent of prescribed enteral feeds (Briggs, 1996; Adam and Osborne, 1997; McClave et al., 1999; De Beaux et al., 2001). Giving only half a prescribed antibiotic regime would be considered unacceptable, yet giving only half of prescribed nutrition appears to be condoned.

Nutrition can be significantly improved through good teamwork and communication between the various professionals involved (Kinn and Scott, 2001), but nurses have a valuable role in identifying patients at risk of malnutrition, assessing nutritional needs, and initiating action. Depending on individual patients' needs, that action may be provided through the nursing staff themselves, or through other healthcare professionals such as dieticians. This chapter focuses on the knowledge nurses in practice need in order to assess and provide nutritional support, not on the more specialised aspects that other healthcare professionals may undertake.

Malnutrition

Healthy body stores can compensate for moderate starvation before using body protein for energy. Once stores have been exhausted the body uses alternative sources of energy, breaking down body fat and protein for energy.

Breakdown of body protein (catabolism) causes muscle wasting, including respiratory and skeletal muscle. With prolonged starvation, 5 per cent of muscle may atrophy each day (Marieb, 2004), with each day's atrophy taking 1 week's nutrition to reverse (Horwood, 1990). Until replaced, wasted respiratory and skeletal muscle is likely to cause prolonged problems with breathing and mobilising, both of which predispose to extended illness and hospitalisation, with more risk of complications and higher mortality. Starvation reduces the metabolism (van den Berghe, 2000), so delaying tissue repair; it also reduces immunity, exposing patients to greater risks from infection.

Nitrogen balance

Nitrogen is a major source of amino acids, used to produce body proteins. Body protein (muscle) building requires sufficient nitrogen. When protein is broken down, nitrogen is lost from the body. An average healthy adult metabolises 20–30 g of protein daily (Guyton and Hall, 2000). Each gram of nitrogen provides 6.25 g of protein, creating 30 g of lean body mass (Hudak *et al.*, 1998). Loss of 1 g of nitrogen similarly represents the loss of significant amounts of lean tissue. Therefore, if nitrogen loss:

■ Exceeds supply, catabolism (muscle breakdown) occurs
■ Equals supply, then existing body tissue is maintained
■ Is less than supply, anabolism (muscle building) occurs.

In health, the only significant loss of body nitrogen occurs as urea and other chemicals in urine, so the nitrogen balance can be reliably calculated by comparing the nitrogen intake in food with the nitrogen loss in 24-hour urine collections. Critical illness increases nitrogen loss from other sources, such as wound exudate and diarrhoea, so 24-hour urine collections become increasingly unreliable as patients become more critically ill.

Energy

Nutrition should ideally balance the energy supply with energy expenditure. Nutritional energy is usually measured in calories (c) or kilocalories (kcal). Energy can also be measured in joules (J) or kilojoules (kJ).

A healthy 70-kg man has a resting energy expenditure of about 1,650 kcal each day, while manual labour, which greatly increases energy consumption, may increase the daily energy expenditure to 6,000–7,000 kcal (Guyton and Hall, 2000). Critical illness similarly significantly increases the energy demand. Scott *et al.* (1998) suggest that critically ill patients may need 1,700–2,500 kcal each day, but needs vary greatly, making this difficult to calculate. There are formulae for calculating energy requirements, but patients requiring this level of nutritional support should be referred to dieticians.

The two main sources of energy are sugars and fats. Diets, whether oral, enteral or parenteral, usually mix both sources.

Sugars

Sugars include carbohydrates, which are metabolised into sugars. Blood sugar needs insulin to be able to cross cell membranes. Inside cells, mitochondria metabolise the sugar into adenosine triphosphate (ATP), the energy used by all cells. Sugar provides much ATP while producing relatively little metabolic waste (carbon dioxide, acids, water), and is therefore the best single source of energy in critical illness.

Intravenous infusions of glucose 5% provide a large amount of 'free water' that crosses cell membranes to provide intracellular hydration. However, 1 litre of glucose 5% contains only 836 kJ; a single bar of chocolate usually provides more energy than a 24-hour regime of 3 litres of glucose 5%.

Fats

Fat provides useful energy. Although obesity is endemic in Western society, causing much ill health, critical illness is not an appropriate time to begin dieting. In health, the body can only use 5 mg/kg per minute of glucose (Scott *et al.*, 1998). For someone weighing 70 kg, this provides about 2,000 kcal/day, which may not meet the needs of critical illness. However, critical illness may limit glucose-derived energy to 3 mg/kg per minute (Scott *et al.*, 1998), so most critically ill patients need energy supplements from non-glucose (i.e. fat) sources.

Fat metabolism produces significantly more waste products (carbon dioxide, metabolic acids, water) than glucose, potentially worsening:

- Respiratory problems
- Acidosis
- Oedema.

Translocation of gut bacteria

The intestines normally contain many bacteria – commensals that, in health, help to digest food. Critical illness can turn gut commensals into blood pathogens. Normally, endogenous infection from gut commensals is prevented by villi (finger-like projections into the gut), which both increase the surface area for the absorption of nutrients and produce protective mucus and immunoglobins. Ischaemia or shock rapidly (within minutes) damage the gut defences, enabling gut bacteria to translocate into the blood.

Blood from the gut drains to the liver, where specialised machrophages called *Kuppfer cells* destroy pathogens. However, ischaemia also compromises liver function (see Chapter 26), exposing the lungs and other organs to infection from gut-derived pathogens. With the other risk factors from critical illness (e.g. immobility, shallow breathing), chest infection may follow. Absence of enteral nutrition significantly increases the risk of pneumonia (Zarzaur *et al.*, 2000).

Lack of food causes gut atrophy, further impairing the gut barrier function (Welsh *et al.*, 1998; Guzman and Kruse, 2001), leading to sepsis (Moore *et al.*, 1992), inappropriately excessive inflammatory responses and lung injury (Harkin *et al.*, 2001; Kudst, 2003). Providing enteral nutrition prevents gut atrophy and significantly reduces the risk from endogenous infection and the risk of damage to other organs (Fukatsu *et al.*, 2001), even if the nutrition absorbed is insufficient to meet energy demands.

Enteral nutrition

Where oral diets prove impossible or inadequate, tube feeding into the gut is both the safest and the cheapest alternative. However, patients who are being enterally fed may experience problems from lack of gastric acidity, and diarrhoea.

Gastric acidity

Food dilutes the stomach's hydrochloric acid, but between meals the gastric pH returns to below 4. Continuous enteral feeding constantly dilutes the gastric acid. Hydrochloric acid is a strong acid, creating a hostile environment for bacteria between the alkaline environments of the upper and lower gastrointestinal tracts. Constant dilution of gastric acid therefore facilitates bacterial colonisation.

Resting feeds allows gastric acidity to return to its normal level. The optimum rest period between enteral feeds remains unclear, although it should be long enough for the stomach to empty. Many critically ill patients have reduced gut motility, prolonging gastric emptying. Lee *et al.*'s (1990) study recommended resting feeds for 8 hours. Anecdotal reports vary from resting for 1 hour in every 6 to a single rest period each day (usually overnight) of 4–8 hours, without significant differences in infection. Physiologically, it makes sense to rest the gut overnight, when body metabolism is lowest.

Diarrhoea

Diarrhoea is caused when there is more fluid entering the bowel than the bowel can absorb during transit time. Therefore, increased water entering the gut or the decreased ability to absorb fluid can result in diarrhoea. Likely causes of diarrhoea include:

- Antibiotics
- Excessive gut fluid
- Hypoalbuminaemia
- Sorbitol
- Contamination of feeds.

Passage of faeces through the colon usually takes about 12 hours. This delay is partly caused by the presence of gut commensals (harmless bacteria). However, antibiotics destroy gut bacteria, thereby increasing the likelihood of diarrhoea. Diarrhoea occurs in only 3 per cent of enterally fed patients not receiving antibiotics, compared with 41 per cent of enterally fed patients receiving antibiotics (Guenter *et al.*, 1991).

Adult gastrointestinal tract secretions exceed 9 l each day. Additional volume from both enteral feed and drugs may cause excessive volume in a malabsorbing gut.

Gut absorption is partly affected by osmotic pressures. High osmotic pressure attracts water. Normally, gut osmotic pressure is low, while capillary blood osmotic pressure is relatively high. This draws water from the gut into capillary blood. Blood osmotic pressure is created mainly by albumin (the main plasma protein), but blood albumin levels are usually low with critical illness, so critically ill patients usually absorb less gut water (Payne-James and Silk, 1992).

Sorbitol, used in many drug elixirs, has a high osmotic pressure. Sorbitol is not absorbed, so patients receiving nasogastric drug elixirs may retain more water in their gut, or even draw additional water into it.

Contaminated feeds may cause diarrhoea. Feeds may be contaminated during manufacture, although this risk is low; feeds are more likely to be contaminated when opened (e.g. cross-infection from colonised hands or equipment). Enteral feeds are designed to provide nutrients for the body; if contaminated, they provide an ideal medium (nutrients, room temperature, and standing for a number of hours) for bacterial growth. The design of feed-giving sets has improved to help maintain closed systems, but giving sets are often handled by various staff, and are exposed to the many virulent bacteria colonising most wards. Feeds should be treated aseptically, and closed giving sets handled as cleanly as possible.

Although enteral feeds increase the volume of gut fluid, they should not cause diarrhoea in health unless given excessively fast (>275 ml/h) or very rich (>2 kcal/ml) (Adam and Osborne, 1997); neither is likely in practice, so enteral feeding should not cause diarrhoea. Discontinuing enteral feeds to stop diarrhoea is treating the symptom rather than the problem.

Giving drugs to reduce gut motility facilitates the absorption of more water, and so reduces diarrhoea. However, diarrhoea removes gut pathogens, so slowing down motility also facilitates more translocation of gut bacteria into blood. Bulking agents do not prevent diarrhoea (Payne-James and Silk, 1992), and so cannot be recommended.

Aspirate

Aspirate volumes indicate absorption. As the gut produces more than 9l each day, aspirates of up to 200 ml after 1 hour's rest should be tolerated (Adam and Osborne, 1997). If larger volumes are aspirated, gut motility can be increased with drugs (e.g. metoclopramide, low-dose erythromycin).

Discarding gastric aspirate means removing:

- Gastric acid
- Electrolytes
- Feed.

This can cause possible metabolic alkalosis and electrolyte imbalances. Aspirate of up to 200 ml should therefore be returned to the stomach.

Tubes

When patients cannot take oral diets, nasogastric feeding tubes are easiest to insert. Although wide-bore tubes (e.g. Ryles®) are easier both to insert and to aspirate from than fine-bore tubes, they are liable to cause inflammation, erosion and haemorrhage of the upper airway and gastrointestinal tract (Bettany and Powell-Tuck, 1997). Therefore, with prolonged gastric tube feeding, wide-bore tubes should be replaced as soon as reasonably possible. Whichever type of tube is used, marking the tube entry site (or recording the position if the tube is already pre-marked) enables staff to detect any migration of the tube (Metheny, 1993).

Total paralytic ileus prevents enteral feeding. However, paralytic ileus is more often partial, affecting the stomach but not the ileum (Kennedy, 1997). Most nutrients are absorbed in the ileum, so feeding directly into the small bowel can provide effective nutrition. This can be achieved through using naso-jejunal or percutaneous jejunostomy tubes. However, infection risks should be weighed against their benefits.

Patients attempting to remove nasogastric tubes usually do so either because they do not understand the purpose of the tube and it causes irritation (either to their visual field or their skin), or they have consciously decided they do not wish to be fed (usually from a wish to terminate their life). In the first case, removing visual and facial irritation by replacing nasogastric with percutaneous gastro-stomy (PEG) tubes may be beneficial, provided patients will not also attempt to tear out the PEG tube. However, if patients have decided they do not want to be fed, they may consciously remove any alternative tube (PEG, central venous feeding line), causing additional trauma to their body. Forcing treatment on patients against their wishes is also assault (with a few specific exceptions under the Mental Health Act), and individual risk assessment is therefore necessary before replacing removed tubes.

Bowel sounds

Bowel sounds are caused mainly by air swallowed during eating (Raper and Maynard, 1992), so if little air is swallowed, bowel sounds may be absent. Patients receiving tube feeds or not being fed at all are unlikely to swallow much air. Therefore, although the presence of bowel sounds indicates gut motility, the absence of bowel sounds does not necessarily indicate paralytic ileus. Feeding should not therefore be delayed until bowel sounds are heard.

Parenteral nutrition

Whenever possible, patients should be fed enterally. Total paralytic ileus, or treatments, may necessitate resting the gut. Gut surgery does not necessarily cause total paralytic ileus, so is not a contraindication to enteral feeding (Lewis *et al.*, 2001; Steed *et al.*, 2002). Providing nutrition parenterally (intravenously) is preferable to starvation. However, disadvantages of parenteral nutrition include:

- Expense
- Gut atrophy and translocation of gut bacteria from non-use of the gut
- Infection risks (from intravenous cannulation and the infusion being feed given for 24 hours).

Parenteral feeds contain concentrated glucose (range 10% to 50%), which may cause thrombophlebitis. Hypertonic solutions damage veins unless the blood flow is sufficient to dilute the solution rapidly. Parenteral feeds may be central or peripheral.

Central feeds should always be given through central venous lines (e.g. Hickman's, internal jugular, peripherally inserted central catheter). Peripheral feeds contain a weaker solution of glucose, so may be given into a large peripheral vein (e.g. brachial), but should not be given into small veins (e.g. those in the hand or foot).

Parenteral feeds containing fat and glucose are white; those containing only glucose are clear. In addition to glucose and (usually) fat, feeds also contain a range of other nutrients which should be individually prescribed for each patient, with prescriptions checked against the bag label before administration. Nutrients may be damaged by exposure to light, so bags, especially of clear (non-fat) feeds, should be covered.

Large volumes of intravenous glucose may exceed the pancreas' ability to produce insulin, so blood sugar should be monitored regularly (e.g. 4-hourly). If it is elevated, continuous sliding-scale insulin infusion is usually prescribed.

Peripheral parental nutrition is usually only suitable for short-term use, as patients often develop thrombophlebitis despite the relatively low glucose concentrations. Peripheral nutrition can only deliver limited energy (up to 2,000 kcal/day) in moderately large volumes (minimum 2 l), so is unsuitable for patients needing high-energy diets or fluid restrictions (Scott *et al.*, 1998).

Parenteral nutrition is better than no nutrition, but it is a last resort, and should be avoided whenever patients can be fed through other routes. When parenteral nutrition is necessary, small amounts (20–30 ml/h) of enteral feed may prevent complications from gut atrophy and translocation of gut bacteria.

Nutritional assessment

Patients needing complex nutritional assessment should be referred as soon as possible to dieticians. However, patients are usually seen first and most often by nursing staff, who are therefore best placed to initially assess nutritional needs, and so prevent further muscle wasting.

Visual observation may indicate:

- Dehydration
- Undernourishment
- Obesity.

Loss of subcutaneous fat (leaving loose skin) often indicates malnutrition. Some muscles, such as the biceps, can be felt, indicating muscle wasting. However, muscle and fat wasting may be masked by oedema.

Patients and/or relatives should be asked about diet, although problems may be denied. Weight loss may indicate malnutrition, although oedematous patients will gain rather than lose weight. Ketonuria indicates catabolism of body tissue. Patients' conditions may also suggest dietary problems. For example, breathless patients are often malnourished because eating exacerbates their breathlessness; alcoholics are often malnourished because, while alcohol supplies carbohydrates (energy), it contains few other nutrients. Seeing what patients eat (e.g. from returned plates) and recording their dietary input is a simple, but often neglected, nursing observation.

Implications for practice

- Many patients admitted to hospital are malnourished
- Hospitals often fail to provide adequate nutrition
- Length of illness, morbidity and mortality all increase with malnutrition
- Nutrition often needs good multidisciplinary teamwork, nursing having a valuable role in assessing and identifying problems, and monitoring and co-ordinating care
- Patients unable to eat an oral diet should whenever possible be fed enterally
- Before stopping/reducing enteral feeds, consider other factors that may affect gut motility, and if possible treat the problem rather than stopping the feed
- Feeds should be resumed with aspirates of up to 200 ml, and aspirate should be returned to the stomach
- When enteral feeding proves impossible, parenteral nutrition should be provided
- Whatever type of nutrition is used, potential complications should be assessed, and care provided to minimise risks to patients.

Clinical scenario

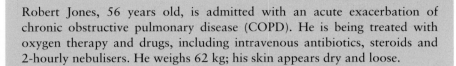

Robert Jones, 56 years old, is admitted with an acute exacerbation of chronic obstructive pulmonary disease (COPD). He is being treated with oxygen therapy and drugs, including intravenous antibiotics, steroids and 2-hourly nebulisers. He weighs 62 kg; his skin appears dry and loose.

1   How would you assess Mr Jones' nutritional needs? From reading this chapter, are there any additional means of assessment you could use?

2   Identify the options for nutrition. List the benefits and risks of each.

3   Devise a care plan to minimise the risks identified. Include how to monitor Mr Jones' nutrition to meet any changing needs.

Bibliography

Key reading

Much is written about nutrition; the Department of Health and various influential bodies frequently produce major reports, the latest of which is *Essence of Care* (DOH, 2001b).

Scott *et al.* (1998) provides a useful handbook for practice. Articles such as those by Kennedy (1997) and Say (1997) provide reliable nursing reviews. Methany has written many authoritative articles about nasogastric feeding; her 1993 article is included in the reference list.

Further reading

Kinn and Scott (2001).

Chapter 7

Acute pain management

Philip Woodrow and Sarah Coulling

Contents

Learning outcomes

After reading this chapter you will be able to:

- Understand the physical and psychological effects of unrelieved pain
- Assess acute pain effectively
- Understand the benefits, limitations and problems of widely-used analgesics.

Fundamental knowledge

Nerve conduction.

Introduction

'Pain is an unpleasant sensory and emotional experience associated with actual or potential tissue damage or described in terms of such' (International Association of the Study of Pain, 1979: 249). This popular definition clearly accepts pain as being a physical and emotional phenomenon; a multidimensional experience rather than simply a measure of sensory intensity.

Pain is a complex phenomenon, indicating some problem, and often causing further physiological, psychological and social problems such as:

- Sleep loss
- Side effects of pain and treatment
- Delayed recovery
- Financial costs to the patient and the health service
- Chronic pain syndromes
- Anxiety, depression and distress
- Loss of social and work roles
- Loss of confidence in healthcare providers.

Benefits of relieving pain are therefore:

- Humanitarian
- Psychological
- Physiological
- Organisational.

Reducing complications associated with poor acute pain management also enables earlier discharge (McCaffery and Pasero, 1999; Macrae, 2001). Much has been written about pain management, but nursing management of acute pain remains poor, partly due to limited knowledge (Royal College of Surgeons/Royal College of Anaesthetists, 1990; Royal College of Anaesthetists, 2000), insufficient staffing, and time factors (Schafheutle et al., 2001).

Pain may be acute (self-limiting) or chronic (beyond the expected time of healing). There is some overlap between causes and management of the two, but also significant differences. This chapter focuses on the physiology, psychology and assessment of and the key aspects of care for acute pain, briefly discussing common pharmacological approaches. However, patients admitted with acute problems may also suffer from simultaneous chronic pain (e.g. arthritis). Nurses should therefore assess the person as a whole, rather than focusing on apparently obvious causes. Specialists in acute and chronic and cancer pain, employed by most hospitals, can provide valuable resources for both patients and staff.

Stress response

Pain triggers the stress ('fight and flight') response (Puntillo and Weiss, 1994), causing:

- Sodium and water retention (oedema)
- Insulin antagonism (hyperglycaemia)
- Tachycardia (increased myocardial work and oxygen consumption)
- Increased peripheral resistance (poor perfusion)
- Hypertension
- Tachypnoea
- Immunosuppression.

Other physiological effects that may prolong recovery or prove fatal to acutely ill patients include:

- Atelectasis due to reluctance to breathe deeply
- Delayed wound healing from ischaemia
- Opportunistic infection due to immunosuppression
- Increased demands on the heart and risk of myocardial ischaemia (particularly in patients whose cardiovascular systems may already be compromised)
- Deep vein thrombosis and pulmonary embolism from immobility and cardiorespiratory changes
- Sore skin and risk of pressure sores from poor peripheral perfusion and immobility
- Nausea, vomiting and ileus from decreased gastrointestinal activity.

Prolonged unrelieved pain also puts patients at risk of developing ongoing chronic pain symptoms as their central nervous system becomes over-sensitised ('wind up') (Macrae, 2001).

Psychosocial factors

Pain is the sum of both the reception of nerve impulses and cognitive perception. Nurses should consider the wide range of psychosocial factors that are thought to influence a person's perception and tolerance of pain, including:

- Culture and religion
- Gender
- Emotional state.

Culture and religion

Cultural background influences how individuals perceive and react to pain, so in multicultural societies pain assessment should include cultural/religious influence as part of holistic care (McCaffery and Pasero, 1999). Although patients may experience a similar condition or surgical procedure, pain responses may differ according to their cultures. Pain is individual, but pain perception and expression is also influenced by culture, and varies between cultures. Some (e.g. Western) cultures value 'the magic bullet remedy', as they have become more medicalised, less tolerant and search for ways to eliminate pain; whereas other (e.g. Eastern) cultures value finding a meaning for their pain (Illich, 1976; Kodiath and Kodiath, 1992; Carr, 1997). The word 'pain' is derived from *poena*, the Latin for punishment. Questions such as 'What have I done to deserve this?' suggest that many people regard pain as a punishment. Others consider that pain has positive qualities, providing spiritual and moral atonement – 'God's will'.

Responses to pain may be stoic or emotive. Stoic patients may express pain and other emotions less, tending to 'grin and bear it' while withdrawing socially. Emotive patients are more likely to verbalise their expressions and feelings. Expressive behaviours are typical of Hispanic, Middle Eastern and Mediterranean backgrounds, while Northern Europeans have a greater tendency to be stoic. In the UK, adults born before the NHS was formed may have been expected to suffer rather than incur medical bills.

Gender

Gender differences regarding the perception of pain are unclear, possibly reflecting gender stereotyping rather than gender itself. Studies are contradictory, although they suggest that women tend to express symptoms more than men, who prefer to remain stoic or 'macho' (Rafferty *et al.*, 1995).

Emotional state

Emotions can both augment and result from pain. Patients with increased emotional distress report more pain. Previous painful experiences can influence perception and the sense of control over a situation. Positive experiences may build confidence and empowerment, whereas negative ones may bring fear, uncertainty and helplessness, making pain worse (Hawthorne and Redmond, 1998).

Negative psychological feedback can lead to defence mechanisms such as aggression, depression and withdrawal. If allowed to persist, this could cause symptoms of post-traumatic stress disorder, such as:

- Chronic anxiety and depression
- Insomnia
- Irritability
- Memory impairment.

(Geisser *et al.*, 1996)

Assessment

Assessing pain is complex, as pain involves both reception and perception, which creates significantly different levels of pain between different individuals. Pain should not therefore be compared between different patients with the same condition. McCaffery's famous claim that 'pain is whatever the experiencing person says it is, existing whenever the experiencing person says it does' (McCaffery, 1965: 95) emphasises the need to assess each patient individually, especially if pain is denied. Patients may under-report or fail to report pain because they:

■ Do not want to appear 'weak'
■ Think busy staff have more important priorities
■ Expect to suffer pain
■ Have not been fully informed about options for managing their pain.

(McCaffery and Pasero, 1999)

Pain indicates a problem. Problems may be physiological and/or psychosocial, but should be assessed and, where possible, managed. Problems may require further medical investigation, so should be reported. Although analgesia may mask symptoms, modern sophisticated diagnostic tests and equipment (Attard *et al.*, 1992) make it unnecessary and inhumane to allow patients to remain in pain just to facilitate medical diagnosis.

Nurses underestimate patients' pain, largely due to lack of education (Seers, 1987; Field, 1996; McCaffery and Ferrell, 1999; Manias *et al.*, 2002), although with the availability of a wide range of tools the documentation of assessment is improving (Lynch, 2001; Schofield, 2003).

Nurses should fully and objectively assess their patients' pain experience, remembering patients' individuality, expectations, the location and intensity of pain, and other influencing factors. Various pain assessment tools have been devised for adults in acute pain. Simple descriptive tools (e.g. 0–3 graded – none, mild, moderate, severe) that ask patients to rate their pain on rest and on movement, such as coughing and touching the opposite side of the bed, parallel the WHO (1996) Analgesic Ladder (Figure 7.1). The 0–3 tool (Figure 7.2) is popular because it is easily understood by patients and, if consistently used by different

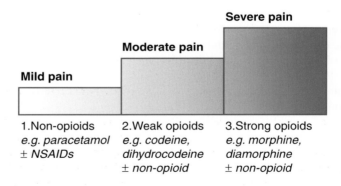

Adapted from the WHO Analgesic Ladder (1996)

Figure 7.1 **WHO analgesic ladder**

The 0–3 pain score
0 = None at rest or on movement
1 = None at rest, slight on movement
2 = Intermittent on rest, moderate on movement
3 = Continuous at rest, severe on movement
Movement: ask patient to cough, observe facial expression and/or ask patient to try to touch the opposite side of the bed

Figure 7.2 **The 0–3 pain score**

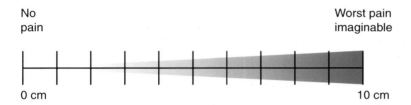

No
pain

Worst pain
imaginable

0 cm   10 cm

Figure 7.3 **Visual analogue scale**

staff, can hasten the provision of analgesia (Macintyre and Ready, 1996; Turk and Melzack, 2001). Visual analogue scales (VAS) can measure pain intensity: for example 0 = no pain, to 10 = worst pain imaginable. Patients plot their score along a 10-cm rule to signify their perceived level of pain (see Figure 7.3). VAS, however, do not measure pain both at rest and on movement (Turk and Melzack, 2001). With semiconscious or confused patients verbal assessment may be unreliable or impossible, necessitating reliance on non-verbal methods in assessing for distress, including:

- Sudden hypertension and/or tachycardia
- Facial expression
- Position and other body language
- Interaction with, or information from, visitors.

(Hawthorne and Redmond, 1998)

Interpretation of these signs as sole indicators of pain alone is, however, subjective, and therefore of limited value (Briggs, 1995) – for example, ill patients are often hypotensive, so increased blood pressure may be misinterpreted as restoration of homeostasis rather than a sign of pain. Pain can stimulate parasympathetic nerves, resulting in hypotension, while illness or treatments causing central nervous system depression, or even paralysis, may prevent visual signs appearing.

Pain may also be referred to other parts of the body. Referred pain usually results from two or more sites sharing the same nociceptors (sensory nerves that

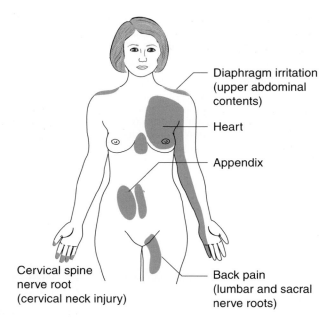

Figure 7.4 **Referred pain**

transmit pain). Figure 7.4 shows some areas where referred pain may be felt. Because pain is individual, nurses assessing pain should consider whether it might be referred, originating from a different site than the one indicated by the patient.

Pharmacological approaches

Acute pain management usually requires analgesics, often opioids. Analgesics should be individualised to patients, considering:

■   Any known drug sensitivity
■   Renal/hepatic function
■   Toxic effects of drugs
■   Potential interactions with other drugs or treatments
■   Whether adverse effects of the drugs used, such as respiratory or cardiovascular depression, will significantly complicate diseases
■   If prolonged use is anticipated, whether accumulation may cause significant problems
■   Administration protocols for analgesia
■   Monitoring of its effectiveness
■   Observation for side effects.

Combining non-opioid (e.g. paracetamol, NSAIDs) with opioid analgesics which act on the central and peripheral pain pathways simultaneously (WHO, 1996;

McCaffery and Pasero, 1999), creates an 'opioid-sparing' effect, achieving similar relief with smaller amounts of opioid. Lowering opioid doses reduces their adverse and unpleasant side effects (see below).

Opioids

Opioids act on specific opioid receptors found mainly in the brain and spinal cord, with some in peripheral tissue, and are particularly effective for inflammatory nociceptive pain following surgery. Common side effects associated with most opioids include:

- Nausea (the most common)
- Respiratory depression
- Sedation
- Constipation
- Urinary retention
- Pruritis
- Dysphoria
- Hypotension.

(Macintyre and Ready, 1996)

Anti-emetics, laxatives and other treatments to reverse or minimise side effects may be needed. Naloxone reverses the effect of opioids such as morphine, diamorphine, fentanyl and pethidine. While naloxone reverses serious side effects, such as respiratory depression, it also reverses analgesia, so pain management should be reviewed. Naloxone has a shorter half-life than opioids, so further doses may be needed to prevent the return of serious side effects.

Opioid-induced nausea and vomiting can be debilitating, leading to dehydration and electrolyte imbalance. Causes are probably multifactorial, but often include opioid stimulation of the vomiting centre (Golembiewski and O'Brien, 2002). After surgery, the incidence of nausea and vomiting is three times higher in women than in men, and is more likely to occur if blood pressure falls by more than one-third and if patients are anxious (Jolley, 2001). It is rarely caused by gastric contents, so giving metochlopramide to increase gut motility is unlikely to provide relief (Wigfull and Welchew, 2001). Anti-emetics that act on the vomiting centre (e.g. ondansteron, prochlorperazine, cyclizine) are more effective, and may be given prophylactically to high-risk groups regularly and even in combination with each other (Strunin *et al.*, 1999).

There are subtle differences between the opioids used in acute pain management (Macintyre and Ready, 1996; Australian NHMRC, 1999; McCaffery and Pasero, 1999). Whichever opioid is chosen, patients should receive sufficient analgesia to achieve comfort with minimum side effects. Many patients and clinicians are anxious about opioid addiction, leading to opioid analgesia frequently being prematurely discontinued (Carr, 2000), but when given for acute pain management in hospital opioids rarely (<1 per cent) cause addiction (Porter and Jick, 1980; McCaffery and Pasero, 1999).

Morphine

Morphine may be administered orally, rectally, intramuscularly, subcutaneously or intravenously. Used since pre-Roman times, it remains the most valuable opioid for severe pain – the 'gold standard' by which others are judged. Doses can be titrated according to individual patient variation; analgesia may be reached at high doses. There is no dose beyond which additional analgesia is not obtained (ceiling effect). Locally agreed protocols offer algorithms that allow further doses to be given safely within defined parameters (such as boluses every 5 minutes for intravenous and hourly for intramuscular and oral preparations) (Oxford Pain Research Trust, 2003). High doses cause fewer side effects if given orally, because of first-pass metabolism in the liver (Macintyre and Ready, 1996).

Diamorphine

Diamorphine may be administered orally, subcutaneously, intramuscularly, intravenously, epidurally, intrathecally or intranasally. Derived from morphine, it is highly lipid-soluble, so crosses through fatty subcutaneous tissue, myelin sheaths and the blood–brain barrier easily (Pinger *et al.*, 1995), giving fast and effective pain relief. It is more potent than morphine, causing less nausea and hypotension with equivalent doses, and is quicker-acting.

Fentanyl

Fentanyl may be administered intravenously, epidurally, intrathecally, intranasally, as a lozenge or transdermally. A synthetic opioid, it causes little histamine release (Eddleston *et al.*, 1997), so is useful for patients who are sensitive to morphine. However, its effectiveness is unpredictable, making titration difficult. Fentanyl derivatives, including alfentanil, sufentanil and remifentanil, are most commonly used in day-case surgery or as continuous infusions in critical care units. Fentanyl patches are licensed for chronic malignant pain.

Pethidine

Pethidine may be administered orally, subcutaneously, intramuscularly or intravenously. It is now seldom used, as it has a very short effect (2–3 hours), produces the long-lasting neurotoxic metabolite norpethidine, is highly addictive, and provides no greater pain relief than morphine (McQuay and Moore, 1998). Its use is limited to patients with a proven allergy to morphine.

Codeine/dihydrocodeine

Codeine and dihydrocodeine may be administered orally, rectally or intramuscularly. These weak opioids can be useful as part of combination therapy, but on their own are unlikely to relieve severe acute pain. They are synergistic with paracetamol and are available in combined preparations which are effective as alternative analgesia after surgery or trauma, when parenteral opioids are no longer required (McQuay and Moore, 1998).

Tramadol

Tramadol may be administered orally, intramuscularly or intravenously. It is a weak opioid, but also relieves pain by inhibiting chemical transmission through the pain pathway. It is useful for moderate but not severe pain (Budd and Langford, 1999). Although causing less respiratory depression and sedation than stronger opioids, it often provokes nausea, and in older people can cause confusion.

Patient-controlled analgesia and epidural techniques

Intravenous patient-controlled analgesia (PCA), epidural PCA (PCEA) and continuous epidural infusions are effective techniques for administering strong opioids for severe pain, typically morphine via IV PCA and fentanyl or diamorphine via epidural (epidurals are usually combined with a local anaesthetic such as bupivacaine). Giving patients control of administering their own opioids, within maximum (preset lock-out) limits, usually achieves better analgesia than traditional intramuscular opioid regimes, and is preferred by patients (Snell *et al.*, 1997). Epidural analgesia can even eliminate severe pain, exposing patients to fewer problems from the adverse effects of unrelieved pain, and hastening recovery (McLeod *et al.*, 2001).

Risk management

Many risks can arise from using PCA or PCEA; for example, there is a greater risk of opioid side effects with IV PCA, and there are specific risks connected with epidurals, which are related to the opioid, the invasive catheter (dural puncture, haematoma, abscess, misplaced catheter – patchy or no sensory block) and to the local anaesthetic (cardiovascular and central nervous system toxicity, urinary retention, total spinal analgesia, motor blockade, sympathetic blockade – hypotension). Risks are reduced by:

- Local protocols and clinical guidelines concerning equipment, drugs, personnel, training, documentation, administration, monitoring, discontinuation, requirements and for management of complications
- Informed patient consent and careful selection based on risk/benefit analyses for example, for PC(E)A, patient dexterity and understanding
- Specific infusion devices and patient monitoring charts
- Sufficient staff competent to local standards
- Designated Acute Pain Service Support and out of hours cover
- Adjunct non-opioid analgesics, an anti-emetic and naloxone prescribed alongside PCAs and epidurals.

       Royal College of Surgeons/Royal College of Anaesthetists, 1990; Clinical Standards Advisory Group, 1999; Royal College of Anaesthetists, 2000.

Monitoring and documentation

Vital sign monitoring (heart-rate, BP, respiratory rate, oxygen saturations), pain, nausea and sedation levels should be frequently scored at intervals. In addition, for epidurals, peripheral sensation and motor strength should be closely monitored (Macintyre and Ready, 1996). A quarter of epidurals fail to provide effective analgesia, often due to catheter misplacement (Ballantyne *et al.*, 2003), so close patient monitoring is essential according to local protocols

Specific charts designed to document PCA and epidural observations should be used as good professional practice, and to comply with medico-legal documentation requirements. These charts should demonstrate an evaluation of the analgesia and detection for the onset of any side effects. Particularly useful are charts that combine: the prescription protocol, troubleshooting guidelines and monitoring tables.

Discontinuation

PCAs and epidurals can remain in place for 72 hours or more. Periodic infusion line and filter changes should be carried out according to local infection control guidelines. Unfortunately, PCAs are often withdrawn too early (Ng *et al.*, 2000). The decision to step down from strong opioids to weaker opioids should be made with the patient according to his or her level of pain, the decreased need for strong opioids, and whether alternative routes for analgesia have been identified. PCA and epidural infusions should be stopped but not removed until satisfactory alternative analgesia has been established. Removal of epidural lines can cause complications, so should be aseptic and, if the patient is anticoagulated, should usually only occur when clotting time is normal. Staff removing epidural lines should follow local hospital protocols and guidelines.

Non-opioids

Paracetamol

Paracetamol may be administered orally, or rectally; intravenous preparations will also soon be available. It is recommended on all parts of the WHO (1996) Analgesic Ladder as a sole agent for mild pain, and in combination with a non-steroidal anti-inflammatory drug (NSAID) and/or opioid for moderate to severe pain, where it also has an 'opioid-sparing' effect. Its site of action remains unclear, but it is thought to work on the central rather than peripheral nervous system. Paracetamol is well tolerated, although hepatotoxicity occurs in over-dosage (Macintyre and Ready, 1996).

Non-steroidal anti-inflammatory drugs

NSAIDs may be administered orally, rectally, intravenously or intramuscularly. All NSAIDs have an opioid-sparing effect when given in combination with opioids. Useful for pain caused by inflammation, they inhibit the action of the enzyme cyclo-oxygenase 2 (cox 2), which is necessary for the production of the inflammatory mediator prostaglandin, released in response to tissue injury. Unfortunately NSAIDs also inhibit cyclo-oxygenase 1 (cox 1), which is necessary for the production of prostaglandins. Prostaglandins protect the bronchial and gastrointestinal mucosal linings and renal perfusion, and facilitate platelet aggregation. Consequently, conventional NSAIDs (e.g. ibuprofen) may cause:

- Bronchoconstriction (wheezing) in 5–20% of aspirin-sensitive asthmatics
- Renal failure when there is impaired renal function, poor urine output or a low blood pressure (renal perfusion)
- Bleeding when the patient is anticoagulated or has underlying bleeding disorders
- Gastric ulceration and bleeding, especially in patients with a history of gastrointestinal problems.

Effects on prostaglandin are systemic, potentially causing generalised thinning of the gastrointestinal mucosa, regardless of the administration route.

NSAIDs should only be used for a short time because of the risk of side effects (Macintyre and Ready, 1996). A new generation of selective cox 2 NSAIDs (e.g. celecoxib, rofecoxib, paracoxib) claim to cause less gastrointestinal irritation, less platelet aggregation, and so less disruption to clotting time; however, their use should still be avoided with impaired renal function or low blood pressure (Fitzgerald and Patrono, 2001).

Non-pharmacological pain management

Non-pharmacological approaches can enhance well-being, release endogenous opioids and reduce the effects of stress (catecholamines, steroids). They also may reduce the quantity of opioids needed. Despite many clinicians being unconvinced by the research evidence, these are popular approaches used commonly in chronic pain management. Acute pain usually necessitates powerful drugs, but additional therapy may be provided through Transcutaneous Electrical Nerve Stimulation (TENS) and other complementary therapies (e.g. hot/cold pads, aromatherapy, therapeutic massage), as well as ensuring patient comfort (e.g. positioning) and relieving anxieties (reassurance, relaxation, distraction).

Comfort

Although much pain experienced by acutely ill patients is caused by their underlying illness/diseases and/or treatments, general discomfort can also lead to pain. Providing comfort whenever possible should be fundamental to nursing, and includes:

- Smoothing creases in sheets
- Relieving prolonged pressure

- Turning pillows over
- Reducing temperature if patients feel uncomfortably warm
- Placing limbs in a comfortable, well-supported position
- Reducing noise and light
- Touch, explanations, reassurance and empowerment strategies.

Implications for practice

- Pain is a complex phenomenon involving both physiological transmission of pain signals and cognitive interpretation
- Pain is individual to each person, so should be assessed individually
- Promoting comfort and alleviating/minimising pain is fundamental to nursing care
- Acute pain management often necessitates opioid drugs, but additional ways to manage pain should be included where appropriate
- Nurses should evaluate the effectiveness of pain relief to optimise its effect and minimise its complications
- Most acute hospitals employ specialist pain-control clinical nurse specialists, provide evidence-based protocols and facilitate training – so use local resources.

Summary

Pain is a complex phenomenon, involving both physiological transmission of pain signals and cognitive interpretation. Pain is culturally influenced and individual to each person, so should be assessed individually. Promoting comfort and achieving effective pain management is fundamental to nursing, yet many patients continue to suffer unnecessary pain. Understanding its physiological and psychosocial effects, together with pharmacology of drugs used, enables nurses to plan effective pain relief. Acute pain often needs opioids, although non-opioid drugs can provide useful synergy with opioids, and non-pharmacological approaches should also be considered. Evaluating and documenting the effectiveness of pain relief helps to optimise its effect and minimise its complications.

Clinical scenario

Mr Michael Newberg, aged 73, had an elective Hartmann's procedure 2 days ago. Due to insufficient staffing levels, his fentanyl and bupivicaine epidural infusion was discontinued and the catheter removed overnight; he was prescribed regular codeine 60 mg with paracetamol 1 g at 6-hourly intervals with as-required intramuscular morphine 10 mg. On the morning ward round he admitted feeling pain, and was given a morphine injection. He also identified shoulder pain, for which he has since been given a heat pad. Now, 2 hours following the morphine injection, his respiration rate is only 10 breaths per minute.

1 How would you assess Mr Newberg's pain? Identify the strengths and limitations of your preferred methods of assessment.

2 Evaluate the likely benefits and adverse effects of the various post-operative analgesics provided so far for Mr Newberg.

3 Identify changes for managing Mr Newberg's pain, together with the reasons for your recommendations and how you would evaluate their effectiveness.

Bibliography

Key reading

McCaffery and Pasero (1999). McCaffery's definition of pain is familiar to most nurses, but her work on pain management remains seminal, and is presented accessibly in this text.

Wall and Melzack (1999). Since developing the gate control theory of pain, Melzack and Wall have been widely recognised as leading authorities. This text provides a comprehensive resource.

Hawthorne and Redmond (1998). Excellent British text; captures the holistic nursing perspective. Especially useful in identifying myths and misconceptions, and assessment of patients' total pain experience.

Further reading

Macintyre and Ready (1996).
Stannard and Booth (1998).
Melzack and Wall (1988).
Moore *et al.* (2003).

Chapter 8

Death and dying

Philip Woodrow

Contents

Learning outcomes

After reading this chapter you will be able to:

- Identify the human needs (patients, families, friends and staff) involved when caring for patients dying on the High Dependency Unit
- Promote individualised care which meets the patient's needs
- Increase awareness of when and how treatment should be withdrawn
- Understand the needs for follow-up care.

Introduction

Acute care aims to provide treatments and cures for people with critical, often life-threatening, illness. However, inevitably not all patients will survive. This chapter explores three main themes surrounding death on critical care areas:

1   Attitudes of nurses and other staff toward death. Some staff need support following the death of patients. While patients may not be admitted for terminal care, life-saving treatment can become futile, unethical and unkind.
2   Treatment, including:

■   When and how such decisions should be made
■   What should be withdrawn and what should remain or be provided as part of palliative care.

3   Needs of patients, family and friends during and after terminal care. While the growth of the hospice movement has improved bereavement care, death in acute wards may be sudden, leaving people little time to adjust to impending loss. This creates unique needs that cannot always be met by theory and practice drawn from areas specialising in palliative care.

Death is largely a taboo subject within society, many people being reluctant to discuss it. Manley (1986) vividly contrasts differing social attitudes by placing a fifteenth-century deathbed scene of a dying person surrounded by his family and priests, with a photograph of a dead patient in ICU surrounded by modern technology but without a living person in view. Many researchers are understandably cautious about approaching bereaved families in case they increase or revive their distress. Research-based evidence is therefore limited both in quantity and sample sizes, making findings more than usually tentative.

In this chapter, 'family' includes all relatives, whether by blood, marriage or common law. Much material can also be extended to anyone close enough to the patient to be affected by their death. Family care is discussed further in Chapter 11.

Death – a medical failure?

Prolonging life, rather than allowing patients to die, sometimes becomes the unreasonable option. However, when to alter from life-sustaining to life-withdrawing treatment is debatable, value-laden and fraught with ethical, moral and sometimes legal dilemmas. Death has traditionally been viewed as a medical failure (Sprung, 1990). Medical and nursing perspectives have traditionally been contrasted as cure versus care. While this is potentially oversimplistic, especially as the roles of doctors and nurses increasingly overlap and medical undergraduates receive greater input into quality of care, nurses may consider prolonging a person's life to be immoral/unethical, and consider that their own status and professionalism are undermined if their views are ignored or over-ridden.

Support for staff

Death of patients can cause distress to nursing staff as well as families (Farrell, 1989). Nurses and family may experience similar emotions, including guilt (Spencer, 1994). Nurses may try to avoid showing their feelings to patients or families. For some, this may be a coping mechanism; others are concerned to remain 'professional'. However, families need honesty from health professionals (Parkes, 1996), and can gain more support if they are aware that staff are also upset (Finlay and Dallimore, 1991).

Support from peers or professional counsellors may help nurses to cope (Spencer, 1994). Peer support could be informal or structured, through debriefing or reflective sessions. Jackson's (1998) survey of bereavement follow-up services for families found that 21 per cent of nurses did not wish to contact bereaved families. There may be various reasons for this, including unresolved grief.

Death is a topic often avoided in Western society, but few nurses can avoid witnessing it. Therefore, including death and bereavement as part of each nurse's professional development can help nurses both to cope themselves, and to provide support to help families cope.

Withdrawing treatment

This term implies withdrawing life-prolonging treatment. When further life-prolonging treatment becomes inappropriate, comfort and dignity should become the focus of care.

The decision to withdraw treatment should be made by a team, ideally including the patient. Nurses can and should be involved in decision-making, so need sufficient knowledge and confidence to participate appropriately.

The practice of withdrawing treatment varies between hospitals and doctors, and is sometimes influenced by the demand for beds (Cook *et al.*, 1995; Ravenscroft and Bell, 2000). Critical illness may prevent patients from participating in decision-making, and less critically ill patients may not always be involved (Morrison, 1994), so UK nurses cannot become complacent either that patients have consented to withdrawing/withholding treatment, or that their consent is necessarily valid. Involuntary passive euthanasia has become a reality of contemporary health care; treatments are withheld or withdrawn in full knowledge that doing so will result in imminent death. Nurse advocacy requires nurses to ensure that decisions in which patients cannot (or do not) participate are in the patient's best interests and reflect the patient's, rather than the nurse's or someone else's, values. However, nurses' values may not necessarily reflect those of patients they are 'advocating' for, and therefore nurses should be cautious about assuming what others would wish. Advance directives can usefully indicate patients' wishes, but these are often either not made or not obviously available.

Quality of life

'Quality of life' is frequently cited when considering whether treatment should be stopped or denied. Ravenscroft and Bell (2000) found only one of all thirteen intensive care units in West Yorkshire assessed quality of life before, and only three following, admission. While this probably reflects practice elsewhere, this survey assumes that:

- Quality of life is quantifiable
- Current tools provide suitable measurements.

Definitions of 'Quality of life' vary significantly between different authors (Farquhar, 1995), making its measurement problematic (North, 1995). Quality of life does not necessarily correlate with measurements of health (Covinsky *et al.*, 1999), and should not be used to determine healthcare provision (Aksoy, 2000).

Time out 8.1

Image you are critically ill, having been diagnosed as having a life-threatening illness. When asked by you, the doctor states that you have only a 20 per cent chance of survival.

1 Would you wish life-prolonging treatment to be given?
2 At what point would life change from being acceptable to unacceptable? Identify an appropriate percentage figure.
3 List any factors that might alter your decision.

Discuss this exercise with some colleagues at work and compare differing values.

Science cannot ultimately *know* the chances in each individual case. Assuming life is worse than death is also value-laden; no-one knows what death is like (Aksoy, 2000).

Pain

Pain is the main cause of requests for euthanasia (Emmanuel *et al.*, 2000). If there is any doubt about the patient's comfort, pain relief should be provided (British Medical Association, 2001). However, nurses' assessment and management of pain is often poor (see Chapter 7). Many bereaved families consider the analgesia provision for their loved one could have been improved (Danis, 1998).

A unique experience

Whatever personal beliefs and values each nurse may hold, death of patients is an inevitable part of nursing in almost any speciality. Family and friends of the patient are unlikely to have seen as many people die as, and will have known the patient longer and more intimately than, the nurse. Therefore, however caring nurses are, experiencing bereavement is likely to be unique to family in a way it cannot be to the nurse. This almost inevitably places nurses outside the intimate circle of grieving.

Death, dying and bereavement are individual processes, so no discussion can hope to provide prescriptive solutions to meet all needs. However, terminal care is the last care anyone can receive during his or her lifetime. When death becomes inevitable, nurses should strive to make the process of dying as comfortable and positive as possible.

Sudden death makes relatives feel they have lost control of their lives and are unable to change the situation (Wright, 1991). Nurses should therefore help the family to regain control and power, while giving them the freedom to express their feelings and face the pain of death (Wright, 1991). Families need both practical advice and information, such as how to make funeral arrangements, and someone to talk to (Hall and Hall, 1994). Nurses may be able to provide either of these, or can arrange contact with other professionals, such as chaplains and patient liaison officers. Providing printed information, such as the Department of Social Services' booklet *What to Do after Death*, can be particularly helpful, as grieving relatives may not remember everything they are told.

Breaking bad news and witnessing suffering can cause stress (Wright, 1996; Farrell, 1999), so understandably many staff feel uncomfortable with taking on this role. Doctors' communication with families is often inconsistent (Ravenscroft and Bell, 2000) and could be improved (Danis, 1998). Nurses' communication is probably similarly variable. Staff trained in counselling skills are likely to be able to support relatives more effectively; however, families often trust particular members of staff, and may value that member of staff speaking with them. For the bereaved family, the nurse's interpersonal skills are more important than his or her professional rank (Finlay and Dallimore, 1991). Staff should therefore try and find out what the family has already been told, both to avoid inconsistencies and to try to ensure that relatives are given sufficient information to meet their needs.

Responses to death may also be affected by cultural influences, such as religion, and nurses should therefore be sensitive to cultural needs. Hospital switchboards can usually provide contacts for advice about various religions. There are also various publications about specific religions and cultures, which offer useful resources for ward staff.

Grief

Cognitive and emotional dissonance about death is widespread. Everyone knows we are mortal and therefore must all die, but many people emotionally deny the prospect of their own death or the death of those near to them. Therefore, many people are unprepared for the emotional reality of death.

Guilt is probably the most painful aspect of grief (Kubler-Ross, 1970). Bereaved relatives often seek reasons for the death. However irrational, they

often blame themselves for causing or contributing to the death. Nurses can profoundly affect how relatives respond to bereavement (Coolican, 1994). Whenever
possible, families should be informed honestly and clearly about the impending
death of their loved one so that they may begin grieving (Eastland, 2001).

Sudden death

Death on acute areas is often sudden. With severe acute diseases, death is more
likely to be relatively quick even when it is expected. Grieving is, however, a long
process, and relatives are unlikely to reach a stage of acceptance before a sudden
death. With sudden death, the bereaved may need more support but often receive
less (Yates *et al.*, 1990). The time immediately surrounding sudden death is
crucial in determining families' ability to accept death and deal with the crisis
(Lindermann, 1994), partly because disbelief can be very strong (Jackson, 1996).

Anticipating events, or imagining what happened if they were not present, is
often worse for relatives than the reality (Ellison, 1992). Viewing the body after
death helps the grieving process (Ashdown, 1985; Cathcart, 1988), providing an
opportunity to 'say goodbye'. However, critical illnesses and their treatments can
be very disfiguring, so nurses should make the body appear as normal as possible.
With neonatal deaths, photographs are normally placed in patients' notes so that
any family later regretting not viewing the body can at least see what it looked
like. Although this practice is not widespread within adult nursing, Cathcart
(1988) suggests that it should be considered. When family intend to view their
loved one's dead body, nurses can help to prepare them by describing what to
expect (e.g. skin colour, expression) and any equipment (e.g. tubes and dressings)
that remains in place.

This traumatic situation can be made worse by relatives being prevented from
seeing their loved one after death. Families may feel 'cheated' if they are not
allowed to see and touch the body (Ellison, 1992). Up to half the people contacting a branch of CRUSE (a voluntary group for bereaved family) did so because of
feelings of anxiety and anger towards hospitals, doctors and nurses (Ewins and
Bryant, 1992).

Not for resuscitation

The medical team, ideally with agreement from the multidisciplinary team and
with the patient's consent, should identify patients who would not benefit from
cardiopulmonary resuscitation. Decisions not to resuscitate should be clearly
recorded, following local policies. Most Trusts have a clear pro forma for 'do not
attempt cardiopulmonary resuscitation' orders.

Follow-up

As grief is a process, relatives need ongoing support. Bereaved relatives usually
value being contacted by nurses who cared for their loved one (Jackson, 1998),
and bereavement programmes can help survivors to cope (Burke and Seeley,

1994). While condolence cards are a well-accepted form of support (Burke and Seeley, 1994), reactions to bereavement will be individual, and so a few people may find them insincere. The best time for sending condolence cards is debatable; most authors recommend after 2–6 weeks (Wright, 1991; Jackson, 1996); Kubler-Ross (1991) recommends 1 month.

Implications for practice

- Nurses should be actively involved in decisions about whether to prolong or withdraw active treatment
- Measuring quality of life is problematic; currently there is no absolutely reliable tool to measure it
- Patients' wishes should be considered and, whenever possible, their informed consent obtained
- Withdrawing active treatment does not mean withdrawing care; terminal care should provide comfort and maintain dignity
- During and following death, the family, friends, and often staff, need support, individualised to each person's needs
- Families value follow-up support from wards where their loved one died
- A system should be maintained for contacting families following bereavement; evidence for the best time for follow-up is 2–6 weeks
- Interpersonal skills of nurses are more valued by families than their professional rank.

Summary

Acute hospitals are designed to provide life-supporting treatments, but not all patients survive. Death is not a medical failure, but the inevitable end of each person's life. Nurses should strive to meet the needs of patients and their families, and actively participate in decisions about prolonging or withdrawing active treatment. Once active treatment is withdrawn, care should focus on comfort and dignity.

Bereavement is likely to be traumatic for family, friends and, sometimes, staff. Nurses should therefore provide support to families during bereavement, including practical information and space to express their emotions. Families value being able to see the body of their loved one.

Quality bereavement care can ease the trauma, but not remove it. Families usually need prolonged support, which hospitals can often initiate. The needs of staff should also be supported. Because reactions to loss are individual, any of the various support structures identified in this chapter may be valuable for both staff and family.

Clinical scenario

Mr Albert Jones was admitted following a myocardial infarction and thrombolysis in A&E. Since taking early retirement 3 years ago at the age of 58, he and his wife have been able to travel more, including visits to their only son and his family, who live 350 miles away.

Mr Jones' condition has stabilised sufficiently to return to a medical ward. However, his cardiac function is poor, and he becomes very breathless on exertion. His chances of survival to discharge are estimated at best to be 10–20 per cent. The medical team has suggested withdrawing treatment.

1 Identify your role as nurse advocate for Mr Jones. What factors would influence your views of whether treatment should be withdrawn?

2 Consider the likely needs of Mr Jones' family up to the time of his death.

3 Reflect on follow-up facilities available in your ward, hospital, and local area. How far do these meet the needs suggested by evidence-based practice?

Bibliography

Key reading

The BMA (2001) provides authoritative guidelines for doctors about withholding and withdrawing treatment. This short book also provides nurses with valuable insights into professional medical guidelines and debates. Classic texts about bereavement include Kubler-Ross (1970), Buckman (1988), Parkes (1996) and Wright (1996).

Further reading

Jackson (1996a, 1998) has reported influential work on follow-up care. Farrell (1999) discusses breaking bad news, while Spencer (1994) explores nurses' own coping mechanisms. Ravenscroft and Bell (2000) analyse decision-making regarding withdrawing treatment.

Chapter 9

Cultural issues

Mary Tilki

Contents

Learning outcomes

After reading this chapter you will be able to:

- Understand the significance of cultural awareness
- Demonstrate knowledge and sensitivity when caring for patients from minority ethnic groups
- Provide culturally competent nursing care for the critically ill patient.

Introduction

Critical care areas in many cities are increasingly caring for significant numbers of people from minority ethnic groups. Evidence from Census 2001 (http://www.statistics.gov.uk 2003) shows that 7.9 per cent of the UK population is from minority ethnic groups, although the proportion is much higher in certain areas. There is evidence of poorer health among this group, with excesses of heart disease and stroke, and a high incidence of diabetes and mental ill-health (Nazroo 1997). There is some evidence that people from minority ethnic groups have difficulty accessing and are less satisfied with their GP (Rudat, 1994). There is also evidence of lower rates of referral for investigation or for surgery (Shaukat *et al.*, 1997). Many of these problems result in crises for the individual and ultimately in the need for high dependency care. Despite this, there is an absence of research on the needs of people from minority ethnic groups in critical care settings.

This chapter is based on the Transcultural Skills Development Model (Papadopoulos *et al.*, 1998). This model proposes that the ability to care competently and safely for people of different cultures, depends on practitioners being culturally aware, having knowledge of different cultures and using sensitive interpersonal skills to assess and deliver nursing care. The components of the model are used to demonstrate the meaning of cultural competence for nurses in high dependency areas and for the patients who are nursed there. In the absence of empirical research, this chapter draws upon the experiences of nurses in critical care settings.

Cultural awareness

There is a tendency in the UK to think of issues of race, culture and ethnicity in terms of skin colour. However, everybody is a product of their culture, and ethnicity relates to the group with which they identify or are identified with. There are many white minority ethnic groups all over Britain, both as settled communities and as newly arrived immigrants. British people too identify with different cultures or regional identities, with Londoners, for example, feeling different to people born in Liverpool or Newcastle.

Census 2001 shows that in addition to those born abroad, increasing numbers of people born in the UK consider they have dual identity, identifying with the culture of parents born elsewhere as well as being British. This reflects the way in which families raise children in their own cultural heritage, often within distinct ethnic communities in different parts of Britain. There are also increasing numbers of people with mixed heritage who identify with the culture of one or both parents as well as their British birthplace.

Cultural labels such as 'Asian' or 'African' presume a heterogeneity that does not exist, and mask the diversity of origin, religion, language or social position in these groups. Equally, it is important to remember that culture and ethnicity are dynamic, changing over time and adapting to different places and situations. They are influenced by the time, experience and place of birth and settlement, as well as differences based on gender, age, socio-economic status and education. Individuals also adhere to different aspects of culture, adopting them to differing degrees and in differing situations.

Cultural awareness is very important in high dependency settings, as professionals work under pressure and are required to make speedy decisions. It is easy under such conditions to make assumptions about individuals or groups and to neglect the diversity within them. It is also possible that differences are seen as problems when in reality they are just alternative beliefs or practices that can often be accommodated without too much effort.

Time out 9.1

The health of people from many minority ethnic groups is worse than that of the population as a whole (Acheson, 1998).

1 Identify the different cultural groups comprising the geographical area in which you work.
2 Consider the particular health problems experienced by each group and reflect on how these might impact on the knowledge and skills required by critical care nurses.

Cultural knowledge

Knowledge of the health profile of particular cultural groups is pertinent to nurses in high dependency situations. Poverty, income and housing are not discussed here, although acknowledgement is given to their role in poor health and potential impact on recovery or rehabilitation (Acheson, 1998). Although some culture-specific disorders exist, people from minority ethnic groups experience the same illnesses as the rest of the population, but often more excessively. The data on some groups are absent, but there is evidence of high mortality from coronary heart disease in Asian and Irish people (Harding and Balarajan, 1996). The incidence of hypertension is particularly high among Caribbean, Asian, African and Irish men and women. This also contributes to increased levels of stroke, and may be exacerbated by high rates of diabetes in Caribbean and Asian communities. Accidents and occupational injuries are common in all manual groups, especially the Irish. There are also high levels of mental illness among minority ethnic groups, and the high incidence of attempted suicide in some groups is relevant for critical care areas.

There is a high use of GP services by people from minority ethnic groups, but low levels of satisfaction with the care received (Rudat, 1994). Some people from minority ethnic groups fail to use services because they are not aware of what is available. However, language barriers, concerns about cultural sensitivity, and experiences of hostility and humiliation may have a greater role to play (ALG, 2000). Research demonstrates lower levels of referral for consultation, investigation, coronary revascularisation, heart and renal transplantation among people from minority ethnic groups (Shaukat et al., 1997). Such institutional racism fails to identify and treat illness early and therefore contributes to physiological crisis, which in turn creates psychological stress. Critically ill people and their relatives feel vulnerable anyway, but this is exacerbated for people from minority ethnic groups who may feel badly treated but are unable to challenge it through lack of knowledge or limited language ability.

People from many cultures hold health beliefs based on a combination of culturally shaped ideas, medical and lay messages about the causes of ill-health or ways of managing illness. However, some groups see ill-health as a punishment or a difficulty to be endured in this life for reward in a later one. Others believe illness to be caused by spirits or curses. There may therefore be tensions between such cultural beliefs and contemporary health care, but it is important that nurses understand and respect them and incorporate them where possible into care and treatment.

Nurses must be aware of the importance of food in recovery from illness. If food or fluids are restricted, this must be carefully explained to the patient and family. Every culture believes certain foods to be therapeutic or avoided in illness. In some cases this relates to ideas of hot and cold, with a 'hot' illness relying on 'cold' food and vice versa. What constitutes hot or cold does not necessarily relate to temperature or spiciness, and foods are classified differently in different cultures. The family may wish to provide culturally appropriate food for their relative, and unless this is inappropriate for physiological reasons they should be enabled to do so. In the absence of adequate provision of ethnic food in hospitals, providing familiar and palatable food can be therapeutic for the patient and beneficial for the family.

There may be tensions regarding the balance between rest and mobility. People from all cultures believe rest will aid recovery from illness, and by implication more serious illness requires more rest. The complications of bed rest invariably require early mobilisation, but unless this is clearly explained, patients may perceive they are not being cared for properly.

Control of pyrexia may cause anxiety to people from other cultures. The natural tendency of many people is to keep warm when they have a high temperature, but nurses take active measures to cool the body. The need for specific cooling procedures must be carefully explained to the patient or family. Maintaining modesty is highly important and, as in the case of all patients, shivering must be prevented.

Ideas about nursing differ from one culture to another. While nurses are generally valued and respected in the UK, nursing is a low-status occupation in many parts of the world. Patients will appreciate the kindness and efficiency of a nurse, but will not necessarily expect a high level of knowledge, or the ability to make clinical decisions or give information. They may either insist on seeing a doctor, or feel disgruntled if unable to communicate with one. The gender of the nurse may be a problem, and it is often unacceptable for male nurses to care for female patients. Male patients may feel more confident when cared for by men, and can be embarrassed when female nurses have to carry out intimate procedures. However, assumptions must not be made, and the ability to communicate in the same language or to share in a cultural or religious background may be more important than gender differences.

Family and gender roles differ across cultures and may be misunderstood in critical care settings. The presence of a large number of visitors may be frustrating for nurses who do not understand the importance of the family in illness and hospitalisation. In many developing countries the family provides hospital care, and, apart from being the only care available, there is an obligation on relatives to be present to encourage and support the patient. In the interests of safe access to all patients it is important to negotiate with the family. Clear access must be balanced against the potential for psychological distress caused by limiting visitors.

Seeking permission, making decisions and gathering or giving information are important aspects of high dependency care which rely on the family if the patient is too unwell to participate. However, it is the norm in some cultures that decisions are made jointly by the family or male relatives in particular, rather than by the individual patient. Patients may therefore be reluctant to make a decision without reference to the wider family. It is important to respect these cultural norms, but to be alert to the fact that in some situations patients may not be totally happy with decisions made on their behalf.

Cultural sensitivity

Knowledge of cultural beliefs, customs and related social factors can reduce the risk of cultural insensitivity. This aspect of transcultural care relies on good inter-personal skills, the recognition of differing norms and mores, and a commitment to respecting them. Respect is a complex phenomenon, shown in different ways ranging from the correct form of address to accepting and working with very different beliefs and values. Patients and family members will respect a nurse who admits not knowing but asks how an individual should be addressed, how a name is pronounced, or for clarification of cultural conventions.

Respect is demonstrated by adhering where at all possible to customs regarding interaction between men and women, and between people of different ages. Eye contact is interpreted as a mark of respect, honesty and evidence of listening in the UK. In many African, Asian and other societies, respect for elders or people in authority is demonstrated by looking away, and nurses may interpret this as unwillingness to communicate, as dishonesty or as withdrawal.

Building trust with people who have experienced hostility or persecution is not easy, but is an essential part of nursing. It requires nurses to challenge their own stereotypes and to be sensitive about the questions they ask and in particular how they ask them. It can be enhanced when nurses take the trouble to learn a few words in the language of the patient, address patients by their correct title, and adhere to conventions regarding eye contact and body language as much as possible.

Although a patient may have used English as a second language for many years, the ability to use it may be impaired during serious illness. Similarly, relatives who communicate reasonably well under normal circumstances often have difficulty under stress. The importance of interpreters cannot be overstated, but it is worth remembering that a person may understand more than their level of spoken English suggests. This can both help and hinder, since they may get the gist of a conversation or simple instructions but have little comprehension of important information. Equally, fairly fluent spoken English can mask a low level of understanding. Continuity of care can often reduce stress, encourage non-verbal communication and increase understanding of commonly used words or gestures.

Nurses must be sensitive to the differing ways in which concern, grief and pain are expressed across cultures. Although there are geographical, generation and class differences, people in Northern and Western Europe tend to be stoical and avoid expressing physical or emotional pain openly. In contrast, people from Southern and Eastern Europe, Asia and Africa express physical and emotional pain more overtly through crying, rocking and beating their chests. This can evoke anger from staff intolerant of what they see as hysteria, and it can earn the disapproval of other patients or families who are struggling with their own pain in a stoical manner.

Respect is shown when nurses either know or attempt to find out about the patients' beliefs and values, and their adherence to particular religious codes and practices. Although it is important to recognise the differences that characterise a culture or religion, it must not be supposed that all members of a group hold the same ideas or uphold them to the same extent. Nurses must recognise the importance of religious beliefs and practices in time of distress, and facilitate opportunities for support from ministers or for personal prayer.

Nurses may feel uncomfortable when a patient or family believe that illness is caused by spells, curses, spirit possession, or punishment by a deity. While there may be clear evidence of pathological causation, the beliefs of the individual must not be trivialised or scorned, but must be accepted and understood. In many cases conventional treatment will be acceptable to a person with supernatural beliefs, providing it is not incongruous with religious requirements or cultural expectations. In other cases, it may mean supporting the right of the patient to decline certain aspects of treatment or care.

Time out 9.2

Patients who require high dependency nursing are highly reliant on accurate assessment, speedy diagnosis and effective treatment. However, it is possible that these aspects of safe critical care are jeopardised by a lack of understanding of the person's culture. Reflect on situations with the potential to assess inaccurately, misdiagnose, or treat a patient inappropriately because of limited understanding of culture.

Cultural competence

Culturally competent care relies on accurate assessment and diagnosis. This requires the avoidance of stereotypes, understanding differences in language, and manifestations of illness, and being able to work with differing beliefs and values. Presumptions of alcohol use among Irish people, and drug abuse among Caribbean men, and disbelief regarding the experiences of persecution among refugees are just some of the stereotypes that cloud the assessment and diagnosis of people from different communities. Nurses commonly assume that people of Mediterranean, Caribbean, African and other origins have a low pain threshold, and therefore deny or delay the use of analgesia. They fail to understand differences in socialisation, whereby people express pain more overtly. Equally, there is a danger that the stoic response of Japanese, Chinese and Northern European people to physical and emotional pain is misunderstood.

While high dependency units use a range of technological devices to monitor blood pressure and oxygen saturation, nurses will occasionally have to care for patients without such assistance. Nurses are generally unskilled in observing skin colour and detecting shock, anaemia or cyanosis in patients with black skin. Cyanosis in particular is a very late sign, and the lack of skill in observing for it may mean that the patient's condition deteriorates significantly before being noticed. It is best observed in the mouth, lips and nail-beds, as they tend to be pale or pink even in very dark-skinned people and readily show cyanosis.

It can be also be difficult to identify bruising, petechiae, purpura and other lesions in black skin. Pressure-sore risk tools that rely on the detection of redness are largely invalid for people with black skin. The identification of wound infection or monitoring of wound healing is equally complex. Nurses must rely more on indices, such as temperature, suppuration and evidence of granulation, but must take responsibility for developing their skills with help from colleagues who are more skilled or who have practised in other cultures.

Nurses are accountable for their own performance, but also share responsibility for that of their co-workers. It is incumbent on them to challenge racist attitudes, language and practices among colleagues and patients. It is particularly important to address institutional discrimination that denies patients culturally sensitive care. Interpreting services, acceptable diet, or facilities for religious observance are not added extras to be provided if funding allows; they are essential aspects of quality care, and are central to physical and psychological health.

Nurses must recognise the racism experienced by colleagues and confront stereotypical attitudes, unwitting prejudice and racist banter. They must challenge patients, relatives or others who racially abuse staff, and support colleagues who complain of racial harassment. They must take every opportunity to learn from peers who belong to other cultures, and enable them to understand the cultures of this society.

Implications for practice

- Nurses must be aware of the tendency to see the patient through the perspective of the majority culture, nursing, or the organisations within which they work, rather than through the patient's culture
- There is evidence that the needs of patients from different cultures are not adequately met; this largely reflects a lack of understanding of values, beliefs, customs and practices within different cultural groups
- Language is an important barrier to effective nursing care, but misunderstandings about different ways of showing respect, gender and family roles, customs relating to eye contact and touch are equally significant
- Different expressions of emotional and physical pain coupled with stereotypical assumptions about patients from different cultures carry the risk of misdiagnosis and inappropriate assessment, and endanger life.

Summary

It is important to remember that culturally competent care means high-quality care for all patients, and that many aspects of such care have minimal financial costs. Even those with cost implications may be beneficial in improving diagnosis, increasing the effectiveness of treatment, speeding recovery, and reducing complications and length of hospital stay. In addition, being able to deliver more effective care and enjoy good relationships with patients from different cultures can be a significant source of job satisfaction for nurses.

Clinical scenario

Mrs Gulten Ibrahim, a 62-year-old Turkish Cypriot Muslim woman and a recently diagnosed asthmatic, is admitted during the holy month of Ramadan with acute bronchospasm. She is unwilling to use her inhalers between sunrise and sunset, although her family understands the need to break the fast of Ramadan for medication during illness.

What strategies can be negotiated by nursing staff to protect the patient's immediate and ongoing safety while respecting her religious beliefs as much as possible.

Bibliography

Key reading

MacLachlan (1997), Papadopoulos *et al.* (1998) and Holland and Hogg (2001) are three sources of information that are relevant to nurses working in various clinical areas. They address conceptual issues and relate them to the care of clients from a range of different cultures.

Suggested reading

Acheson (1998).
ALG, 2000.

Chapter 10

Health promotion

Tina Moore

Contents

Learning outcomes

After reading this chapter you will be able to:

- Appreciate the reasons for adopting a health promotion role (when applicable)
- Analyse critically the current practices in relation to health promotion
- Discuss the different meanings of health and describe health promotion models
- Acknowledge opportunities within your own practice setting to implement concepts of empowerment and partnership.

Introduction

As part of the care package there is either an implied or contractual obligation for nurses to undertake and participate in health promotion (DOH, 1999a). Health promotion should be viewed as an integral part of most care activities rather than as a separate or 'add on' activity.

The shift from the traditional illness-focused care to health-related care is not occurring (Benson and Latter, 1998). Instead, health promotional activities are usually limited by their unstructured, haphazard, *ad hoc* approaches, and are far more likely to be opportunistic and limited to information-giving (Whitehead, 2000). Nurses appear to have difficulty in conceptualising a health-promoting role, particularly in relation to acutely or critically ill patients. Health promotion may still be viewed by nurses working in hospitals as predominantly an activity for well people, and thus primarily a concern for community nurses or health visitors.

Health promotion can start before the onset of critical illness. Some patients undergo planned treatment that will make them acutely or critically ill afterwards, and pre-planned visits to a critical care unit or pre-assessment clinic can provide health promotion both before and after treatment.

Due to the severity of their illness, patients may not have the capacity or desire to be involved in health promotion. However, once they have passed the 'critical phase' of their illness and are assessed as 'competent' (see Chapter 41), health promotion should begin. Opportunities for health promotion within critical care exist, but many are missed, possibly resulting in some patients feeling unprepared for discharge to the general ward.

This chapter will largely focus upon the prerequisite for health promotion activities – i.e. creating a culture that is able to facilitate this.

Time out 10.1

1 Write down your overall understanding of health promotion.
2 What does the concept mean to you?
3 Now read the following section, and compare your definition with those given below.

Definitions of health promotion

A number of interpretations of health promotion are evident. Health promotion is referred to as a group of activities that help to prevent disease and improve health and well-being (Naidoo and Wills, 1998). It is the process of enabling people to increase control over, and to improve, their health (WHO, 1986).

Definitions of health promotion are broad and potentially unhelpful within clinical practice due to their lack of strategic direction, particularly in relation to the acutely or critically ill patient. There are now several documents produced by the government to offer direction in health promotion – for example, *Saving Lives: Our Healthier Nation* (DOH, 1999b), and the National Service Framework. However, these documents still fail to consider this group of patients.

Conceptualisation of health in its broadest sense must occur if a health promotion model is to be followed adequately. This should incorporate a holistic view (physical, mental, social and spiritual) (Kiger, 1995) and is a developmental process. Such an approach should be adopted within critical care (see Chapter 2). For example, patients recovering from the acute effects of diabetic ketoacidosis (newly diagnosed) will need to accept the fact that they are now diabetic (this involves exploring beliefs and values). Social values and how diabetes may affect their lifestyle should be considered before educating them about diet. Education regarding blood glucose monitoring, insulin administration and avoiding hypoglycaemia concerns the physical aspect.

Two main theoretical perspectives on health promotion exist (Green and Raeburn, 1990): the first places emphasis on political, sociological or systems factors in health; whilst the second emphasises personal and small group decision-making, psychological factors, and the methods of health education. A combination of these two perspectives appears to be the aim of health promotional policies and practices (Green and Raeburn, 1990). These two perspectives can be in contradiction – for example, if a patient's social and political conditions are unchanged, health promotion efforts are potentially wasted. Sociological and political influences need to be addressed first.

Foundations for health promotion are built upon empowerment and partnership (Macleod Clark, 1993). These features include holism, equity, participation, collaboration, individualisation, negotiation, facilitation and support. A 'sick nursing' approach is distinguished by interactions that are dominating, generalised, prescriptive, reassuring and directive (Macleod Clark, 1993). All nursing interactions have the potential to be health promoting; however, the culture of the clinical setting should foster a facilitative environment before health promotion activities can begin.

Initially, critically ill patients will require a 'sick nursing' approach. However, unhealthy dependency is encouraged if this approach continues when patients are in the recovery phase of their illness.

Time out 10.2

With particular reference to level-2 patients, what type of health promotion activities occur within your practice setting?

Health promotion models

Descriptive models identify the diversity of existing practice, but make no judgments regarding which kind of practice is preferable (see, for example, Tannahill, 1985). Analytical models are explicit about the values underpinning practice, and often prioritise certain kinds of practice over others. Downie *et al.* (1996)

proposed a model in which health promotion is viewed as efforts to enhance positive health and prevent ill-health, through the overlapping spheres of health education, prevention, and health protection.

There are various approaches to health promotion: health behaviour approaches rely on social psychology and communication theory; the educational approach has education theory underpinning it; epidemiology theories underpin the medical approach; sociology and organisational theories underpin the social change approach; and social psychology and the humanities theory underpin the empowerment approach.

Nurses need to have knowledge of the appropriate model to use, depending upon the patient's needs. An amalgamation of these theories may be used. For example, if a patient is admitted for treatment of exacerbation of asthma (through continual smoking), and has tried to stop smoking on a number of occasions without success, health promotion can be offered in relation to:

- Discussing the issues with the patient (psychology theory)
- The effects of smoking on the body (education theory)
- The effects' affect on others, social implications such as restricted areas, social isolation (social theory)
- Providing information (facts and figures) regarding diseases contracted through smoking and asthma caused through smoking (epidemiology theory)
- Planning a strategy to give up smoking (organisational theory).

Health assessment should be used as a starting point for planning any health-related programme. It is assumed that patients expect to participate more in making decisions about their health care, and that they also want to learn about how to maintain and improve their health (Clarke, 1991). This appears not to be the case with all patients – for example, critically ill patients' priority relates initially to being alive (Moore, 1998) – who hence adopt the 'patient role'. This may indicate that patients need to get used to the idea of being in hospital, particularly when admitted as an emergency or following a relapse in their illness. Health promotion should be a gradual process, starting with empowerment and the shifting of control.

Empowerment

Time out 10.3

Think about your own beliefs and values, and those of the staff you work with, in relation to health promotion within your area of practice. Write down your answers.

We will return to these later.

Approaches to care can be paternalistic, where healthcare professionals know what is in the best interest of 'their' patient. Paternalistic care is often characterised by authoritarian, prescriptive, persuasive, protective and generalised

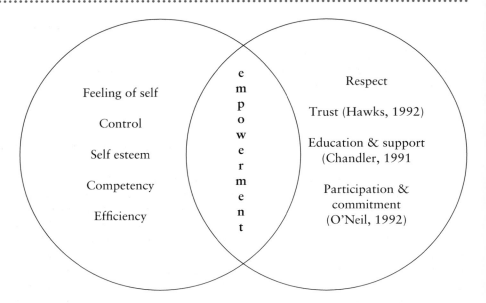

Figure 10.1 **Components of empowerment**

information being given by the 'expert' to the 'ignorant' layperson. Currently, the need for an empowering, client-centred and collaborative approach is emphasised.

The WHO (1986) definition of health promotion suggests improving and increasing the patient's control. Enhancement of control can be achieved through empowerment. Reports and guidelines from the government repeatedly emphasise this process.

Within practice, the term 'empowerment' has been used inappropriately (Rodwell, 1996), often dictated by perceptions/understanding of the concept.

The process of empowerment is a developmental one, increasing the shift of power and control to patients by increasing their knowledge and skill and ability to participate. Key features of empowerment (Figure 10.1) include:

- The need to clarify individuals' beliefs and values about themselves, health, and health-influencing behaviour (Downie *et al.*, 1996). For example, patients who are admitted with uncontrolled hypertension should be encouraged to articulate what hypertension means to them, what affect it has on them, and how they can change their lifestyle and dietary habits.
- A requirement to foster empowerment through raising self-esteem, beliefs about self-efficacy and the acquisition of life skills (Tones, 1991) in patients, for example by constant reassurance and by allowing them time to make decisions relating to how they will adapt or change their lifestyle etc. Nurses should not dictate to patients what they should be doing.
- A partnership model of communication (Downie *et al.*, 1996) – i.e. communicating *with* patients, not *at* them.

Time out 10.4

Go back to the list you made in Time out 10.3. Do you think that what you have written relates towards empowering patients, or encouraging unnecessary dependency?

Autonomy versus paternalism

(Chapter 12 provides definitions and further discussion regarding autonomy.)

History has outlined the nurse's role as nurturing dependency within the patient, particularly the acutely or critically ill. This behaviour stemmed from the needs of society, and from nurses' own interpretation of their role. Today there is a shift in health and social values, indicating that patient dependency should be reduced and autonomy enhanced. There will always be situations in critical care that indicate paternalistic actions, and in such situations acting paternalistically is regarded as a duty – consider, for example, a patient who is in hypovolaemic shock, requiring invasive monitoring and aggressive fluid replacement while very anxious and still suffering from the psychological trauma of being admitted to the ward as an emergency. There is a thin dividing line between respecting a person's autonomy on the one hand and being open to the charge of negligence or failure of duty to care on the other (Tingle and Cribb, 1995).

A nurturing and caring environment is necessary for the promotion of autonomy; not one of inappropriate paternalism. There must also be willingness and consent of both the nurse and the patient. Nurses need to respect patients' individual capacity for growth and self-determination. The process of empowerment is a developmental one, increasing the shift of power and control to patients by increasing their knowledge and skill and ability to participate.

Power versus control

Before attempting to enhance patient autonomy, nurses must be willing to relinquish their control of the nurse–patient relationship and allow the patient to make more decisions. The attitude that 'nurses know best' fosters a sense of dependency. Patient participation should be encouraged (at any level), and nurses need to be prepared to accept that patients may make decisions that are different from those that might be decided for them. This can only occur if the nurse assumes that health belongs to the individual (i.e. the patient), who is therefore responsible for his or her own health. Owing to the nature of critical care, this may in many instances be difficult to achieve.

Instead of the healthcare provider giving up power, passive clients should be actively encouraged to participate in health care (Strickland and Strickland, 1996). This may prove to be difficult, as some patients are socialised in the tradition of the medical model and expect to be told what to do by the expert. Waterworth and Luker (1990) suggest that some patients do not want to be actively involved in decisions about their care. In these situations, gradual facilitation by constant involvement in the decision-making process should be encouraged.

Partnership

While the idea of a nurse–client partnership is appealing, current nursing literature is unclear about the elements and processes in such a partnership in acute or critical care settings. This lack of clarity is hardly surprising, as definitions of partnership differ in scope and vary according to the context of the partnership and types of partners (Gallant *et al.*, 2002). Such inconsistency makes it difficult to find common ground to communicate about partnership, but Box 10.1 indicates the values forming the basis of partnership.

Box 10.1   Values forming the basis of partnership

- Co-operation (Courtney, 1995)
- Commitment to sharing responsibility, risk, power and accountability (Gillies, 1998)
- Open and respectful acknowledgement of what each partner brings to the relationship (LaBonte, 1994)
- Positive attitudes towards clients and the willingness to relinquish the status and privilege associated with being a nurse (Munro *et al.*, 2000)
- Belief in empowerment and actively encouraging the client's involvement in decision-making (Strickland and Strickland, 1996)
- Interpersonal skills of respect, trust, authenticity and courtesy (Malloch and Porter-O'Grady, 1999)
- Self-awareness, preconceptions about the other, anxiety, ways of knowing and learning, competency and success in other interpersonal relationships
- Freedom to choose a partnering relationship
- Power sharing and negotiation (Gallant *et al.*, 2002).

Once the patient's condition permits, the nurse should assume a facilitative role, acting as a resource person and providing health promotion in a non-judgmental way. For success, both patient and nurse must commit to the roles required in partnership. In partnership, the nurse brings nursing knowledge and clinical experiences, while the client brings experiential knowledge about health and managing health concerns.

Nurses can promote patient partnership by:

- Maintaining the relationship
- Reinforcing patient progress
- Supporting decision-making
- Assisting the patient to learn new knowledge and skills.

Implications for practice

- Nurses need to assess patients' potential for requiring health promotion information
- Nurses must trust patients' ability to make decisions and accept responsibility and act for themselves
- Health might not be an important concern for many patients, either through severity of illness or lack of interest or motivation.

Summary

Health promotion activities should start as soon as the patient's condition allows and does not have to involve complicated processes. Prerequisites to facilitate partnership and empowerment need to be in place before health promotion attempts are successful.

Clinical scenario

Mrs Linda Thomas, a 44-year-old single parent with three pre-teen children, was admitted with bowel obstruction and underwent small bowel surgery involving colectomy and formation of a temporary colostomy. She was admitted to critical care for stabilisation and was intubated for less than 24 hours. She progressed from level 3 to level 2 care after 2 days. Mrs Thomas's main complaints were poor appetite, lack of sleep and abdominal discomfort.

1 Describe the model of health promotion and type of partnership appropriate to Mrs Thomas.

2 Outline areas for health promotion. When should health promotion be initiated?

3 What support groups, forums and specialist nurses within your hospital or local area would be useful to Mrs Thomas?

Bibliography

Key reading

Government documents.

Further reading

Benson and Latter (1998).

Chapter 11

Family care

Tina Moore

Contents

Learning outcomes

After reading this chapter you will be able to:

- Identify the needs of family members
- Appreciate the role of the family when caring for the critically ill
- Identify the issues surrounding family-witnessed resuscitation
- Examine critically the current practices in relation to family care
- Acknowledge conflicts within the caring situation.

Introduction

Genuine holistic care demands that nurses meet the needs of visitors and recognise the importance of the impact of visitors upon the patient care given in the critical care environment.

(Priestley, 1999: 27)

Nurses are constantly reminded that they should adopt a holistic perspective in carrying out their role. This holistic perspective includes consideration of members of the patient's family within the context of care. The importance of the role played by family members is an established one (Leske, 1992). The effects of the individual's illness constitute an important part of family life, and are closely related to the health status of its members (Weeks and O'Connor, 1994). The family can also be a significant source of information about the patient.

This chapter explores the role of the family within the context of critical care, and considers whether that role should include witnessing resuscitation. Conflicts arising from such a situation will also be highlighted.

Definitions of a family

There have been many attempts to define the concept of family, with very little consensus (Nock, 1992). Traditional definitions of family (extended and nuclear) are no longer viewed to be the norm. Indeed, many sociologists believe that there is no longer one type of family life. The concept of family has become broader to include one-parent families, unmarried couples living together, children from previous relationships coming together as one unit, and single-sex families (gay and lesbian). Bell and Wright (1990) offer a broad definition of the family, stating that the family is 'who the client says it is', thus respecting the patients' perspective and also indicating that family membership is not necessarily a blood relationship. Thus, the concept of family also includes 'significant others'.

Wright and Leahey (1994) change the focus from the individual's perspective to that of the family, suggesting that the family is 'who *they* say *they* are'. Robb (1998) reports that this may be a particularly useful definition, and of significant value when the patient is unable to communicate through critical illness. Problems will arise if the patient's views are different (when the patient is in a position to express them). This has implications particularly regarding confidentiality (see later).

Family nursing

Whatever the effects on the health of family members, critical illness in an individual is a catastrophic event that can upset the equilibrium of the family system (Halm, 1990). Family members may display a tendency to ignore their own needs. Assessment, intervention and support must be offered to enable the family to cope with the illness of their loved ones.

There are three levels of family nursing identified by Friedemann (1989):

1   Individually-focused family nursing
2   Interpersonal family nursing
3   Family system level nursing.

Often, within critical care environments, the patient is the sole focus of the nurse's attention. Various reasons may be put forward to account for this:

■   The patient's safety is the priority
■   Patients require a considerable amount of emotional support
■   Tension exists between a holistic approach to care and the nurse's legal duty of care to the patient, which is owed to the patient and not the family
■   Lack of time prevents a focus on the family
■   Nursing critically ill patients can be physically and emotionally exhausting, and this leaves little time or energy for the nurse to meet the needs of the family members.

During the past two decades, studies in relation to critical care environments have been carried out which have identified the needs of the family (Molter, 1979; Dyer, 1997). These studies have been replicated many times, verifying the original findings. Conclusions have been drawn to suggest that family visitors in critical care units whose needs are met can then provide support and be a positive influence in the care of the patient.

Time out 11.1

When caring for the critically ill patient, do you consider the needs of the family?

1   If your answer is 'no', think of possible reasons for this.
2   If your answer is 'yes', what are the main needs you have identified?

Identifying the needs of the family

Blackmore (1996) acknowledged nurses as the main resource to meet the needs of visitors to ICU. However, the results of a study by Quinn *et al.* (1996) suggest that family and critical care nurses differ in their perceptions of how important needs are for visiting relatives. This is consistent with the findings of Forrester *et al.* (1990). This is important, as the perceptions of family needs by the staff often determine which needs get met.

Reasons for dissatisfaction amongst family members include:

■   Lack of information concerning both diagnosis and the consequences of the illness (Malacrida *et al.*, 1998)

■ Lack of moral and psychological support before death (Malacrida *et al.*, 1998). (Malacrida's research needs to be viewed with some caution, as the opinions of the relatives were sought after recent bereavement. This may have influenced the findings. However, the results are consistent with other research on the topic.)
■ Not being involved in the decision-making processes
■ Healthcare professionals not being open and honest
■ Feelings of frustration
■ Powerlessness.

(Fulbrook *et al.*, 1999)

Family needs identified include:

■ To feel there is hope (Wilkinson, 1995; Burr, 1998)
■ To be honestly informed (Molter, 1979)
■ To be reassured that the patient is receiving the best possible care
■ To be reassured concerning the patient's future
■ To be relieved of anxiety
■ To be sure of being notified should the patient's condition deteriorate (Forrester *et al.*, 1990)
■ To be treated with empathy and compassion
■ To feel secure
■ To be with their loved ones (Meyers *et al.*, 2000)
■ To receive honest, consistent and understandable information (Burr, 1998).

Supporting the family

Quinn *et al.* (1996) indicate that the needs of the family are either forgotten or ignored. Nurses must ensure this does not happen. Priestley (1999) appeals to nurses to rethink the priorities within their role, and indicates that holistic nursing care is a priority.

As nursing staff are in a position of providing 24-hour patient care, they should strive towards creating an environment that is supportive to holistic practice and is family-sensitive. Within this environment nurses can design and implement strategies to meet the needs of family members, but only when they have accurately assessed these needs and their relative importance for family members (Forrester *et al.*, 1990). O'Malley *et al.* (1991) concluded that nurses' responses to the needs of the family are affected by their perceptions of importance, the time available, the environment, and the ability to meet the need.

If nurses are to promote holistic care, they should identify the needs of the family and support its members during a stressful period. This can be achieved by consistently assessing the family, providing appropriate intervention, and evaluating its effectiveness. By supporting the family, it becomes empowered. If visitor stress can be reduced, this may actually reduce the stress on nurses (Dyer, 1991).

Family-sensitive care indicates that nurses and relatives need to develop a rapport and respect for each other. This can be accomplished through effective communication channels, giving new information and reinforcing information already given. Relatives should not be bombarded with unnecessary jargonsitic information. Content should be adequate to enable them to understand what is happening and put them in a position to be able to ask questions.

Timely assessment by nurses and the implementation of appropriate interventions are essential for the functioning of a family system in crisis (Appleyard *et al.*, 2000). Family members could be encouraged to be involved in actual care delivery at a very basic level – for example, assisting with basic hygiene needs, emptying urine bags etc. However, not all family members have the ability or motivation to be involved, and therefore nurses should carefully assess their ability. Relatives need to feel that they are contributing positively in some way (Burr, 1998), and this involvement should not be denied. Family members' interaction with and support of the patient is a way of demonstrating their love and concern, and constitutes an aspect of care that only they can provide (Burr, 1998). Achieving a balance between over- and under-involvement in therapeutic relationships may prove to be difficult.

Families like to have a 'presence' within the critical care unit (Burr, 1998). This presence is related to 'being with' the patient, having emotional as well as a physical presence. It involves connectedness and bonding. Humanistic practitioners are personally involved (Walters, 1995). Nurses should act as effective role models in talking to and touching the patients, as many relatives feel awkward talking to someone who is unconscious.

Supporting the family as well as the patient may prove to be stressful for some nurses. Staff need supporting through mechanisms such as clinical supervision, case conferences, effective practice education, and training. Nurses must be aware of both their important role as a resource for meeting relatives' needs and their responsibility to implement those needs.

Time out 11.2

What are your views in relation to family-witnessed resuscitation? Consider arguments for and against.

Family-witnessed resuscitation

Traditionally, family members have been excluded during resuscitation interventions. This issue has been the subject of a longstanding debate, which is both controversial and ongoing.

Arguments in favour of family-witnessed resuscitation include the following (appears mainly from the family's perspective):

- It gives a feeling of the family helping and supporting the patient
- It shows that everything possible is being done (Meyers *et al.*, 2000)
- It helps with the grieving process and the coming to terms with death (Adam, 1994; Robinson *et al.*, 1998)
- It lessens the family's feelings of guilt (we should have done more)
- It assists in the closure of shared life (Hanson and Strawser, 1994)
- It reminds healthcare professionals of the patient's personhood

■ It helps relatives with a sense of 'connectedness' (Meyers *et al.*, 2000)
■ Exclusion of the family may devalue death to a clinical procedure or a failure of treatment, rather than being a unique human event that touches the lives of others (Hatchett, 1994)
■ Relatives may have already been involved in pre-hospital resuscitation, either directly or as a witness (Ardley, 2002).

Arguments against family-witnessed resuscitation include the following (appears mainly from the health care professional's perspective):

■ It inhibits a slightly relaxed atmosphere (coping strategies of the staff). Staff feel they are always having to be on guard.
■ There is the fear that relatives could become disruptive and interfere with resuscitation efforts
■ It is distressing for relatives (Eichhorn *et al.*, 1996), particularly with invasive procedures
■ The environment is too cramped and there is not enough room for spectators
■ Staff cannot provide enough support to relatives and patient at the same time
■ Staff feel apprehensive about saying or doing something to offend relatives
■ Staff fear being viewed as incompetent (Schilling, 1994)
■ It breaches patient confidentiality
■ Relatives may be unable to cope (Higgs, 1994)
■ It hinders the grieving process
■ Relatives cannot be prepared.

Conflicts within care

When allowing family members to witness resuscitation attempts, or indeed when encouraging family involvement in care, a conflict automatically rises between maintaining patient confidentially and the advocacy role of the relatives. It is suggested throughout the Nursing and Midwifery Council *Code of Professional Conduct* (NMC, 2002a) that nurses should also act in the capacity of an advocate for the patient, promoting and safeguarding his or her interests. Potentially, the advocacy role of the nurse may come into conflict with the advocacy role of the family members.

Patients have a legitimate expectation that the information they give and information about them will be kept secret. This is one of the fundamental principles of health care, and confidentiality has been described as central to preserving the human dignity of the patients. There is therefore potential for breaching the patient's right to confidentiality if a family member witnesses the resuscitation. Lack of written policy on this issue compounds these conflicts.

Supporting the family during witnessed resuscitation

■ If family members request to witness resuscitation there should ideally be agreement of all concerned with the resuscitation that they are comfortable with such presence

- Members should be briefed about the process and given continuing support during the process by a trained person
- Members should be fully informed
- Members should be counselled immediately after the event
- Members should be able to enter and leave when they want to, and have the right to change their minds about the decision to be present
- Members should be involved in the decision-making processes
- Pastoral care should be available if indicated or requested
- Professionals should react with compassion and understanding (Baskett, 1994)
- Relatives should be offered a bereavement programme (Eichhorn *et al.*, 1996)
- Debriefing and support for staff should be available, as many find it difficult to become emotionally detached from the relatives
- There is a need for healthcare professionals to be trained to work in public as death becomes a public event (Baskett, 1994).

Implications for practice

- Holistic care involves caring for relatives as well as the patient
- The nursing process approach to care delivery should extend to the family
- Nurses should provide a sensitive, compassionate approach to family members
- It is important to assess the ability and motivation of family to be involved in the basic provision of care
- Nurses (particularly junior) need support in caring for relatives
- Discussions regarding family-witnessed resuscitation need to be facilitated at a local level.

Summary

Holistic nursing involves caring not only for patients but also for their families, in the broadest sense of the term. Needs of the family predominantly include psychological needs in relation to their loved ones (i.e. being kept informed through open and honest communication channels, and being close to their loved ones). Family members can be supported through giving honest, understandable information, and allowing/encouraging their participation in patient care. Family-witnessed resuscitation remains under debate, each perspective having valid reasons.

Clinical scenario

Monica Sinclair is the wife of Nigel (36 years old), who was admitted 2 days ago following an episode of uncontrolled blinding headaches. He is unconscious, and his blood pressure is fluctuating between 100/70 mmHg and 180/110 mmHg. Monica is constantly at her husband's bedside. Occasionally other members of the family visit. She is very anxious and constantly tearful, and indicates that she is unsure of what is happening to her husband.

1   Identify Monica's needs and suggest ways of meeting them.

2   Consider any conflict between meeting Monica's needs and those of her husband.

3   Nigel's condition deteriorates and eventually he dies. Evaluate the situation with Monica, and suggest what type of intervention she should now receive.

Bibliography

Key reading

Belanger and Reed (1997) challenges all nurses to take the care of the dying one step further.

Eichhorn *et al.* (1996) provides guidelines for supporting relatives during and after witnessed resuscitation.

Further reading

Fulbrook *et al.* (1999) reports on an insider's perspective of being a family member of someone who is critically ill. The insider's perspective is that of a nurse working in critical care.

Albarran and Salmon (2000).

Chapter 12

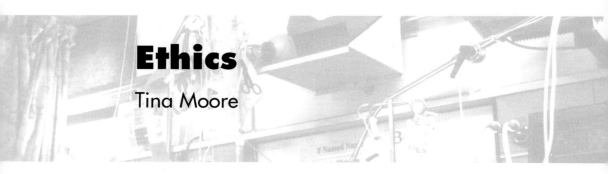

Ethics

Tina Moore

Contents

Learning outcomes

After reading this chapter you will be able to:

- Demonstrate an understanding of the need to be aware of the ethical issues and their importance in clinical practice as a guide in the provision/framework of care
- Identify actual and potential ethical situations relating to the critically ill patient and suggest strategies for resolution/ coping
- Develop an awareness of your own beliefs and values during exposure to clinical situations
- Apply ethical principles as a guide in the provision/framework of care.

Introduction

Due to the complexities of critical care nursing, ethical considerations have become an integral part of care. As a direct result of conflicts within care, nurses are now more exposed to ethical dilemmas. Conflicts can arise from situations involving withholding treatment, deciding when the burdens of further therapeutic measures outweigh the benefits, limited resources, and deciding entry criteria to critical care units. Ethical issues can also arise from the usage of complicated technology, the vulnerability of patients and the complex decision-making processes.

Many critically ill patients are unable to act autonomously, and therefore rely on healthcare professionals (particularly nurses) to make decisions for them. Consequently, there is a risk of initial decisions being made mainly in relation to patients' ailments and not necessarily in their best interest. Healthcare professionals may think they are making decisions in the best interest of patients, but sometimes this is not the case (see Miss B, p. 105). Clinical decisions, whether made by the patient or by a healthcare professional, may not be generally acceptable, and thus can create a sense of uneasiness and possibly resentment.

Due to its complexity, ethical decision-making is not an easy process. Nurses must develop a clear understanding of ethical considerations in order to ensure that the care they provide is morally and legally acceptable. Some ethical issues have already been discussed in Chapters 1 and 2, and this chapter is designed to build upon that content. The concept of advocacy is not discussed; this is included in Chapter 1. An opportunity will be created for nurses to examine their own values and beliefs in relation to nursing the critically ill. The intention is not to provide answers (this would be considered morally wrong), but to create an awareness and wider understanding of some of the fundamental issues faced by nurses within critical care.

Time out 12.1

1 Write down your understanding of the term 'ethics'.
2 How do you think ethics relates to health care?
3 Make a list of ethical 'ground rules' you consider appropriate for nurses.

Nature of ethics

To appreciate ethical dilemmas, the meaning of ethics and its relationship to practice should be examined. The term ethics, derived from the Greek *ethos* relates to the philosophical study of the moral values of human conduct and the rules and principles that govern it (how we should behave). Ethics is the practical application of moral philosophy.

Determining exactly what is right from what is wrong is very difficult (what may be seen to be right for one person could be wrong for another). Ethical values directly relate to beliefs concerning what is right and proper, as opposed to what is effective or desirable. A clinical decision to withdraw treatment may be viewed as the most effective way to reduce prolongation of life, but might not be right in relation to the patient's quality of life (e.g. effects of dehydration). Nurses may face situations where the patient's belief of what is right conflicts with their own beliefs – for example, a Jehovah's Witness refusing a life-saving blood transfusion. Nurses should not force their own values onto others, but should try to understand and appreciate the perspective of others.

There are two main approaches to ethics: non-normative (descriptive) and normative (prescriptive). Non-normative ethics describes standards of behaviour, i.e. the *actual* behaviour without the use of prescriptive guidelines causing individuals to act in a certain way. This is usually culturally determined, and fails to consider influencing factors.

Normative ethics relates to what *ought* to be, prescribing how people should behave, without reference to how things actually are. The 'ideal' behaviour is based on specific values and principles, which define what is right and wrong, and incorporates the theories of ethics discussed below. Each ethical theory section contains an ethical action/guide. The *Code of Professional Conduct* (NMC, 2002a) sets out what is considered to be 'ideal' professional behaviour.

Ethical theories

Consequentialism (utilitarianism)

This involves the ethical merit of an act that is best determined by the consequence it produces – i.e. the person assesses competing values in terms of likely and intended results. In essence, 'the ends can justify the means'. Actions are deemed right and good when they produce benefit, pleasure or happiness, or prevent harm, pain or unhappiness. The action is judged on the outcome (consequences). The decision-maker is required to consider and predict the likely consequences of the contemplated action (weighing the good the act will produce against the harm it may cause). The aim is to produce the greatest possible balance of benefits (good) over burdens (harm). The motivation of the person involved in the action is considered important. Not all decisions that are made consciously attempt to produce the most useful outcome.

Consider the case of Miss B (Miss B v Secretary for Health, March 2002), who had sarcoma of her C2 (cervical vertebrae) and as a result was paralysed from the neck down and ventilated. She was fully conscious and deemed to be of a competent mind. Her prognosis was extremely poor. She decided to take legal action to have all treatment stopped, including ventilator support, thus ending her life. In balance, life on the ventilator was viewed as a living torture to this lady. She wanted to die with dignity, and thus ending her life was good in comparison to the harm she suffered. This scenario clearly illustrates the consequences of freedom from suffering (evil) and being allowed to die with more dignity (benefits). The High Court Judge, Elizabeth Butler Sloss, ruled that Miss B had the right to end her life and die with dignity.

Deontological (duty-based)

This theory believes that people have an absolute duty to do the right thing under all circumstances, and what is 'right' has nothing to do with the actual consequences. The *Professional Code of Conduct* (NMC, 2002a) reflects this view. The foundation of morality is the ability to act rationally (a rational being is free to act out of principle and to refrain from acting out of impulse or the desire for pleasure), but is an individual whose beliefs and values contradict deontological beliefs and values irrational?

From a deontological perspective, it would be considered wrong to bring about Miss B's death prematurely; this would constitute an act of killing. Life is seen to be sacred and should be preserved. Conflicts can arise between the duty of healthcare professionals and respect for patient autonomy – i.e. those patients who want to end their lives and the healthcare professional who want to save it.

Rights-based

Autonomy is a crucial concept within this theory (see p. 110 for further information). Autonomy demands respect for the individual rights, and rights are seen as being justified claims that the individual (or groups) can make upon others. The Human Rights Act (1998) sets out the articles of the European Convention of Human Rights (discussed further on p. 107).

Patients' rights and the rights of others may be in conflict, e.g. the right to refuse treatment versus the right to give safe and competent care.

Ethical principles

Ethical principles cannot address all situations, but may help to clarify the issues involved.

There are four main ethical principles:

1 Autonomy
2 Nonmaleficence – the obligation not to inflict harm intentionally and not to engage in actions that risk harming others (could be argued as impossible within health care)
3 Beneficence – actions are intended to benefit and prevent harm
4 Justice and fairness – treating everyone equally.

Beneficence, justice, autonomy, veracity (truthfulness) and respect for persons are characteristics that all nurses must have in order to be ethical (Beauchamp and Childress, 2001). Within clinical practice, conflict arises between the principles. Consider, for example, nonmaleficence and beneficence – a patient may be complaining of considerable pain and require analgesia (via injection), but while the administration is viewed as beneficial the injection will cause harm (skin puncture).

The principle-based approach to problem solving has been criticised as being too abstract and complex to be helpful in reality (Edwards, 1996). Edwards suggests an alternative, i.e. situational ethics, which determines the decision-making processes to be unique to each situation. Nurses should view each situation as unique and consider other influencing factors (e.g. patient's prognosis and quality of life). Each moral problem should be regarded positively.

Nurses are often exposed to situations that involve complex networks of conflicting influencing factors, and may find therefore this approach useful. However, some decisions may be more favourable to one person than another. Primarily, responsibility is to the patient (duty of care). This approach requires an experienced practitioner who is able to identify clearly the issues within a given situation.

Time out 12.3

1 Consider any tension/conflict that may occur between the four ethical principles.
2 How can these tensions/conflicts be overcome?

The Human Rights Act (1998)

Box 12.1 illustrates articles of the Human Rights Act (1998) applicable to nursing. (The author's commentary appears in italics.)

> **Box 12.1   Human Rights Act (1998): summary of articles pertinent to health care**
>
> The Act came into force on 2 October 2000. It gives further effect to the fundamental rights and freedoms in the European Convention of Human Rights. Now cases can be heard in a UK court or tribunal instead of the European Court of Human Rights in Strasbourg.
>
> Article 2 – **right to life** – everyone's right to life should be protected by law. *(Advanced Directives could be considered here).*
>
> Article 3 – **prohibition** – no one shall be subjected to torture or to inhumane or degrading treatment or punishment. *(Links have been made to certain aspects of care and torture as demonstrated by the writings of Dyer, 1995).*
>
> Article 5 – **right to liberty and security** – everyone has the right to liberty and security of person. *(Unlawful detention should not apply within health care; patients admitted to hospital have the right to discharge themselves unless they were brought in under the Mental Health Act, 1983).*
>
> Article 6 – **right to a fair trial** – everyone has the right to a fair trial. *(This can be interpreted as patients not being prejudged).*
>
> Article 9 – **freedom of thought, conscience and religion.** *(These should be respected and processes put in place to enable this to happen).*
>
> Article 10 – **freedom of expression.** *(Patients have the right to express their opinions, irrespective of the opinions of healthcare professionals).*
>
> Article 14 – **prohibition of discrimination.** *(Patients should not be discriminated against in relation to sex, race, colour, language, religion or political opinion).*
>
> Article 17 – **prohibition of abuse of rights.** *(Patients should have their rights respected and upheld).*
>
> *Issues arising from the Human Rights Act to be considered include:*
> - *When one person's right impinges on the rights of another*
> - *Where there is a conflict of rights (from one person or more than one)*
> - *Whether it is possible to prioritise individual rights.*

Time out 12.4

Reflect on a 'difficult' situation that you have experienced.

1 Describe the main features arising from the situation
2 Discuss how the issues were managed
3 Describe the decision-making processes
4 Were any ethical concerns considered before making a decision?

Ethical decision-making

Making ethical choices is seldom straightforward, particularly when related to complex situations such as emergency admissions, the severity of patient illness, and not having enough information to make a quality decision. Emotions can sometimes influence the decision-making processes (consider, for example, a patient who is repeatedly admitted following multiple overdoses and who has in the past stated that she no longer wishes to live).

Many of the moral dilemmas experienced by nurses are of an interdisciplinary nature. Nurses have numerous and, at times, competing obligations to various stakeholders with varying beliefs and values, and are often expected to balance commitments to all involved. This concept reinforces our obligation to make all reasonable efforts to foresee possible consequences and take reasonable steps to avoid unjustified harm to others (Navran, 1996).

Most ethical decisions have to be made in the context of professional, social and economic pressures that can sometimes challenge ethical goals and conceal or confuse the moral issues. Ethical decision-making refers to the process of evaluating and choosing among alternatives in a manner consistent with ethical principles. These ethical principles are considered to be the ground rules of decision-making.

A conflict of values, both internal (individual) and external (others) may make nurses unsure of how to act, and as a result they may not take any course of action. Noticing the ethical issues and being committed to acting ethically is not always enough. In complex situations, reasoning and problem-solving skills are also necessary.

Ethical decision-making model

When faced with an ethical issue, nurses should approach the situation logically and systematically in order to enable rational and ethically sound decisions. Where rationality exists, decision-making can be justified. An ethical decision-making model may help with this process.

Navran (1996) suggests an ethical decision-making model that enables decisions to be both generic and specific in nature, allowing the individual to consider as many influences as possible.

There are six steps:

1 *Define the problem and describe why the decision is necessary.* Identify what is and what should be. Gather as much relevant/factual information as possible, involving all concerned. Assess the nature of the problem. Involve all concerned.

2 *Identify alternatives.* Identify as many alternatives as possible, and be open to new solutions.

3 *Evaluate the alternatives.* Consider the positive and negative consequences of each alternative. Within the critical care environment, it is rare to find one alternative that completely resolves the problem. Personal perceptions, biases

and predispositions influence the evaluation. Self-awareness is required, and the implications for others must be considered. Include the assessment of PLUS, and assess the ethical impact. Consider whether the solution will create new problems. The ethical component uses the acronym 'PLUS':

- **P** – Policies (decisions should reflect local national professional policies, procedures and guidelines)
- **L** – Legal (decisions should reflect the law of the land and professional law)
- **U** – Universal (as far as possible the decision should conform to the principles/values of the organisation and individuals, including the patient)
- **S** – Self (examination of one's own beliefs and values in relation to the situation/decision).

4 *Make the decision.* A definition of the problem, a list of alternatives and a rationale to the proposed solution are necessary. A consultation period is required. If a consensus is not forthcoming, the definition of the problem needs to be agreed first. People must share a common definition of the problem for internal logic to lead them toward a commonly acceptable solution.

5 *Implement the decision.*

6 *Evaluate the decision.* Consider whether the result of the situation resolves the problem.

(After Navran, 1996)

Withdrawing/withholding treatment

Confusion may exist over the aim of withholding treatment. 'Withholding' refers to never initiating a treatment, whereas 'withdrawing' is concerned with stopping a treatment once it has been started. It may be emotionally more difficult for healthcare professionals to withdraw than to withhold. However, it is legally and professionally acceptable to end treatment (withdraw) for sound moral reasons (British Medical Association, 2001).

'Do not attempt to resuscitate' (DNAR) is sometimes mistaken as 'do not treat'. DNAR means 'do not resuscitate', but underlying problems should be treated in an attempt to enhance the quality of life left and reduce the patient's suffering.

Factors that should be considered when withdrawing treatment include the following:

- Caring for relatives and patients should take priority over the inappropriate preservation of life
- There must be consensus on the withdrawal of treatment (after considering ethical/moral legal factors)
- The patient should be free from pain and suffering (withdrawing some treatment, e.g. fluids, may have a detrimental effect in terms of suffering)
- Effective communication with the patient's family and other healthcare staff is vital.

(British Medical Association, 2001)

Patient autonomy

This principle is grounded ultimately in the integrity of the person and his or her ability to make decisions. The action of an autonomous person is intentional, taken with understanding and without controlling influences that determine actions. Autonomy is to do with self-determination rather than other-determination (Tingle and Cribb, 1995).

Some patients do not automatically become dependent and unthinking when they become critically ill. Novice and advanced-beginner nurses may be preoccupied with pathology and medical treatment, with areas such as information-giving, communication, recovery and rehabilitation possibly being neglected. Some patients are clearly unable or do not want to be autonomous. Brearley (1990) indicates that even in situations where passivity is the only option, information is vital for the purpose of consent and in some cases to enhance the patient's feeling of personal control.

Paternalism may be appropriate under certain conditions, particularly in the instances where patient safety is affected. In such situations, acting paternalistically is regarded as a duty: it is assumed that the patient desires health. However, paternalism can sometimes be contradictory to maintaining and promoting patient autonomy.

Autonomy should not be imposed. Patients need to be given the choice to execute their autonomy. It can be quite difficult to focus on the assessment of what the patient *can* do as opposed to what the patient cannot do, but is crucial in the restoration of patient autonomy.

In the ideal situation, appropriate dependency is merely the precursor to a restoration of autonomy (Campbell, 1990). Problems develop when dependency is unnecessarily prolonged, and then there is a risk that actions became paternalistic and nurses may find it difficult to separate acceptable beneficent acts from unacceptable paternalistic ones.

Implications for practice

- Nurses need to be aware of their own beliefs and values, and how they influence the care they provide
- The patient has a right to receive legally and morally accepted standards of care
- Nurses should attempt to understand/appreciate the perspective of others, particularly if different from their own
- Ethical guidelines may be useful in providing a framework for morally guided care
- Healthcare professionals should be involved in case conferences to discuss issues, etc.

Summary

Within clinical practice, ethical dilemmas can create a complicated, messy approach to care. Ethical considerations need to be acknowledged and discussed. By analysing situations through discussion and reflection, ethical awareness can be achieved.

Bibliography

Key reading

Edwards (1996) provides further consideration of an alternative approach when taking into account ethical issues.

Further reading

Beauchamp and Childress (2001).

Part 2

Pathophysiology and treatments

Chapter 13

Neurological assessment

Vikki Howarth

Contents

Learning outcomes

After reading this chapter you will be able to:

- Use the Glasgow coma scale correctly
- Identify those patients at risk of deterioration
- Understand the best practice whilst carrying out neurological observations
- Increase your awareness of the interpretation of all sections of the neurological observations.

Fundamental knowledge

- The 12 cranial nerves.

Introduction

Neurological complications occur in over half of all critically ill patients, and these may affect their outcome as well as their length of stay (Vespa, 1998). Following any neurological insult, nursing assessment is vital in order to measure progression or deterioration. Most nurses should be familiar with a neurological assessment chart, which should include four distinct sections:

1   The Glasgow coma scale (GCS)
2   Pupil reaction
3   Vital signs
4   Limb responses.

It is important for all four categories to be completed in order to gain a complete picture of the patient's condition.

The Glasgow coma scale

The Glasgow coma scale (Teasdale and Jennett, 1974) is a simple tool to use. It has been utilised as a prognostic device during immediate assessment following a head injury. Patients displaying a lower score have a poorer prognosis (Waldmann and Thyveetil, 1998).

The GCS gives practitioners an internationally accepted format that assists communication, minimises user interpretation, and rapidly detects changes in the patient's condition. The GCS measures the degree of consciousness under three distinct categories:

1   Eye opening
2   Best motor response
3   Verbal response.

These categories are further divided, and each of the subdivisions is awarded a score. All the scores are added to give a total score. The maximum score for the conscious, alert individual is 15, whereas the lowest possible score for the deeply unconscious patient is 3. A score of 8 and below should give cause for concern. However, all patients should be closely monitored for signs of deterioration (see Figure 13.1).

Factors influencing assessment should be noted – for example, the effects of sedatives and spinal injuries, severely shocked patients, and those in the post-ictal phase (following an epileptic seizure). Patients with a spinal injury should be assessed using facial movements only.

NEUROLOGICAL OBSERVATION CHART

Patient name:
DoB:
Hospital No.
Ward: ·
Consultant:

DATE:

TIME:

Eyes open	Spontaneously	4
	To speech	3
	To pain	2
	None	1

C=Eyes closed by swelling

Best verbal response	Orientated	5
	Disorientated	4
	Inapprop. words	3
	Sounds only	2
	None	1

T=Endotrach. tube or tracheostomy
D=Dysphasia

Best motor response (record best arm)	Obeys commands	6
	Localize pain	5
	Normal flexion	4
	Abnormal flex	3
	Extension	2
	None	1

P=Paralysed

COMA SCALE TOTAL

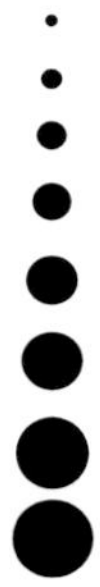

Pupil diameter guide (mm):
1
2
3
4
5
6
7
8

BLOOD PRESSURE AND PULSE

230
220
210
200
190
180
170
160
150
140
130
120
110
100
90
80
70
60
50
40
35
30
25
20
15
10
5

TEMPERATURE °C
39.5
39.0
38.5
38.0
37.5
37.0
36.5
36.0
35.5
35.0
34.5
34.0
33.5
33.0
32.5
32.0

Respiration

PUPILS	Right	Size (mm)
		Reaction
	Left	Size (mm)
		Reaction

+=reacts
−= no react
Sl=Sluggish

LIMB MOVEMENT	ARMS	Normal power
		Mild weakness
		Severe weakness
		Flexion
		Extension
		No response
	LEGS	Normal power
		Mild weakness
		Severe weakness
		Flexion
		Extension
		No response

Record right (R) & left (L) seperately if there is a difference between the two sides

P=Paralysed
#=Fracture

Figure 13.1 Neurological assessment chart

Time out 13.1

Think about the patients you have nursed who required assessment and monitoring through a GCS.

1   What was the underlying reason for this type of monitoring (medical condition)?
2   Describe your assessment using this tool.

Applying painful stimuli

Painful stimuli should only be applied if patients are not responding to speech or touch. Any method should not be applied to such an extent as to leave patients bruised or their dignity compromised. Although applying strong painful stimuli to patients can be distressing to many nurses, the results of this seemingly crude test can have major implications for patients and their treatment.

Any stimulus should start with a low level of force and be increased gradually until a response is either activated or regarded as being absent.

Central pressure (such as sternal rubbing) assesses arousal, whereas peripheral stimuli (such as nail bed pressure) measure awareness. Box 13.1 illustrates how and where to apply stimuli.

Box 13.1   How and where to apply painful stimuli
■ *Nail bed pressure*. Pressure is usually applied with a pen alongside the nail (never onto the nail bed, as this can cause permanent damage). ■ *Trapezius pinch*. The trapezius muscle is a broad, flat, triangular muscle that covers the back of the neck and the shoulders; 5 cm of this muscle should be pinched and twisted gently. ■ *Pressure at jaw margin*. Do not apply this stimulus if the patient has sustained facial injuries, or if a basal skull fracture is suspected. Pressure should be applied at the jaw margin, just in front of the earlobe. ■ *Sternal rub*. Knuckle pressure is applied to the sternal notch. This can cause bruising, and should not be used in patients who have chest trauma. ■ *Supra-orbital pressure*. Pressure is applied to the supra-orbital notch. Pressure should *not* be applied onto the orbit itself, and should not be used on patients with facial injuries or to assess the eye-opening response.

Time out 13.2

Try the above tests on yourself, and then reflect on the amount of force required on a patient.

Eye opening

- *Spontaneous eye opening* (score 4). This should be observed before the patient is directly approached or spoken to. The presence of spontaneous eye opening indicates a state of arousal, but does not always indicate that the patient is aware of the surroundings.
- *Eye opening to speech* (score 3). The patient should be initially approached when speaking in a normal tone of voice. This may be increased to elicit a response, as the patient may have a hearing defect. In this case, a gentle hand on the patient's shoulder or arm should elicit a response. The patient may be responding to voice alone and not the content of the request, and therefore this test may not be a good indication of cognitive assessment.
- *Eye opening to pain* (score 2). As mentioned, this test should not be assessed using a supra-orbital rub, as this will stimulate a grimace response. Application of nail bed pressure, or sternal rubbing, should be used to stimulate a response.
- *No eye opening* (score 1). This is scored following the application of painful stimuli. If the patient has significant peri-orbital swelling, inhibiting eye opening, the letter C (closed) or S (swollen) should be recorded on the chart.

Verbal response

Good verbal response indicates both arousal and awareness, and can demonstrate cognitive function. This communication may only take place following arousal, which may require an auditory or sensory stimulus. Influencing factors, such as difficulty in hearing, language barriers or culture differences (e.g. a patient new to the UK may not know who the Prime Minister is) need to be considered when conducting this assessment.

- *Orientated response* (score 5). The patient can communicate knowledge of time, place, person, current season, year, Prime Minister.
- *Confused response* (score 4). This is identified by the patient's ability to talk in sentences, but the content of his or her speech is disorientated to the above questions.
- *Occasional words* (score 3). Here, occasional words are used rather than sentences, and make little sense of the context of questioning.
- *Incomprehensible sounds* (score 2). Sounds are initiated with either painful or auditory stimuli. The response consists of moans and groans only.
- *No verbal response to pain or sound* (score 1). If the presence of an endotracheal or tracheotomy tube renders the patient unable to vocalise, the letter T (tube) should be recorded on the chart.

Best motor response

Due to the presence of spinal reflexes occurring in the patient's legs, when measuring the GCS *arm* and *facial* responses only should be recorded.

■ *Both sensory input and cognition* (score 6). The patient is asked to either stick out the tongue or lift the arms and touch his or her nose. Avoid asking the patient to squeeze your hand, as this is a primitive response and does not always indicate cognition.

■ *Localising toward a stimulus* (score 5). With the presence of any brain injury, the patient may no longer respond to a verbal request, and therefore the response to painful stimuli must be ascertained. This is a purposeful movement toward the source of discomfort. By applying supra-orbital notch pressure or a jaw margin rub, the patient should raise the hand to beyond his or her chin. The patient may also be witnessed trying to remove uncomfortable apparatus, such as an endotracheal tube.

■ *Flexion to pain* (score 4). This is observed when the patient makes a flexion of the elbow following nail bed pressure, but is too weak to localise this toward a central stimulus.

■ *Abnormal flexion* (score 3). This is a flexion of the elbows accompanied by spastic flexion of the wrist. This decorticate movement is an abnormal sign, and suggests a degree of cerebral damage.

■ *Extension to pain* (score 2). This occurs when there has been an insult to the brain stem. The arms will straighten, and sometimes internally rotate at the shoulder, elbow or wrist.

■ *No response to deep pain* (score 1). This indicates severe brain stem impairment.

Pupil size and reaction

Pupil reaction is undertaken by the second and third cranial nerves because of their long intracranial pathway. Pupil diameter is measured in millimetres, and the normal range is 2–6 mm. Pupils should be round in shape and equal in size bilaterally. Most neurological assessment charts have a guide to pupil size.

The pupils should be examined initially in moderate lighting conditions; this usually necessitates the dimming of overhead lighting. The size, shape and equality of both pupils should be noted. Direct and indirect pupil reactions to *bright* light should then be ascertained on both pupils. A direct response is observed as a constriction of the pupil when directly illuminated. The indirect response (or consensual reaction) is the simultaneous reaction of the other pupil. The light source should be introduced from the outer aspect of each eye, towards the pupil; the pupils should constrict briskly. This is recorded as a plus (+) sign on the chart. Once the light source is removed, the pupils should dilate back to their ambient state. Patients should not be positioned where light will directly be upon them (e.g. facing a window).

If the reaction is sluggish, unequal or absent, this should be recorded and reported immediately. Lesions causing compression of the third cranial nerve will cause an irregularity in pupil size and reaction.

Vital signs

Temperature

Temperature recordings are traditionally underestimated during neurological assessment. Disruption of the temperature-regulating centre in the hypothalamus can manifest itself as either hypothermia or pyrexia. An increase in temperature causes increased metabolism, and this reaction increases the by-product carbon dioxide, which is a potent vasodilator (see Chapter 27). Pyrexia may also indicate the presence of infection; therefore full microbiological screening should take place to identify and correctly treat any pathogens.

Hypothermia is defined as a core temperature below 35°C, and can manifest in patients with a damaged hypothalamus or brain stem. However, for proper assessment to take place, particularly if brain stem testing is anticipated, hypothermia must be treated and controlled using active warming techniques.

Pulse

Bradycardia is present in the compensatory phase of a raised intracranial pressure (ICP), and should therefore be reported immediately. This is caused by mid-brain compression. If it is associated with a hypertension and decreasing GCS (Cushing's response), this indicaties tentorial herniation. If this is not treated rapidly it will lead to herniation of the lower cerebellum through the foramen magnum, and sudden death (Sutcliffe, 1997).

Blood pressure

The vasomotor centre in the brain stem controls blood pressure. The presence of ischaemia in this area, resulting from a raised ICP, causes the triggering of Cushing's response (see Chapter 27). In an attempt to maintain perfusion, increasing intracranial pressure triggers an increase in arterial blood pressure. Elevation of the arterial blood pressure increases cardiac output and pulse pressure.

Hypotension is rarely characteristic of brain injury alone, except in the terminal stages of herniation. Hypotension is more often due to hypovolaemia following multiple injury and inadequate resuscitation (Withington, 1997). A full examination should take place in order to identify further areas of injury, such as intra-abdominal bleeding or bony fractures. This is particularly important in the young, who will compensate for hypovolaemia for longer than the elderly.

Respirations

The brain requires a constant supply of well-oxygenated blood. If this supply is disrupted for more than a few minutes, permanent ischaemic neuronal damage will occur. Early respiratory disorders are a common cause of ischaemic damage resulting in a significant fall in GCS. If the GCS score continues to decrease there is a loss of protective reflexes (e.g. cough and gag), which can lead to further ischaemia.

Breathing is initiated and controlled in three main areas of the brain: the brain stem regulates the automicity of respiration; the cerebellum synchronises and co-ordinates the muscular effort of respiration; and the cerebral hemispheres regulate any voluntary control over the normal respiratory pattern. During the early, acute stages of a raised ICP, with pressure inflicted on the cerebellum and cerebral hemispheres, the respirations slow, indicating respiratory function at the brain stem level only. If ICP is left unchecked, and the brain stem becomes altered, the respirations will become rapid and noisy prior to terminating.

Limb responses

Assessment of all four limb responses is undertaken to identify a focal deficit. This deficit could be caused by nerve pathway damage, or by the compression of brain tissue as a result of a rising ICP or a space-occupying lesion. Assessment is more straightforward in the semi-recumbent co-operative patient. The patient should be asked to perform extension and flexion movements against an antagonistic force supplied by the assessor. The less co-operative patient can be observed and assessed using involuntary movements. Although this is a less objective measure, encouragement and reassessment of collaboration should be performed prior to each evaluation.

Determination of mild or severe weakness is performed by judging the strength of the patient response against opposing pressure, and by asking the patient to lift individual limbs from the surface of the bed. A mild weakness is indicated if the assessor can easily push the limb back onto the bed. Movements of the limb, without the inability to overcome gravity to raise the limb, indicate severe weakness. A full range of movements should be assessed to gain a clear picture of the patient's condition. If the patient is not responding to a verbal request, a reaction to pain should be sought.

When measuring the GCS, the 'best response' should be recorded. The GCS is not a tool to measure a focal deficit, and therefore it is not necessary to record the difference between the left and right responses. It is also important to remember that the arm and facial responses only should be recorded when assessing GCS.

Implications for practice

- Nursing should monitor trends relating to patient data, rather than noting isolated observations
- The accuracy of the GCS is dependent upon the assessor using it and interpreting it correctly
- Patient dignity should be maintained throughout the assessment process.

Summary

Neurological assessment using the GCS is familiar to most nurses, irrespective of clinical setting. The GCS, although an internationally used tool, is subject to bias variability, and therefore the same nurse should, wherever possible, be involved in the assessment/monitoring phases.

If conducted properly, the GCS can indicate deterioration or improvement in the patient's condition. However, the tool should not be reduced to just numbers; that is not its purpose (Hanley, 1997). Nurses, indeed all healthcare professionals, should describe the patient's condition as a whole, not just relying on a numerical score.

Clinical scenario

Mrs Mary Hinds is a 46-year-old lady who has been admitted to the critical care unit following a sub-arachnoid haemorrhage. Her past medical history includes hypertension, for which she normally takes Atenalol 50 mg daily. Her initial results on admission are:

GCS   E3 V2 M4=9
B/P   156/87
Pulse 93 bpm
CVP   5 mmHg
Temp   36.7°C

1   Explain why the GCS is the tool of choice in this assessment, and state what the score represents.

2   Write down how you would conduct a neurological assessment on Mrs Hinds, using the GCS.

3   Interpret Mrs Hinds' assessment data. What do they indicate?

Bibliography

Key reading

Dawson (2000).
Hanley (1997).

Further reading

Ellis and Cavanagh (1992).
Waldmann and Thyveetil (1998).

Chapter 14

Respiratory assessment

Tina Moore

Contents

Learning outcomes

After reading this chapter you will be able to:

- Assess the patient's respiratory status appropriately and correctly
- Identify signs of hypoxaemia
- Identify signs of hypercapnia (carbon dioxide retention)
- Initiate appropriate nursing intervention in a patient who is experiencing respiratory difficulties

Fundamental knowledge

- Respiratory physiology, gaseous exchange, carriage of gases.

Introduction

Deterioration in a patient's respiratory function is one of the major causes of critical illness and accounts for one of the main reasons for admission to the critical care unit. The primary purpose of respiratory assessment is to determine the adequacy of oxygen transportation. After undertaking a full and systematic assessment, a nurse is in a unique position to act upon findings from the data collected and ensure that appropriated medical/nursing intervention occurs (Cox and McGrath, 1999). This chapter identifies issues regarding respiratory assessment, and the implications in relation to respiratory failure and treatment.

Time out 14.1

1 Think about how you assess a patient's respiratory status. What 'type' of patients do you conduct this assessment on?
2 On your next shift, count how many patients have respiratory problems. How many of these patients have their respiratory function recorded on an observation chart?
3 List other respiratory observations made by nursing staff (e.g. peak flow measurements).

Respiratory assessment

Wherever possible, the same nurse should be involved in the assessment/monitoring of the patient's respiratory status for the duration of a shift. This will enable the identification of subtle as well as overt changes. Depending on the severity of respiratory impairment, history-taking may be limited and observational skills will therefore need to be relied upon. During assessment, significant factors that influence the patient's respiratory function should always be taken into consideration, including:

- Pregnancy. Fluid retention is caused by increasing oestrogen levels, resulting in oedema. Progesterone levels rise six-fold through pregnancy (Lumb, 2000) and have a significant effect on the control of respiratory and arterial blood gases. In addition, enlargement of the uterus in the third trimester causes the diaphragm to be misplaced, thus affecting lung expansion.
- Obesity. If obese patients are poorly positioned in bed, this may cause an impediment to lung expansion.
- Circulatory factors. Pulmonary oedema and anaemia both affect respiration.
- Environmental influences. Exposure to the cold, for example, may cause shivering, thus distorting assessment findings.

Patients should be positioned upright wherever possible, with their head bent forward and arms crossed in front of them. This position may be difficult for some patients who may need support, as in leaning over the bedside table. This position not only facilitates lung expansion, but also enables access to the anterior and posterior thorax. Alternative positions may distort findings and will need to be acknowledged when interpreting data. If indicated, remove patients' clothing, as this may act as a barrier, again distorting findings. Some patients may be aware that their respiratory function is being assessed and this may lead to a subconscious response that influences their breathing. Generally, respiratory assessment can be broken down into four areas – inspection, palpation, percussion and auscultation. Nurses do not perform percussion as a mode of respiratory assessment unless additional training has been undertaken (see Chapter 28).

Inspection

Rate

The respiratory rate should be counted for one full minute, and categorised into one of the following:

- Eupnoea ('normal' rate of 10–18 per min) (Darovic, 2002a)
- Tachypnoea (greater than 18 per min), which is usually the first indication of respiratory distress; possible causes include anxiety, pain, cardiac-related (e.g. left ventricular failure), circulatory problems (e.g. anaemia)
- Bradypnoea (less than 10 per min), which could indicate increased intracianial pressure, depression of the respiratory centre, narcotic overdose (e.g. opiates), severe deterioration in the patient's condition
- Hypopnoea (abnormally shallow respirations), which may vary with age.

Rhythm

The normal respiratory rhythm has regular cycles, with the inspiratory phase being slightly longer than the expiratory phase. The ratio of respiration to pulse rate in the healthy adult is 1:4. As a rule of thumb, the rhythm varies between men and women. Men tend to breathe predominantly from their abdomen or diaphragm, whereas women have a tendency to breathe via their thorax or costal muscles. Sleeping patients tend to breathe via their abdomen. Nurses need to be aware of this difference, as there is an assumption that an increase in respiratory effort relates to the use of abdominal muscles. This could lead to a wrong diagnosis. Altered rhythms indicate an underlying disorder, e.g. Kussmaul breathing (rapid deep respirations due to the stimulation of the respiratory centre in the brain caused by metabolic acidosis) occurs in diabetic ketoacidosis. Cheyne-Stokes respirations (periods of apnoea alternating with periods of hypoxia) could indicate left ventricular failure or cerebral injury, and are sometimes seen in the end stage of life.

Quality of breathing

Normally, there is symmetry in chest movement. Failure of the chest wall to rise adequately may indicate fibrosis, collapse of upper lobes of the lung, or bronchial obstruction. It may also indicate severe pleural thickening, which can cause flattening of the chest wall anteriorly and diminished respiratory effort. The legacy of previous thoracic surgery may be highlighted by the presence of old scars.

Degree of effort

The use of accessory muscles (sternocleidomastoid, scalenus, trapezius) may suggest that the patient has difficulty in breathing. The patient may suffer from orthopnoea or even platypnoea (shortness of breath when sitting upright). Patients who have difficulty in expiration may indicate abnormalities of lung recoil and/or airway resistance (e.g. emphysema, pulmonary oedema, asthma). Increased inspiratory effort can indicate upper airway obstruction (e.g. anaphylaxis, epiglottitis). Tracheal deviation may indicate pneumothorax, possibly induced through treatment.

Expiration may be prolonged, as seen in asthma or emphysema, and the influence of the severity of breathlessness on the restricted activity should be noted. Some patients may breath through 'pursed lips' on expiration.

Skin colour

Cyanosis (particularly central), occurs when large amounts of unsaturated haemoglobin are present, and may be detectable when the oxygen saturation of arterial blood drops to between 85 and 90 per cent (Lumb, 2000). However, this is subject to considerable variability. Cyanosis is often difficult to appreciate in artificial lighting, unless quite gross, and is best seen on the lips and under the tongue. Cyanosis can easily be missed, and requires diligence in observation and assessment. Prolonged hypoxaemia can lead to erythrocytosis and produce a ruddy appearance. Particular caution needs to be taken when assessing skin colour in patients with dark pigmented skin. In anaemic patients there may be insufficient haemoglobin, producing a blue colour in the mucous membrane.

Deformities

Clubbing of the finger digits occurs as a result of a chronic condition, over a long period of time. This may be indicative of hypoxaemia from pulmonary or cardiovascular disease.

Deformities of the posterior thorax can affect the quality of breathing. The anterior/posterior diameter of the chest should be compared with the side-to-side diameter; if the anterior/posterior diameter is approximately double this indicates a 'barrel chest' (caused by emphysema). Spinal deformities such as kyphosis also influence lung expansion.

Mental status

A reduction in the patient's level of consciousness or an altered mental status may indicate hypoxaemia. Symptoms include inappropriate behaviour, drowsiness and confusion. Assessment of patient's mental status needs to be conducted with care, as some patients feel a sense of suffocation and become very frightened and anxious but are not hypoxic. Language barriers and cultural approaches to disorders and diseases also need to be considered when assessing patients.

Secretions

Sputum is a useful indicator of lung pathology, for example:

- Frothy white (sometimes blood-stained) sputum indicates pulmonary oedema
- Bloody sputum (haemoptysis) indicates pulmonary embolism
- Blood-stained sputum indicates pneumonia, abscess, aspiration
- Green and purulent sputum indicates a lung infection
- Green and thick sputum indicates pneumonia
- Yellow/green and copious sputum indicates advanced chronic bronchitis
- Black sputum indicates smoking (tar)
- Old blood in the sputum indicates TB, lung cancer.

Palpation

Palpation is used to assess bilateral movements of the chest/diaphragm. It is also used to assess surgical emphysema. The palm of the hand (which should be warm) is placed on the chest to feel for any vibrations. The depth of inspiration and expiration may be more pronounced in some patients when a hand is placed on the anterior thorax.

Auscultation

Assessment of breath sounds should form part of the nursing assessment. Knowledge of the different types of breath sounds is important to aid description and diagnosis. Without a stethoscope, normal breathing should be quiet. Normal breath sounds are described as vesicular, bronchovesicular and bronchial.

- Normally, vesicular sounds (low-pitched, low-intensity – described as 'soft and breezy') can be heard over most of the lung fields
- Bronchovesicular sounds should be heard anteriorly near the mainstem bronchi and posteriorly between the scapulae; sounds are more moderate in pitch and intensity
- Bronchial sounds are high-pitched, loud and hollow sounding, and are normally heard over the larger airways and the trachea. If bronchial sounds are heard in other areas, this could indicate consolidation of lung tissue as in pneumonia (consolidated lung tissue transmits sounds better than air).

Abnormal breath sounds, known as adventitious sounds (crackles, indicating pulmonary oedema; wheezing, indicating asthma and pleural friction rubbing) should be listened for. Normally, obstruction of the airways by bronchospasm or swelling causes wheezing. Stridor (high-pitched sound) usually occurs on inspiration, and is caused by laryngeal or tracheal obstruction; this requires immediate attention.

Crackles may be fine, medium or coarse:

■ Fine crackles are high-pitched, and are heard at the base of the lungs near the end of inspiration
■ Medium crackles are lower in pitch, and are heard during the middle/latter part of inspiration
■ Coarse crackles are loud, bubbling sounds that are heard on both inspiration and expiration.

Respiratory failure

The older person is at increased risk in developing respiratory failure due to underlying pulmonary disease, loss of muscle mass and other co-morbid conditions (Sevransky and Haponik, 2003).

Respiratory failure is a syndrome in which the respiratory system fails in one or both of its gas exchange functions – oxygenation, and carbon dioxide elimination (Sharma, 2003). Therefore, respiratory failure exists when the lungs cannot fulfil their primary function of maintaining adequate gas exchange at rest or during exercise. This condition can be acute or chronic. Blood gas disturbances occur as a result of ventilation–perfusion (V/Q) inequality, inadequate alveolar ventilation, or a combination of both (see Chapter 16).

Unventilated alveoli results in vasoconstriction, which then diverts the perfusion to ventilated alveoli, resulting in the collapse of a lung.

There are two types of respiratory failure: type 1 (oxygenation) and type 2, ventilatory.

Type 1 respiratory failure

This type of respiratory failure occurs when there is hypoxia without carbon dioxide (CO_2) retention. It occurs in diseases that increase the fluid barrier in the alveoli or interstitial tissues. Most pulmonary and cardiac conditions can cause type 1 respiratory failure, pulmonary oedema and chronic obstructive pulmonary diseases being the more common causes. Carbon dioxide levels in the blood remain normal because it is far more soluble than oxygen (O_2), so it can continue to perfuse across such oedematous tissue. As a result of alveolar hypoventilation the $PaCO_2$ then rises, resulting in a fall of PaO_2. Respiratory failure that develops slowly allows renal compensation with retention of bicarbonate, often resulting in a near normal pH. A change in the pH of the blood together with an increase in carbon dioxide effects the saturation of haemoglobin.

Type 1 respiratory failure is defined as PaO_2 <8 kPa; $PaCO_2$ <6 kPa (British Thoracic Society, 2002).

Clinical features

Dyspnoea arising from respiratory diseases, particularly acute, is often associated with anxiety and panic, which exacerbates the symptoms. Respiratory causes of breathlessness may be divided into those resulting from disease of the airway, of the lung parenchyma, of the pulmonary circulation, and of the pleura and chest wall. Airway disease usually causes a pattern of airflow obstruction, as in asthma and emphysema (Seaton *et al.*, 2000; see Chapter 15).

Diseases that affect the lung parenchyma usually cause a steadily progressive type of breathlessness with a restrictive pattern of lung function, e.g. alveolitis, alveolar cell and metastatic carcinoma.

Early indicators of hypoxaemia include:

- Irritability, clouding of consciousness, confusion
- Restlessness, anxiety, fatigue
- Cool and dry skin
- Increased cardiac output/tachycardia as a result of stimulations of ventilation via the carotid chemo-receptors, also causing headache.

Immediate indicators include:

- Confusion/aggression
- Lethargy
- Tachypnoea
- Hypotension
- Cardiac dysrhythmias – bradycardia.

Late indicators include:

- Cyanosis
- O$_2$ saturations of less than 75 per cent
- Diaphoresis (sweating)
- Coma, convulsions
- Cardiac dysrhythmias
- Respiratory arrest.

Pulmonary arteries respond to hypoxia by vasoconstriction, producing vascular resistance and pulmonary hypertension. Right ventricular enlargement or *cor pulmonale* develop later. Nursing care should be directed at preventing the patient from developing late clinical features.

Type 2 respiratory failure

Type 2 respiratory failure is caused by increased airway resistance and reduced lung compliance. Both oxygen and carbon dioxide blood levels are affected, as in acute bronchitis. Alveoli are microscopic and prone to collapse (atelectasis) and therefore produce surfactant to help them inflate. However, production is inhibited by hypoxia, acidosis, poor perfusion, smoking and dry gas, such as unhumidified oxygen.

Oxygen levels are low, and in addition there is inadequate removal of carbon dioxide.

Type 2 respiratory failure is defined as PaO_2 <8 kPa; $PaCO_2$ >6 kPa (British Thoracic Society, 2002).

Clinical features

In addition to the signs of hypoxaemia, the patient may show clinical signs of hypercapnia:

- Irritability, aggression, confusion and coma
- Headaches and papilloedema (CO_2 contains dilatory properties that may result in increased cerebral flow)
- Warm, flushed skin and a bounding pulse (CO_2 on the peripheral vascular smooth muscles of the peripheral circulation may also produce vasoconstriction by sympathetic stimulation).

Management

Identifying the type of respiratory failure is important, as it determines the intervention. Underlying causes of respiratory failure should be treated (e.g. chest infection or trauma).

Hypoxaemia must be treated as the first priority. Administration of oxygen is the fastest and most effective method of treatment, but this will do nothing to improve the $PaCO_2$ and may make it worse (Lumb, 2000). It is therefore essential to ensure that palliative relief of hypoxia does not result in hypercapnia, and arterial $PaCO_2$ should be monitored.

Type 1 respiratory failure may require supplementary oxygen, although some local policies advocate non-invasive ventilation (NIV) therapy. Type 2 respiratory failure will require additional support (e.g. non-invasive ventilation). (Refer to Chapters 16 and 18 for specific content on these treatments.)

Time out 14.2

Revisit your findings from the study conducted in Time out 14.1. After reading this chapter and additional reading, together with colleagues write guidelines for respiratory assessment relating to your area of practice.

Implications for practice

- A comprehensive assessment of the patient's respiratory status should be performed
- Assessment should be used to identify potential respiratory problems
- Early intervention is essential in order to improve the prognosis of patients who have identified respiratory problems.

Summary

Deterioration of respiratory status is one of the major reasons for admission to a critical care unit. Therefore, comprehensive respiratory assessment should be performed on all patients to highlight actual or potential problems. There are two types of respiratory failure, and common symptoms are found in each. Type 2 failure has the additional symptoms of hypercapnia. The mode of treatment will depend upon the cause.

Clinical scenario

John Ross, 55 years old, has been transferred to the critical care unit from the ward after developing 'respiratory problems'. He underwent extensive abdominal surgery 3 days ago. He looks unwell, and is complaining of severe abdominal pain. He is a known smoker. Ward documentation suggests that John's abdominal pain was never under control, and he always lay in a semi-recumbent position.

John is breathing spontaneously but is dyspnoeic. His respiratory rate is 30 per minute, the pattern is regular but shallow, and he is using his accessory muscles. He has a cough, which is unproductive. He looks pale, and no central cyanosis is present. Auscultation of the lungs indicate reduced air entry at both bases with some coarse crackles in the right mid-zone and widespread mild expiratory wheeze (also heard without a stethoscope).

John's heart rate is variable (atrial fibrillation), with an approximate rate of 120 bpm. He looks pale and clammy. His blood pressure is 160/110 mmHg, and oxygen saturation levels are 87% on 40% oxygen. Blood gas analysis gives PaO_2 of 10.3, $PaCO_2$ of 4.9, bicarbonate base excess.

John responds to verbal instructions but appears drowsy. He feels cold and slightly clammy.

1 Identify the type of respiratory failure

2 What type of nursing/medical intervention will John require?

3 What criteria would you use in order to assess the success of treatment?

Bibliography

Key reading

Cox and McGrath (1999) gives detailed information relating to respiratory assessment.

Lumb (2000) provides more advanced information in relation to respiratory physiology.

Further reading

Most texts relating to intensive care and high dependency care will have appropriate content.

Chapter 15

Acute respiratory pathologies

Philip Woodrow

Contents

Learning outcomes

After reading this chapter you will be able to:

- Understand the main pathologies causing critical respiratory illness
- Provide evidence-based care for patients with these conditions
- Identify patients' needs to junior colleagues.

Fundamental knowledge

Respiratory failure, respiratory monitoring (see Chapter 14).

Introduction

Respiratory failure is classified into two types:

- Type 1 (hypoxaemia + normocapnia; PaO_2 <8 kPa + $PaCO_2$ <6 kPa)
- Type 2 (hypoxaemia + hypercapnia; PaO_2 <8 kPa + $PaCO_2$ >6 kPa)
  (British Thoracic Society, 2002).

This chapter describes pathologies that more often necessitate or complicate adult admission to acute wards.

Exchange of gases in the lungs relies on *ventilation* (volume of air reaching alveoli), *perfusion* (volume of blood in pulmonary capillaries) and *diffusion* (exchange of gases between the two). Respiratory disease can occur when one or more of these are inadequate.

Chronic disease is largely irreversible, needing prolonged (often community) care. However, people with chronic lung disease are particularly susceptible to acute exacerbations from infection or other factors, and therefore chronic obstructive pulmonary disease (COPD), emphysema and asthma are discussed below.

The second part of this chapter focuses on acute conditions:

- Pneumothorax
- Pleural effusion
- Pulmonary embolism.

Acute disease often occurs as a complication of chronic respiratory disease.

This chapter discusses diseases, medical tests and treatments, but with the focus remaining on nursing rather than on medical aspects of care. More detailed discussion of medical aspects may be found in medical texts. Problems experienced by different patients with similar conditions will vary, so care should be individualised to meet each patient's needs.

Chronic lung disease

Chronic obstructive pulmonary disease

COPD is a group of diseases resulting in the common problem of permanent limitation to airflow. Although this group includes conditions such as asthma and bronchiectasis, most people with COPD have chronic bronchitis (85 per cent) or emphysema (15 per cent) (British Thoracic Society, 1997a; Bach *et al.*, 2001).

COPD is under-diagnosed by doctors (Connolly, 1996), being the sixth most common cause of death in England and Wales (Fehrenbach, 2002) and likely to become the third by 2020 (Crocket, 2002), with 85–90 per cent of cases being caused through smoking (Bach *et al.*, 2001).

Although respiratory disease can occur at any age, chronic limitations and disease tend to occur in later life due to changes in body tissue (airways, vasculature or interstitial) that impair gas exchange. Some changes inevitably result from ageing, but healthy ageing alone should not cause respiratory disease (Watson, 2000a). Toxic damage from inhaled pollutants (cigarette smoke, environmental pollutants or other chemicals) causes nearly all chronic respiratory conditions.

People with COPD often develop right-sided heart failure (*cor pulmonale*) and other problems, such as limited mobility, some of which may have little or no direct connection with their COPD. Breathlessness often makes people reluctant to eat and drink, causing malnourishment. At the same time, dyspnoea significantly increases the work of breathing, increasing energy requirements when the energy supply is reduced. Chronic dyspnoea therefore often leads to malnutrition, with sufferers being typically emaciated. Limited airflow causes shallow breathing, making static lung bases a reservoir for developing acute chest infections. Acute exacerbations create additional problems, so care should:

- Maintain the normal activities of living (as far as possible)
- Prevent further complications
- Reverse the acute problem.

Care should be individualised, but likely management includes:

- Oxygen (up to 28% until arterial blood gas measurement has been performed (British Thoracic Society, 1997a), and then titrated and respiratory function monitored according to blood gas results)
- Drugs (e.g. bronchodilators, steroids, antibiotics)
- Ventilatory support (e.g. non-invasive ventilation)
- Positioning (upright to aid diaphragmatic expansion)
- Deep-breathing exercises and physiotherapy
- Monitoring
- Providing as calm an atmosphere as is reasonably possible.

Various medical tests may be performed to measure respiratory function, but probably the most useful is peak flow monitoring (Frausing *et al.*, 2001), which, together with respiratory rate and depth and oxygen saturation, should form part of regular nursing observations for patients with COPD.

With respiratory failure from COPD, the best treatment is non-invasive ventilation (see Chapter 18), which should be used before severe acidosis develops (Lightowler *et al.*, 2003).

Emphysema

Damage to distal airways and alveoli causes permanent distension with loss of elasticity (compliance), so severely impairing the exchange of both oxygen and carbon dioxide. Acute emphysematous damage may be caused by excessive respiratory effort from diseases such as bronchopneumonia, asthma or tuberculosis. Chronic emphysema is usually caused by smoking (Hogg and Senior, 2002). Once diagnosed, damage is irreversible and usually extensive. Interventions for chronic emphysema are largely limited to alleviating acute exacerbations and supporting activities of living. Lung reduction surgery may prolong life.

People with emphysema usually have co-existing COPD, so medical management for the two diseases is similar. However, by the time patients need hospital admission the disease may be nearing its end stage, so while medical management of emphysema and COPD are similar, patients with emphysema may need more psychological and social support.

Asthma

Asthma is a common condition that affects more than five million people in the UK, one in thirteen adults and one in eight children (NAC, 2001a). A Manchester study found that 30 per cent of people over 45 years old had asthma or bronchitis (Renwick and Connolly, 1995). Although UK incidence is particularly high (NAC, 2001b), world-wide rates are increasing (Cates, 2001). Attacks are not usually severe enough to necessitate hospital admission, but one-tenth of people seen in A&E departments are admitted to hospital, with one-tenth of these needing invasive ventilation (FitzGerald, 2001). There are 1,500 deaths from asthma each year, more than one-third being under the age of 65 (NAC, 2001b). Many deaths could be prevented with adequate routine and emergency care (NAC, 2001b).

In people with hyper-responsive airways (Brewin, 1997; Cates, 2001), a trigger (e.g. smoking, pollution, cold air, pet hair, house mites, pollens, moulds, drugs, vigorous exercise) causes:

■ Spasm of bronchiole smooth muscle
■ Oedema
■ Increased mucus secretion.

(Inwald *et al.*, 2001; Roberts, 2002)

Resulting in narrowing and mucus plugging of small airways (Sim, 2002). One-tenth of adult asthma is occupational (Zacharisen, 2002). Typically, airway responses occur on inspiration, trapping air in the lower airways and causing a distinctive expiratory wheeze as air is forced out through very constricted airways. Drugs such as beta-blockers, aspirin and non-steroidal anti-inflammatories (NSAIDs) release mediators that cause bronchoconstriction, so may trigger asthma attacks. Although excessive excitement, fear and anxiety do not cause asthma, they may exacerbate it (Reinke and Hoffman, 2000).

Increased work of breathing (WOB) causes respiratory muscle fatigue (Sim, 2002) and distress/panic. Excessive parasympathetic stimulation on inspiration may cause pulsus paradoxus (a fall in systolic blood pressure of more than 10 mmHg on inspiration) (Sim, 2002), although pulsus paradoxus is not useful for assessing asthma (British Thoracic Society, 1997b).

Oxygen therapy should be commenced at the same time as or before bronchodilators (British Thoracic Society, 1997b), restoring oxygen saturation above 90% (Smaha, 2001). If SpO_2 is below 92%, arterial blood gas should be analysed

(BTS/SIGN, 2003). During acute attacks, 40–60% oxygen should be given (British Thoracic Society, 1997b). Drugs (bronchodilators, steroids) will be given either as inhalers/nebulisers or intravenously. Antibiotics are not routinely given (Sim, 2002).

Asthma attacks are frightening, causing the sufferer to fight for breath. Gas exchange is poor, with hypoxia and hypercapnia. Hypoxia may cause acute confusion. Providing as calm an atmosphere as possible, with information and support, can help to reduce stress. Empowering patients, rather than making them passive recipients of care, can reduce distress. Sedatives that cause respiratory depression, such as morphine, may prove fatal, so should not be given. Instead of trying to treat the symptom of fear, treatment should reverse the asthma that causes the fear (Rees and Kanabar, 2000).

Perspiration and tachypnoea often cause excessive fluid loss, resulting in hypovolaemia (Sim, 2002), so fluids should be given. Sim (2002) recommends giving crystalloids, but where rapid infusion of crystalloids may exacerbate oedema, colloids may be preferred.

With recovery, health education may be needed to help people control their asthma and prevent further attacks (Smaha, 2001), although Paley (2000) found that some asthmatics felt guilty for 'failing' to control their asthma.

Acute lung conditions

Pneumothorax

A pneumothorax is gas or air in the pleural space. The pleura form the two outer layers of the lung, separated by 5–10 ml of pleural fluid. Any damage to the pleura, whether from trauma or disease (spontaneous), may allow extra-pleural contents to accumulate in the pleura, resulting in severe respiratory distress. Fluids in the pleural space, such as blood (haemothorax), cause similar problems to air, so although grammatically incorrect, in practice and in this chapter 'pneumothorax' is used to describe any abnormal volume accumulating between the pleura. Often both air and fluids enter the pleural space with a pneumothorax.

Most pneumothoraces are spontaneous (Mallett and Dougherty, 2000), usually occurring in either otherwise healthy people, often aged 20–30 (Gallon, 1998) or in older people with emphysema (Miller and Harvey, 1993). Various respiratory diseases, such as asthma, cystic fibrosis, chronic bronchitis, TB, pneumonia and carcinoma (Gallon, 1998; Mallett and Dougherty, 2000), can also cause spontaneous pneumothoraces.

Pneumothoraces may be either simple or tension. A *simple pneumothorax* forces the inner pleura inward, reducing lung volume. A *tension pneumothorax* occurs when the ruptured pleura remains open, creating a one-way valve. Each breath in draws more air or fluid into the pleural space (due to negative intrathoracic pressure), but the valve (tension) prevents it leaving on expiration. Tension pneumothoraces therefore create a life-threatening emergency.

Increased intrathoracic pressure on the side of the pneumothorax shifts the lungs and mediastinum towards the other side of the chest (often seen on chest X-rays). This causes cardiac tamponade (Gallon, 1998), where mechanical compression limits ventricular filling, resulting in hypotension, raised central venous pressure, and related symptoms such as breathlessness, poor perfusion and oliguria.

Smaller (<20 per cent) pneumothoraces may spontaneously resolve, but larger ones require needle aspiration or a chest drain. A chest drain creates an escape valve, thereby turning a tension pneumothorax into a simple one.

Pleural effusion

Pleural effusion may be transudative or exudative.

Transudation is caused through either increased intracapillary pressure or reduced oncotic pressure, both of which cause excessive loss of intravascular fluid into the interstitial spaces. Exudation is caused by inflammation (pleurisy), increasing capillary permeability and so loss of intravascular fluid into the interstitial space (Beers and Berkow, 1999). As plasma proteins accumulate in tissues they create an osmotic pressure, which draws further fluid into the intrapleural space (Collins and Benedict, 1996).

Untreated pleural effusions may cause atelectasis (Collins and Benedict, 1996). The person typically suffers severe chest pain on inspiration, is pyrexial, but has a non-productive cough.

Pleural effusions frequently complicate critical illness; Mattison *et al.* (1997) found them in 62 per cent of medical ICU patients. They are usually detected by chest X-rays, providing patients are sitting up.

Underlying causes of pleural effusions should be reversed. Like pneumothoraces, larger (>20 per cent) pleural effusions may be aspirated. Symptoms may require treatment, such as giving oxygen for the hypoxia caused by atelectasis. Inflammation may be reversed with steroids.

Pulmonary embolism

Pulmonary emboli are almost always preceded by deep vein thrombosis (DVT) (Hyers, 2003). Emboli can occlude any blood vessels smaller than themselves. Between 22 and 80 per cent of critically ill patients develop deep vein thrombosis (DVT) (Attia *et al.*, 2001) and efforts should be made to reduce the likelihood by:

■ Using subcutaneous heparin and anti-thrombotic stockings for patients on bed-rest (Perkins and Galland, 1999), which halves the incidence of deep vein thromboses (Attia *et al.*, 2001)
■ Early mobilisation (Martinson *et al.*, 2001).

Emboli flowing into the right ventricle are forcefully ejected into the delicate pulmonary circulation, usually affecting both lungs (Beers and Berkow, 1999). Without perfusion, gas exchange fails. Most (>70 per cent) of pulmonary emboli originate from deep vein thromboses (British Thoracic Society, 1997c), and if large are usually fatal within a couple of hours. Pulmonary emboli cause one-tenth of hospital deaths, and contribute to a further one-tenth of hospital deaths from other causes (Fennerty, 1997). They are one of the commonest causes of sudden death in young adults, and are often only identified at post mortem.

Without gas exchange in affected areas of the lung, blood returns to the left atrium with venous levels of gases ('shunt blood'). Ventilation/perfusion (V/Q) mismatch causes tachypnoea and hypoxia. The person suffers severe chest pain, is likely to be very distressed, and will show various other signs related to these problems, such as restlessness and cyanosis.

Pulmonary emboli may cause:

- Pleural effusion
- Haemoptysis
- Pyrexia
- Tachycardia
- Atrial dysrhythmias
- Distension of neck veins
- Progression to pulmonary infarction within 6–24 hours.

Pulmonary emboli may be diagnosed by various clinical signs and tests, which sometimes fail to show abnormalities. Spinal CT scan is the most accurate test, but V/Q scans and blood tests for fibrin degradation products such as D-dimers are also useful. ECG changes (Hampton, 2003a) show right ventricular and atrial enlargement, best seen in the early chest leads (V1, V2). However, ECG changes vary, and by themselves are non-specific. Blood tests for D-dimers are often useful (British Thoracic Society, 1997c), levels typically being >500 nanograms/ millilitre with pulmonary emboli. V/Q scans are the best way to diagnose pulmonary emboli (Feied and Handler, 2002).

Without treatment, pulmonary emboli are fatal in about half of cases, and are likely to recur in survivors. Initial treatment is oxygen, fluids and bed rest. Pulmonary emboli were traditionally treated with anticoagulants (e.g. heparin 48,000 units IVI over 24 hours). Medical practice is divided about whether thrombolysis increases survival and reduces risk of recurrence (Agnelli *et al.*, 2002) or not (Thabut *et al.*, 2002). Inotropes may be needed, and patients should initially be closely observed and monitored.

Psychological care

Breathing is fundamental to life, so dyspnoea causes distress. Many of the conditions discussed in this chapter may cause haemoptysis. Coughing up blood was for centuries usually a terminal sign of tuberculosis (consumption), and this is so ingrained in our culture that people who may be unfamiliar with the medical label given to their disease may fear their haemoptysis is a death sentence.

Hypoxia can cause acute confusion, making the person feel vulnerable, frightened and potentially paranoid. Offering (honest) reassurance and involving relatives with their care can help patients gain confidence in their care.

Implications for practice

- With dyspnoea, patients should be positioned upright and sitting forward to enable maximum expansion of the diaphragm and intercostal muscles (unless their medical condition contraindicates this position)
- Respiratory failure should be treated promptly and appropriately
- Respiratory acidosis with pH between 7.25 and 7.35 is an indication for non-invasive ventilation
- Severe dyspnoea usually causes an extreme stress response (panic), so good psychological support (explaining, calm atmosphere, honest reassurance) can help relieve some of the distress
- Nurses should actively prevent or minimise complications from respiratory failure, especially encouraging breathing exercises, early mobilisation, and maintenance (as far as possible) of normal activities of living.

Summary

Respiratory disease can be acute or chronic, but people with chronic respiratory diseases are more susceptible to acute exacerbations. This chapter has described the main respiratory conditions that necessitate acute high dependency care. Medical intervention and tests will vary according to precipitating conditions, but fundamental nursing care and monitoring can improve the quality of the patient's life and detect any deterioration or complications early. Yet respiratory monitoring remains the most neglected vital sign.

In addition to fundamental care and observation, certain conditions or treatments may require specific nursing care, such as management of chest drains (see Chapters 17, 18, 19).

Clinical scenario

Mrs Jenny Franks, aged 45, is admitted to your ward with bronchopneumonia. She is known to be asthmatic and a smoker, with no history of chronic obstructive pulmonary disease. She is very anxious about her son, who left home 1 month ago to study at university. She is found outside the ward, having suffered a severe asthma attack while smoking a cigarette. Her respiratory rate is now 45 per min, blood pressure 175/95 mmHg, heart rate 128 bpm. Her oxygen saturation is 83%.

1   List your initial priorities during Mrs Frank's attack. Mrs Franks is prescribed 4-hourly nebulisers of ipratropium and salbutamol, reducing daily doses of initially 40 mg prednisolone. Using a pharmacology text, such as the *British National Formulary*, list the expected effects and potential side effects of these medicines. What observations and other aspects of nursing care might be needed because of these drugs?

2   Drawing on your own experiences, material in this chapter and any other material that you have access to, develop an evidence-based plan of care for Mrs Franks for the first 48 hours following this attack.

3   The day following her attack, Mrs Franks' son arrives unexpectedly on the ward, and appears very frightened and anxious. He has already seen his mother, who has given him vague information about what happened. He asks you for information. What information and other care details would you give to Mrs Franks' son? Justify your decisions.

Bibliography

Key reading

British Thoracic Society guidelines (many currently dating from 1997, as cited in this chapter) remain the UK 'gold standard' for medical management of respiratory disease. The British Thoracic Society's journal *Thorax* regularly prints valuable articles on respiratory medicine.

Further reading

Articles on respiratory nursing frequently appear in the professional press. Brewin's (1997) article on COPD remains useful, although Fehrenbach (2002) is more recent. Gallon's (1998) article is one of the few recent substantial nursing reviews about pneumothoraces.

Chapter 16

Oxygen therapy

Sandra Gallacher

Contents

Learning outcomes

After reading this chapter you will be able to:

- Understand the principles of respiration and ventilation
- Care safely for the patient receiving oxygen therapy
- Understand the factors affecting oxygen uptake and distribution.

Fundamental knowledge

Carriage of gases, gaseous exchange, respiration assessment (Chapter 14).

Introduction

This chapter will discuss the common methods of administering oxygen. Although a brief overview of the processes of respiration and ventilation is given, the reader is recommended to access a dedicated anatomy and physiology textbook for a full discussion of these processes.

With an understanding of normal respiration and ventilation, the need for respiratory support in the critically ill can be addressed. Oxygen administration using a facemask or nasal cannulae will be discussed, in addition to factors that can affect the uptake and distribution of oxygen.

Respiration and ventilation

These terms are often used indiscriminately, but respiration and ventilation are two distinct processes (Breshers and Davey, 1998). Respiration is the exchange of oxygen and carbon dioxide during cellular metabolism (Shuldham, 1998), and occurs in two ways. *External respiration* occurs in the lungs, where exchange of oxygen (O_2) and carbon dioxide (CO_2) takes place. *Internal respiration* occurs in the body tissues. Oxygen moves by diffusion from the blood to the tissues, and carbon dioxide diffuses from the tissues into the blood (Watson, 2000b).

When oxygen delivery is insufficient to meet demand, cells can respire using an anaerobic method. This method of respiration, however, produces lactic acid, which can lead to a metabolic acidosis (Oh, 2003). It is important, therefore, that supplementary oxygen is given to vulnerable patients.

Ventilation refers to the mechanical movement of gas or air through the mechanical movement of the diaphragm, chest wall and external intercostal muscles. The accessory muscles are used during periods of excessive demand, such as vigorous exercise or airway obstruction (Breshers and Davey, 1998).

The critically ill patient may be suffering a disruption of respiration (due to lung disease) or ventilation (as a result of surgery), or both. Respiratory failure can be classified as type 1 (hypoxaemia) or type 2 (hypoxaemia with carbon dioxide retention) (see Chapter 14). It is in this context that respiratory support may be prescribed.

The mechanism of breathing

Breathing consists of two phases, inspiration and expiration. Each phase can only occur following a chain of events and involves a complex system of processes. Any or all of these processes may be adversely affected in the critically ill patient.

Inspiration

The principal muscle involved in this phase is the diaphragm (Shuldham, 1998), which normally does about 70 per cent of the work of breathing. On inspiration, the diaphragm contracts. This results in a flattened, lowered diaphragm, which lengthens the thoracic cavity (Watson, 2000b). The external intercostal muscles contract, lifting the ribs upward and outward and so increasing the depth of the thoracic cavity. This allows for lung expansion. The accessory muscles (trapezius, scalene and sternocleidomastoid) are not used during normal, or quiet, breathing, but assist the elevation of the ribs during maximal, or laboured, inspiration.

Expiration

This is usually a passive process. The diaphragm relaxes and returns to its domed shape. The intercostal muscles relax, returning the ribs to their original position. This forces air out of the lungs.

Factors affecting the mechanism of breathing

Respiratory failure is often complicated by poor lung compliance and increased airways resistance (Shuldham, 1998). This can occur due to smoking, emphysema, asthma or infection, and many other causes have been identified. It is important to remember that, whatever the primary reason for admission, some patients may also suffer from chronic or underlying respiratory disease. Cardiac and respiratory systems are complementary in the delivery of oxygen from the air to the cells and vice versa with carbon dioxide, so any failure of gas exchange and delivery will result in respiratory symptoms. Respiratory monitoring is therefore fundamental to critical illness.

The regulation of breathing

Respiration is controlled by the respiratory centre in the medulla oblongata. The rate and depth of respiration is controlled by a complex system of nerve pathways and chemoreceptors. In health, an accumulation of carbon dioxide in the blood stimulates central chemoreceptors in the large arteries. Impulses are generated, which are carried by the vagus and glossopharyngeal nerves to the respiratory centre. The phrenic nerves stimulate the diaphragm, and the intercostal nerves stimulate the intercostal muscles. However, with chronic hypercapnia, as seen in patients with chronic obstructive pulmonary disease (COPD), the respiratory centres can become desensitised to carbon dioxide.

Ventilation/perfusion mismatch

The efficiency of gas exchange in the lungs is dependent on inspired air reaching the alveoli (alveolar ventilation) and a continuous blood supply to transport oxygenated haemoglobin to the cells. Even in healthy individuals, neither alveolar ventilation nor capillary blood flow is uniform (Brashers and Davey, 1998). In the critically ill, this process can be adversely affected by anything that reduces airflow to the alveoli (perfusion with reduced ventilation), for example:

- Airway obstruction
- Narrowing of the airways
- Respiratory depression
- Pulmonary oedema.

There are also factors that can reduce blood flow to the alveoli (ventilation with reduced perfusion), such as:

- Abnormal circulation (shunts)
- Congestion (as seen with cardiac failure)
- Collapse of lung units (for example pneumothorax)
- Consolidation (associated with pneumonia)
- Occlusion of the pulmonary arteries.

Certain respiratory diseases can affect alveolar ventilation (see Chapter 15). Gases are transported across the pulmonary membrane (Gonce Morton, 1998), and in a healthy adult the total area available for gas exchange is $60\,m^2$. This area can be significantly (and permanently) reduced by emphysema and chronic bronchitis (Holgate and Frew, 2002).

In most cases, the cause of inadequate ventilation or perfusion will be quickly determined and corrected. In cases of suspected pulmonary embolism, a ventilation/perfusion (V/Q) scan may be performed. The purpose of this scan is to assess how much of the lung is receiving oxygenated blood and to measure the blood supply. The V/Q scan also be helpful to determine lung function in COPD, and to identify any abnormalities in the pulmonary circulation (Bushnell, 2003). The results of a V/Q scan can be used in conjunction with other clinical investigations, such as X-rays, to provide a diagnosis (Kaufman, 2001).

Oxygen therapy

Indications

Oxygen is a drug, and should be administered with caution under the guidance of the medical team. The main indications for respiratory support are:

- Type 1 and Type 2 respiratory failure
- Acute myocardial infarction
- Shock of any cause
- Increased metabolic demands (e.g. infections, trauma)
- A reduced ability to transport oxygen (e.g. anaemia)
- Cardiac and respiratory arrest.

The levels of oxygen should be measured for each individual patient, and the simplest way is by pulse oximetry. This indicates the amount of haemoglobin saturated with oxygen as a percentage (Woodrow, 2000).

A more precise measurement, oxygen consumption, can indicate whether or not the body's oxygen requirements are being met (Dolan, 2000a). This can be ascertained from arterial blood gas analysis.

Complications of oxygen therapy

Carbon dioxide narcosis

Carbon dioxide levels directly influence respiration and ventilation. Central chemoreceptors monitor arterial blood indirectly by sensing changes in the acidity (pH) of cerebrospinal fluid (CSF). Carbon dioxide in arterial blood diffuses across the blood–brain barrier into CSF until the partial pressure of carbon dioxide is equal on both sides. Carbon dioxide combines with water to form carbonic acid which dissociates into hydrogen ions that are capable of stimulating the central chemoreceptors. In this way, it regulates ventilation through its impact on the pH of the CSF. If the level of carbon dioxide rises, carbon dioxide diffuses across the blood–brain barrier until carbon dioxide levels in the blood and CSF reach equilibrium. The resulting decrease in pH stimulates the respiratory centre to increase the rate and depth of ventilation.

This situation is slightly different in individuals with chronic respiratory problems, such as COPD. Individuals with chronic respiratory disease lose the acute sensitivity of the central chemoreceptors. Instead, the principle respiratory stimulus becomes a falling level of arterial oxygen (PaO_2). In this situation, delivery of a high concentration of oxygen can cause respiratory depression (Dolan, 2000a). Should this occur, the oxygen should not be abruptly withdrawn, as this could lead to hypoxaemia (Oh, 2003).

Although it is better to err on the side of caution, the number of individuals affected by carbon dioxide narcosis is small – 20 per cent, according to Bateman and Leach (1998).

Oxygen toxicity

It is believed that oxygen directly affects lung tissue (Oh, 2003). Although the exact mechanism is not known, decreasing lung compliance occurs as a result of haemorrhagic interstitial and intra-alveolar oedema (Dolan, 2000a). There is no definitive level of harm, but it is generally believed that administration of oxygen above 50% for more than 24 hours can lead to oxygen toxicity. The nurse is in an excellent position to monitor the patient and ensure that supplemental oxygen levels are reduced as soon as is safely possible.

Discomfort

Oxygen is a dry gas, which dehydrates exposed membranes. Patients receiving oxygen through a facemask will quickly experience a dry mouth and considerable discomfort, which can lead to non-compliance with the therapy. The best way to rehydrate oral mucosa is to give oral fluids. If the patient is nil by mouth, mouth-washes can be used. It should be remembered that mouthwashes refresh but do not clean, and are no substitute for oral hygiene (McNeill, 2000). As a preventative measure, humidification can be added to warm and moisten the oxygen. This is particularly helpful if the patient has a large amount of pulmonary secretion. Humidification will reduce the drying of secretions, so making it easier for the patient to expectorate (Dolan, 2000a). Bateman and Leach (1998) suggest that flows of up to 4 l/min are adequately humidified by the airway. However, increased hydration via oral fluids or intravenous infusion (if the patient is nil by mouth or very breathless) should still be encouraged.

Combustibility

Oxygen is highly combustible, and no smoking should be permitted in its vicinity. Extreme care must be used during cardiopulmonary resuscitation (CPR) if defibrillation is to take place. There is the danger associated with electrical sparks and static electricity.

Oxygen delivery

The primary consideration when choosing the method of administration of supplemental oxygen is that it must be tolerated by the patient. Oxygen therapy must be continuous (Oh, 2003), and patient compliance is essential. The flow of oxygen must be carefully regulated to ensure the desired concentration is delivered. It is also essential that the apparatus or devices used allow for expulsion of carbon dioxide to prevent excessive accumulation.

Oxygen delivery systems are commonly classified as low-flow or high-flow (Dickson, 2002). Low-flow systems are more comfortable, but the delivery of oxygen is affected by the patient's ventilatory pattern. High-flow systems deliver a pre-determined concentration of oxygen, and are less affected by the patient's respiratory pattern.

Facemask

The most commonly used method is the Venturi mask. Venturi masks can be adapted to deliver varying concentrations of oxygen by the use of flow-regulated valves (e.g. 24–35%). Higher concentrations of oxygen require a greater rate of flow. The high-flow system effectively eliminates rebreathing, thus avoiding the accumulation of carbon dioxide. The delivery of oxygen can be affected by dyspnoea, and it is not always possible to guarantee that a fixed concentration of oxygen is being delivered to the patient (Oh, 2003).

Alternatively, a low-flow Hudson mask can be used. Hudson masks have been associated with carbon dioxide retention, as exhaled air can be retained in the facemask (Cooper, 2002). Patients with COPD requiring low concentrations of oxygen are at particular risk of hypercapnia. This needs to be considered when choosing the type of mask to be used (Cooper, 2002).

Via nasal cannulae

A commonly used low-flow device is nasal cannulae (Dickson, 2002). Whilst this method has advantages in terms of increased patient compliance and comfort, it is very difficult to gauge the concentration of oxygen being delivered to the patient. Patients in respiratory distress frequently breathe through the mouth, further reducing the efficacy of this delivery system (Dolan, 2000a). The respiratory rate can also influence the amount of oxygen received by the patient. Hyperventilation will significantly reduce the amount of oxygen delivered to the patient (Cooper, 2002).

Implications for clinical practice

- Respiratory support is common with critically ill patients
- Nurses are accountable for providing safe care, and therefore must be competent in the delivery of care for patients receiving oxygen therapy
- Oxygen is a treatment with complications, and must be regularly reviewed
- Respiratory distress and failure are intensely frightening experiences
- Patients will need education and support to ensure their co-operation with treatment.

Summary

Patients requiring a high level of care will frequently require respiratory support. The 24-hour care provided by nurses places them in a key position to monitor their patients for changes. Reducing oxygen concentrations quickly to reduce the risk of lung damage is vital, and it is the nurses who will be aware of changes in their patients' respiratory status. Patients requiring a high level of care are increasingly being cared for in general ward areas (Brooks, 2000), and all clinical staff need to be able to administer oxygen therapy safely and appropriately.

Clinical scenario

Mr Jones has been admitted to hospital with an ineffective exacerbation of his COPD. Pulse oximitry shows a saturation of 82 per cent, and oxygen therapy is prescribed.

1 How would you explain to Mr Jones why he needs oxygen therapy?

2 Identify complications of oxygen therapy that specifically affect Mr Jones.

3 What action would you take in the event of oxygen toxicity?

Bibliography

Key reading

Cooper (2002).
Dolan (2000a).
Watson (2000b).

Chapter 17

Temporary tracheostomies

Philip Woodrow

Contents

Learning outcomes

After reading this chapter you will be able to:

- Identify why patients with severe respiratory failure may benefit from a temporary tracheostomy
- Understand the problems patients with a temporary tracheostomy may experience
- Recognise the risks created by a tracheostomy
- List emergency equipment, and checks that should be performed at least once every shift
- Develop an evidence-based plan of nursing care for a patient with a temporary tracheostomy.

Fundamental knowledge

Tracheal anatomy, respiratory failure (see Chapter 15).

Introduction

A tracheostomy (a stoma in the trachea) may be temporary, permanent ('silver tube'), or a minitracheostomy.

Patients with acute severe respiratory disease may benefit from formation of a temporary tracheostomy to reduce *dead space*. Permanent tracheostomies are usually formed when part of the airway has been removed due to cancer, and minitracheostomies are currently rarely used. This chapter therefore discusses only temporary tracheostomies.

Tracheostomies may be surgical or percutaneous. Percutaneous tracheostomies are easier to perform, and so expose patients to fewer risks. However, percutaneous stomas may not 'mature' for 7–10 days (Broomhead, 2002), with emergency reintubation potentially creating a false and fatal passage.

Reducing dead space

Exchange of gases only occurs in alveoli. The volume of air remaining between where air enters (normally the mouth or nose) and the alveoli forms the first part of the breath to reach the alveoli. This air, remaining from the last breath, is relatively oxygen poor (often about 15 per cent) and carbon dioxide rich (often about 6 per cent). This volume is called *dead space*.

Normal adult dead space volume is about 150 ml. Healthy adult breaths (at rest) are 300–500 ml, so dead-space air forms a relatively small part of the total volume reaching the lungs. However, with shallow breathing a greater proportion is dead-space air. If breath size is reduced from 450 ml to 200 ml, oxygen-rich air is reduced from 300 ml to 50 ml. This disproportionately large reduction provokes severe respiratory distress/failure. Shallow breath volumes are often consistently lower than 200 ml. For people in respiratory distress, such as those with acute exacerbation of chronic obstructive pulmonary disease (COPD), this change may make the difference between breathing adequately and suffering respiratory failure.

Tracheostomies can halve dead space (Pritchard, 1994), which with shallow breathing significantly increases both the amount of oxygen reaching the alveoli, and carbon dioxide clearance. Reducing breathlessness lessens distress and the work of breathing – oxygen consumption by respiratory muscles. This leaves more oxygen for the rest of the body.

Tube sizes

Normal adult tracheostomy sizes are 7.0, 7.5, 8.0. 8.5 and 9.0 mm diameter. The size is moulded on the outer surface of the flange. If both outer and inner tube diameter sizes are given, the tube size is the outer diameter. Most tubes also print the tube size (more clearly) on the external bladder. Tube size should be recorded clearly in the care notes, but nurses caring for patients with tracheostomies should also check the tube size each shift.

Problems

Tracheostomies may create various problems for both patients and staff, including:

- Communication difficulties
- Nutritional problems
- Impaired cough reflex
- Ulceration
- Infection
- Loss of normal airway functions (humidification, warming, filtering of air)
- Occlusion.

Communication difficulties

Speech is created by air passing through the vocal cords. As tracheostomy tubes are inserted below the vocal cords, they usually prevent sound being formed. Loss of speech isolates patients, so nurses should explain to them that loss of speech is caused by the tube, and that their voice will return following removal of the tube.

Alternative ways to communication include:

- Mouthing words and lip-reading
- Writing boards and pens
- Sign/alphabet boards
- Speaking valves/tubes.

Speaking valves or tubes necessitate the cuff being deflated, so patients must have cough and swallow reflexes, and be able to protect their own airway. Speech therapists should, where ever possible, be included in the multidisciplinary care team.

Speaking valves are one-way valves placed on the tracheostomy opening (see Figure 17.1), which allows air to enter through the tracheostomy but close on expiration. The tracheostomy cuff must therefore be deflated to allow the patient to breathe out. Exhaled air passes around the tube and through the vocal cords, so enabling the person to speak, although their voice may not sound fully normal.

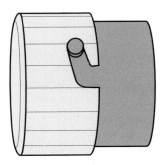

Figure 17.1 **Speaking valve**

Some patients whose tube cuff has been deflated or who have a sufficient leak find that placing a finger over their tube restores their voice. However, human skin is covered with commensals which, in the respiratory tract, could become pathogens, so finger occlusion should be discouraged.

Tubes made with holes in the side ('fenestrated' tubes) allow air to pass through the vocal cords. Fenestrated tubes should have both fenestrated and unfenestrated inner tubes. Fenestrated inner tubes normally remain in place to enable speech. However, suction catheters can pass through the fenestration, damaging airway tissue rather than removing secretions, and therefore, prior to suction, a fenestrated inner tube should be replaced with an unfenestrated one.

Nutritional problems

The oesophagus and trachea are virtually adjacent, so inflated cuffs that surround a tracheostomy tube inevitably place some pressure on the oesophagus. For patients on an oral diet, swallowing can be uncomfortable (rather like swallowing food with a sore throat), making them reluctant to eat solid or lumpy food. Nurses should therefore assess patients' ability to swallow and monitor nutrition, supplementing with liquid or nasogastric feeding if necessary, and involving dieticians.

Impaired cough reflex

An effective cough relies on closure of the glottis. With the glottis closed, pressure increases within the lungs, forcing the glottis to open and expel mucus at up to 500 miles (800 km) per hour (Hough, 2001). This force ensures that airways are effectively cleared.

A tracheostomy tube prevents complete closure of the glottis, so although cough reflexes may remain, coughing may not fully clear secretions and suction may be needed. Remembering individual professional accountability (NMC, 2002a), nurses should assess patients each shift. If patients are unable to cough effectively, suction once to assess from the amount, colour and consistency of secretions whether further suction is likely to be needed either immediately or later during the shift.

Although suction catheter size should be chosen according to the size of the tracheostomy, the only suction catheter sizes that should be available on most adult wards are: FG10, FG12 and FG14.

Suctioning (see Chapter 31) can cause mechanical damage to the delicate airway tissue. For most adult tracheostomies, the FG10 should adequately clear secretions while causing minimal damage. If secretions are very thick, an FG12 may be needed. FG14 catheters are not recommended for use with tracheostomies.

Suction will cause trauma, so the number of passes should be limited, generally to two (Docherty and Bench, 2002). If further suction is needed, then either the patient has copious secretions and may need help of other professionals (such as physiotherapists), or the suction technique is ineffective and the patient needs the help of someone more experienced at performing suction. In either case, it is useful for the nurse to re-evaluate the patient's needs after two passes.

Ulceration

Pressure sores, usually associated with visible skin near bony prominences, can develop wherever sustained pressure exceeds the perfusion pressure of capillaries supplying oxygen and nutrients to that tissue.

Inflated cuffs place continuous pressure on very delicate tracheal epithelium. When pressure sores heal scar tissue remains, which, being inelastic, may cause chronic respiratory limitation. Crimlisk *et al.*'s (1996) literature review found that recommended cuff pressures ranged from 14–30 mmHg, so Mulvey *et al.*'s (1993) recommended 25 mmHg will usually be safe.

Cuff pressure can be measured with a simple manometer (similar to tyre pressure gauges) that attaches to the external bladder. Manometers usually indicate a 'safe' area of pressure. If a manometer is not available, an indication of pressure can be gained by feeling the external bladder, which should be soft enough to be easily squeezed but maintain an inflated shape when released. Cuff pressure should be checked each shift as well as whenever air is removed from or added to the cuff.

Insufficiently inflated cuffs allow air to escape, causing a 'bubbling' at the back of the throat as air passes through pooled saliva. If the patient is receiving supplementary oxygen through the tracheostomy, the percentage may be diluted by any air bypassing the cuff. Secretions at the back of the throat may be aspirated, so should be cleared with a soft suction catheter, passed orally or nasally. Then, using a relatively large syringe (e.g. 20 ml), the cuff should be fully deflated and then reinflated until the leak disappears. Cuff pressure should then be checked, and the amount of air inserted recorded in the patient's notes. If the volume of air needed to inflate the cuff seems excessive this probably indicates that the tracheostomy tube is too small, and this should be reported for an anaesthetist to review.

When tracheostomies are inserted, patients may have tracheal inflammation and oedema from their respiratory disease. As healing occurs, this inflammation and oedema may subside, increasing the airway lumen. Therefore, cuffs may develop significant leaks, potentially enabling the person to breathe, and speak, past the cuff. This is especially likely to happen where inflammation is being actively treated (e.g. with steroids).

Infection

Like most surgical wounds, tracheal stomas should be kept clean and redressed. Dressings should usually be changed daily, or more frequently if soiled, but following stoma formation surgeons will usually prefer dressings to be left undisturbed for 48 hours or longer. Nurses should therefore check the surgical notes before performing the first dressing.

Changing tracheostomy dressings *always* requires two people, standing each side of the patient, to prevent loss of the tracheostomy and possible respiratory arrest. The second person assists by holding the tube, so acts under supervision and need not be a qualified nurse.

Redressing tracheostomies requires:

- A standard dressing pack (including sterile swabs)
- Sterile normal saline (0.9%)
- A sterile tracheostomy dressing
- Tracheostomy tapes.

Dressing is easiest if patients lie supine, as this makes them less likely to cough.

Tracheostomies can also cause damage to skin and other body tissue. Sores may develop around the site of the stoma. These are most likely to be caused by pressure or irritant fluids, and may form a focus for infection from micro-organisms colonising the respiratory tract.

The warm, moist area underneath the tracheostomy flange can easily be colonised by micro-organisms. A swab may need to be sent for culture (MC+S). If large, secretions may need to be removed with a soft suction catheter (e.g. FG10). The stoma should be cleaned thoroughly with saline. Current medical practice varies regarding whether or not tracheostomy flanges are stitched to the skin. If the tracheostomy is stitched to the skin, sterile cotton buds or forceps and gauze may be needed. Buds with loose cotton may leave fibres which could be inhaled, so should be avoided.

Once clean and dry, stomas are covered with a commercially-produced dressing (e.g. Lyofoam®) that has a cross-shaped incision to fit around the tracheostomy tube. If stitched in, forceps may be needed to draw the dressing fully under the flanges. Dressings have a foam and a matt side; the matt side should be placed against the skin.

Two unequal lengths of tape/tube-holder should be used to secure the tube. The shorter length is fixed on the side of the nurse performing the dressing and the longer one on the side of the assistant; this is then drawn underneath the patient's neck and fixed to the shorter holder. Holders should be tight enough to allow two fingers to slide beneath them (Docherty and Bench, 2002), adequately supporting the tracheostomy tube without being uncomfortably tight for the patient.

The change of dressing should be recorded together with relevant observations:

- How clean is the site?
- Colour and amount of secretions?

Loss of normal airway functions

The human airway warms, humidifies and filters the air breathed in. Most of these functions take place in the dead space. Reducing the dead space by up to half significantly impairs all three functions, so artificial alternatives are needed to replace them.

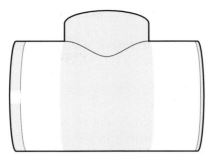

Figure 17.2 **Heat moisture exchange humidifier ('Swedish nose')**

Heat/moisture exchanger (HME) humidifiers (e.g. 'Swedish nose' – see Figure 17.2) reflect warmth and moisture back into the airways, and filter inspired air. Heated water humidification is more effective for the patient, but can cause burns and infection, so is not recommended unless it can be closely supervised.

Inadequate humidification can cause dry, sticky mucus plugs, which may block parts of the lower or upper airway, potentially occluding the tracheostomy and causing respiratory arrest. Saline (0.9%) nebulisers (e.g. 2 ml every 2–6 hours) may help to loosen secretions, but instilling bolus saline with a syringe into the tracheostomy is not recommended (Cook, 2003).

Occlusion

As with any arrest situation, help should be summoned urgently. If suction fails to clear the airway, the tracheostomy cuff should be deflated with a syringe to allow some air to bypass the tube. As much oxygen as possible should be given, preferably 100%.

The tracheostomy tube should be removed, using scissors to cut/remove tapes and any stitches (there is not usually time to fetch a stitch cutter). The tracheostomy tube should be easy to remove. Stomas are usually well formed by 7 days (Bodernham and Barry, 2001), so should provide the patient with a reasonable airway, although a replacement tube should be inserted as quickly as possible. New stomas may collapse quickly, necessitating more rapid insertion of a replacement tube.

Two spare tubes (one the same size as the patient's, and one a size smaller) should be kept near the patient's bedside, together with a pair of tracheal dilators. With a well-formed stoma, a new tube of the same size should be easy to insert. If the stoma is newly formed, appears to be collapsing, or if there is any difficulty with trying to insert a tube of the same size, there are two options:

1   Insert the smaller tube (which can be replaced later in a planned, controlled procedure)
2   Use tracheal dilators (which should be near the patient's bedside) to enlarge the stoma sufficiently to insert the larger tube.

In an emergency, it is usually quicker (and hence safer) to opt for the smaller tube.

Once the patient has a patent airway, a doctor (preferably an anaesthetist) should urgently review the patient.

Emergency equipment

The tracheostomy is the patient's only airway, so emergency equipment needs to be quickly and easily accessible, mainly by the patient's bedside. Items that could be dangerous (e.g. stitch-cutters) should be stored in some other easily accessible place, such as at the nurses' station.

Emergency equipment by the beside should include:

■   Tracheal dilators
■   Spare tubes, one the same size and one a size smaller
■   Suction (ready to use)
■   Suction catheters
■   Syringe (there may be cases where this is safer stored elsewhere).

Other emergency equipment should include

■   Scissors (preferably with one pointed blade)
■   Stitch-cutter (if tracheostomies are stitched in).

Remembering individual professional accountability (NMC, 2002a), staff caring for patients with a tracheostomy should ensure that emergency equipment is easily accessible at the start of their shift, and that suction equipment is working.

Planned removal

Most patients with temporary tracheostomies will recover sufficiently for tubes to be removed rather than replaced with a permanent one. However, removing the tube significantly increases the work of breathing, by up to a third (Chadda *et al.*, 2002). This may result in respiratory distress, necessitating re-insertion of another tube. To minimise this risk, cuffs should ideally be deflated 1 day before removal (Serra, 2000). With fenestrated tubes this should not cause problems, but occluding unfenestrated tubes causes significant airflow limitations, resulting in dyspnoea and necessitating re-opening of the tube. During this time the patient's respiratory function should be closely monitored, and if respiratory distress occurs, the occludor should be removed, restoring patency of the tracheostomy. The patient should be kept fully informed of the plan of care.

Provided respiratory function is adequate with the tube occluded, removal the following day will be similar to the steps described for emergency removal. Because the stoma is likely to have become well formed, and the patient should now be breathing through his or her normal airway, the stoma should be covered with an occlusive dressing that will form a complete seal (e.g. Sleek®). Occasionally laryngeal oedema may cause temporary hoarseness or loss of voice, so patients should be warned of this possibility before removal of the tube.

Implications for practice

- Temporary tracheostomies reduce airway dead space, so can significantly reduce the work of breathing
- The upper airway warms, moistens and filters air; bypassing most of the upper airway therefore creates potential risks and problems
- Although the cough reflex normally remains, tracheostomies weaken the strength of coughs, so patients often need suction to clear airway secretions
- Thick, dry secretions can occlude the tracheostomy, causing respiratory arrest
- Staff caring for patients with temporary tracheostomies should know how to re-establish an airway as quickly as possible
- Emergency equipment should be checked each shift
- Unless the patient is adequately clearing airway secretions, suction should also be performed at least once each shift, near the start, to enable individualised planning of care for that shift.

Summary

Temporary tracheostomies can provide a useful medical treatment for severe acute respiratory limitations, but they create many actual and potential problems for patients. Nurses should therefore know the potential risks created and how to minimise the problems caused by tracheostomies.

Clinical scenario

Mr Thomas Fraser was admitted to hospital 3 weeks ago with a severe acute exacerbation of COPD, initially requiring artificial ventilation in ICU, where a percutaneous temporary tracheostomy was inserted. He is now self-ventilating, but still has the tracheostomy, and has now been transferred to a step-down unit.

1   From reading this chapter, and your own experiences, list actual and potential problems the tracheostomy might cause Mr Fraser. Identify any equipment that will be needed. Where it is not stocked in your own workplace, identify where you could obtain this equipment.

2   Identify nursing observations that should be performed in relation to Mr Fraser's tracheostomy, including frequency of observations. From this book, and any other available sources, identify the evidence base for this aspect of care.

3   Over the following week, Mr Fraser's condition slowly deteriorates. Without non-invasive or invasive ventilation, it is unlikely that he will survive. However, if ventilation is started, his chances of discharge home without it are slim. Unfortunately Mr Fraser is hypoxic and appears frightened, so the multidisciplinary team consider that his ability to make an informed decision is limited. Note your own thoughts about the advantages and disadvantages of whether more aggressive treatment should be initiated. As Mr Fraser's nurse, decide whether, on balance, how far (if at all) you would advocate any escalation of treatment.

Bibliography

Key reading

Review articles on tracheostomies periodically appear in the nursing press. Serra (2002) and Docherty and Bench (2002) are reliable recent examples.

Further reading

General texts, such as Mallett and Dougherty (2000), provide useful supplementary material.

Chapter 18

Bilevel non-invasive ventilation

Philip Woodrow

Contents

Learning outcomes

After reading this chapter you will be able to:

- Identify which patients are likely and unlikely to benefit from non-invasive ventilation (NIV)
- Understand the main differences between CPAP and bilevel NIV
- Explain the main options offered by most bilevel non-invasive ventilators
- Identify safe nursing care of patients being supported by NIV.

Fundamental knowledge

Respiratory anatomy and physiology, respiratory failure (see Chapter 15).

Introduction

Respiratory failure may be either type 1 (oxygenation failure) or type 2 (ventilatory failure) (see Chapter 14). Ventilation is the movement of air in and out of the lungs, so with ventilatory failure there is insufficient volume moving in and out of the lungs. Because carbon dioxide clearance relies mainly on the size of breaths, ventilatory failure results in insufficient exchange of both carbon dioxide and oxygen. The British Thoracic Society (2002) defines type 2 ventilatory failure as an arterial oxygen (PaO_2) below 8.0 kPa together with an arterial carbon dioxide ($PaCO_2$) above 6.0 kPa. Severe type 2 respiratory failure may therefore need ventilatory support. Until recently, this necessitated intubation, invasive ventilation, and usually sedation and admission to intensive care; each of these creates additional risks for patients. Non-invasive ventilation (NIV) offers an easier and safer alternative for many patients with ventilatory failure. The British Thoracic Society (2002) therefore recommends that indications for NIV include:

- COPD with a respiratory acidosis pH 7.25–7.35
- Hypercapnic respiratory failure secondary to neuromuscular disease (e.g. Gullain Barré syndrome) or chest wall deformity (e.g. scoliosis)
- Cardiogenic pulmonary oedema.

Baudouin (2002) also recommends using NIV for severe pneumonia.

There are many types of non-invasive ventilation, all of which may be used in community settings, but in acute hospital settings positive pressure non-invasive ventilation is almost always used. In the past, the main type of positive pressure non-invasive ventilation was CPAP (continuous positive airway pressure). Although still used, CPAP is increasingly being replaced by positive pressure bilevel non-invasive ventilation (bilevel NIV). Bilevel NIV is often called by the brand name of whatever system is used with the hospital (e.g. NIPPY®, BiPAP®). Most bilevel machines can also deliver CPAP by setting the two levels at an identical figure.

With increasing replacement of CPAP systems by bilevel NIV, this chapter focuses on bilevel NIV, but uses NIV to describe both options and the names of each where comments apply mainly or solely to one mode. Unfortunately much evidence for both modes derives from small-scale studies, often with people suffering from chronic sleep apnoea. How applicable such studies are to acute use of NIV remains questionable. Much remains unknown, and many questions are unanswered. However, the British Thoracic Society (2002) guidelines usefully synthesise existing evidence for practice.

Contraindications

Various authors have suggested different contraindications to either CPAP or bilevel NIV, or both. Contraindications listed in the British Thoracic Society (2002) guidelines are:

- Impaired consciousness
- Severe hypoxaemia
- Patients with copious respiratory secretions
- Routine use in acute asthma
- Recent facial or upper airway surgery, facial burns or trauma
- A fixed obstruction to the upper airway
- Vomiting
- Pneumothorax, until a chest drain is inserted.

However, the British Thoracic Society also states that with most of these contraindications NIV may still be commenced provided intubation and invasive ventilation can be rapidly commenced.

Non-invasive positive pressure ventilation

With CPAP, a closed circuit that includes the patient's lungs provides a flow of air (with or without supplementary oxygen) which can only escape through a pressure valve. Therefore, as the strength of the patient's breath weakens towards the end of expiration the valve closes off, sealing the remaining volume within the airways. This:

- Helps to prevent further alveolar collapse (*stabilisation*)
- Opens up collapsed alveoli (*recruitment*)
- Enables gas exchange between breaths and so improves oxygenation.

However, CPAP is often noisy and uncomfortable, it may increase arterial carbon dioxide, and is often poorly tolerated by patients.

Like almost any equipment used in hospitals, different manufacturers provide different options on bilevel non-invasive ventilators. This chapter therefore describes only the main controls, terminology and options. Users should familiarise themselves with equipment used locally. Originally designed for (chronic) domestic rather than (acute) hospital use, bilevel non-invasive ventilators are simple and offer relatively few options compared with the complex invasive ventilators that are used in most intensive care units. Any adjustments to ventilation should usually be based on blood gas analysis.

Bilevel positive pressure ventilation alternates between two pressures, a higher one on inspiration (inspired positive airway pressure – IPAP) and a lower one on expiration (expired positive airway pressure – EPAP). This provides additional support while breathing in, and creates less resistance and discomfort when breathing out, allowing larger volumes to both enter and leave the lungs, and so improving carbon dioxide clearance (Calzia and Radermacher, 1997). For example, CPAP is often commenced at 5 cmH$_2$O, whereas bilevel NIV is often commenced at IPAP of 10 cmH$_2$O and EPAP of 4 cmH$_2$O.

Increasing the difference between IPAP and EPAP increases the *pressure support* for the breath, and so the breath volume and carbon dioxide clearance. However, most people find breathing out against high levels of EPAP uncomfortable, so if more pressure support is needed, IPAP rather than EPAP is usually increased.

With normal unassisted breathing, inspiration involves active muscle movement, and so is normally fairly quick. After a brief pause, or plateau, when the air is held in the lungs, expiration is caused by passive recoil of the respiratory muscles, and so is fairly slow. The inspiratory to expiratory ratio (I:E ratio) is normally between 1:2 and 1:2.5. Some bilevel non-invasive ventilators may have I:E controls; others may allow adjustment of inspiratory (i) time. People with constricted airways, for example from chronic obstructive pulmonary disease (COPD), may benefit from a slow inspiratory time. Conversely, with asthma slower expiratory times are less likely to cause spasm of bronchiole muscle (the British Thoracic Society (2002) recommends avoiding NIV routinely for asthma). People with constricted airways may also benefit from slower *rise time*. Rise time is the amount of time inspiration takes to achieve the preset pressure. Typically, rise time will be set at 50 per cent or 0.2 seconds.

Many bilevel ventilators provide apnoea back-up, so should the patient stop breathing for a pre-set time, the ventilator will initiate breaths. This ability to sense breaths by patients also enables machines to offer a *trigger*. At a preset volume or pressure, the machine senses respiratory effort by the patient, which 'triggers' the machine to support the patient's own effort by adding extra volume into what would otherwise probably be a shallow breath. Trigger modes are more comfortable for patients, as the machine follows their own pattern of breathing rather than making them follow the machine's preset cycle. The trigger mode is also useful if patients have weak respiratory muscles and need to be 'weaned' off the ventilator, as the trigger can slowly be increased to 'build up' the respiratory muscles to the point where they will enable the patient to breath adequate volumes without ventilatory support. Trigger systems often necessitate the use of smooth-bore tubing between the ventilator and the mask, as 'elephant tubing' can cause sufficient air turbulence to auto-trigger the ventilator.

Most bilevel non-invasive ventilators deliver air, and so if supplementary oxygen is needed it usually has to be through ports directly into the face mask or earlier into the circuit.

Masks

For both CPAP and bilevel NIV, masks should be accurately fitted. Most CPAP circuits rely on a near-complete seal against the face, making the masks tight and uncomfortable, and often causing pressure sores. Many bilevel ventilators compensate for leaks in the circuit, which allows masks to fit more loosely and comfortably against the face. Leaking of air up into the eyes should be avoided, as it may cause conjunctivitis (Hillberg and Johnson, 1997; Kannan, 1999). The condition of the patient's facial skin should be observed and recorded both before starting NIV and during its use. Patients should be asked whether the mask causes discomfort. Some discomfort may be unavoidable, but whenever possible nurses should relieve or reduce discomfort, for example by repositioning the mask.

Most manufacturers supply a range of masks. Initially full-face masks will usually be needed (see Figures 18.1, 18.2), but as the patient's condition improves nasal masks can often be useful, provided the patient breathes through the nose and not the mouth. Nasal masks allow patients to eat, drink and talk normally.

Masks are held in place with adjustable headgear, usually placed behind the head and having four straps that fix onto the mask. This headgear can be uncomfortable and cause sores. Most manufacturers supply a range of colours, as different colours can have different connotations in different cultures. For example, in some Muslim North African countries white suggests death (Jonker, 1997).

Commencing NIV

Many patients find NIV, especially CPAP, uncomfortable and distressing. While some patients may overtly refuse it, others may covertly resist its use by removing (or attempting to remove) it frequently. NIV relies on sustained use to provide

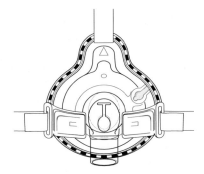

Figure 18.1 **Full face mask**

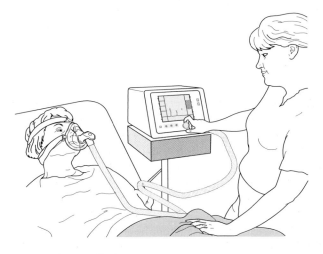

Figure 18.2 **Non-invasive ventilation**

benefits; many practitioners cite a minimum time of 20 minutes to inflate alveoli fully. Therefore, frequent removal provides little or no benefit to the patient, while the distress experienced by the patient causes a stress response (including tachycardia, hypertension, tachypnoea and hyperglycaemia). Russo-Magno et al. (2001) report a non-compliance rate of one-third in people with sleep apnoea.

Approaching the patient with a facemask and NIV headgear may provoke fear. Having explained what NIV can offer, whenever possible patients should be given the mask to hold in their hands and encouraged to place it against their own face

Hypotension

Positive intrathoracic pressure reduces ventricular filling and so, unless other compensatory mechanisms occur, reduces blood pressure. However, problems from reduced perfusion pressure may be offset by improved oxygenation, including to the myocardium. For some patients, NIV improves cardiac function (Sin et al., 2000; Nelson et al., 2001; Yin et al., 2001). Whether these findings are generalisable to other patients may be answered by the current Canadian Positive Airway Pressure for Heart Failure trial (Yin et al., 2001).

At low pressures this effect is usually insignificant, but CPAP above 10 cmH$_2$O can cause significant hypotension (Kiely et al., 1998). Bilevel NIV does not appear to cause significant hypotension (Somauroo et al., 2000). However, when commencing positive pressure NIV blood pressure should be closely monitored, such as setting automated non-invasive blood pressure monitors on 5- or 10-minute cycles for 30 minutes, and using appropriate alarm settings to warn staff about any hypotension.

Gut distension

With swallowing, some air enters the stomach. Because both the trachea and the oesophagus lead off the oropharynx, positive pressure in the upper airway causes more air to be swallowed, and impedes escape of that air back through the oesophagus. As more air accumulates in the stomach, gastric distension causes:

- Splinting of the diaphragm (reducing breath size and making breathing more difficult)
- Discomfort, nausea and/or vomiting
- Flatus (Parsons et al., 2000), if air is not removed.

A nasogastric tube should therefore be passed and left on free drainage to remove gastric air. The bag may need frequent emptying. Anti-emetics and peppermint should be prescribed to relieve discomfort.

Deterioration

Many patients will benefit from NIV, but about a quarter will deteriorate further, necessitating intubation or withdrawal/limitation of treatment. Which patients will deteriorate further is unpredictable (Poponcik et al., 1999), so NIV should be attempted (Jolliet *et al.*, 2001), monitored closely and, if inadequate, replaced by invasive ventilation within 6 hours of reaching optimal NIV settings (British Thoracic Society, 2002). Therefore, commencing NIV should include plans for how far to pursue treatment, and staff and equipment should be available to ventilate invasively as soon as appropriate.

Observation

Non-invasive ventilation is usually commenced because patients cannot adequately breathe by themselves. Therefore, patients receiving NIV should be closely observed. Observations also enable the effectiveness of NIV to be assessed. With improvement, reduction of ventilatory support enables quicker recovery; however, with deterioration, alternative treatments may need to be offered urgently. This necessitates an appropriately staffed and equipped area.

Observation should include:

- Nursing the patient in an easily-observed area
- 'Vital signs' (temperature, pulse, blood pressure, respiratory rate, oxygen saturation)
- Visual signs
- Mental state
- Arterial blood gas analysis.

Some of these observations provide quantitative figures, such as heart rate, whereas others are more subjective, such as depth or comfort of breathing. However, all signs should be actively observed for and recorded. If NIV is effective, most or all of these signs should improve.

The British Thoracic Society (2002) recommends assessing:

- *Chest wall movement.* Unless the person has a specific pathology in one lung, chest wall movement should be bilateral. Unilateral movement may therefore indicate problems such as a pneumothorax.
- *Co-ordination of respiratory effort with the ventilator.* Ventilators that have triggers will co-ordinate with the patient's breathing pattern, but some ventilators are unable to do this. If the patient's and ventilator's patterns conflict, the patient will be uncomfortable, and waste respiratory effort on ineffective breaths. This may indicate that the patient's breathing is sufficient not to need ventilatory support, but if support is still needed, the ventilator may have to be changed.
- *Accessory muscle recruitment.* Breathless patients usually use accessory muscles to help their breathing, especially their clavicular muscles. With improved gases from NIV, use of accessory muscles should decrease or cease
- *Patient comfort.* As respiratory distress resolves, patients should appear generally more comfortable
- *Mental state.* With improved cerebral oxygenation from NIV, patients should be less anxious/distressed, better orientated, and have an improved attention span.

Pulse oximetry indicates oxygenation, so should be continuously monitored for at least the first 24 hours of NIV (British Thoracic Society, 2002). However, oximetry does not measure carbon dioxide. Both type 1 and type 2 respiratory failure cause hypoxia; the difference between the two is that type 2 (ventilatory) failure also causes hypercapnia. Occasionally capnographs are used to measure exhaled carbon dioxide, but the mainstay of carbon dioxide measurement in clinical practice is blood gas analysis (see Chapter 30). Blood gas analysis may be capillary or arterial, and can use indwelling catheters or (sometimes) transcutaneous probes, but currently most acute wards rely on arterial 'stabs'. Whichever means of gas sampling is used, it is the single most important method of assessing respiratory function. Therefore the British Thoracic Society (2002) recommend gas sampling within 1–2 hours of commencing NIV. Having optimised settings, if samples taken 4–6 hours later show little improvement, NIV has failed and should therefore be replaced by invasive ventilation (British Thoracic Society, 2002).

Outcomes

NIV is a useful treatment for ventilatory failure. It enables quicker recovery (Masip *et al.*, 2000) and improves long-term survival (at 1 year) in COPD (Plant *et al.*, 2001), so should be the first-line intervention with respiratory failure in COPD (Lightowler *et al.*, 2003) rather than being used when other options have failed. Elliott (2002) recommends that NIV should be available in all acute hospitals admitting patients with acute respiratory illness. However, this also necessitates constant (24-hour) support for staff managing NIV; the British Thoracic Society (2002) recommends that hospitals providing NIV should have a nurse-led 24-hour NIV service.

Pulmonary oedema

In acute settings NIV is most often used to treat type 2 respiratory failure (Kacmarek, 1999), especially acute exacerbations of COPD. However, CPAP can also help to resolve pulmonary oedema (Pang *et al.*, 1998). A continuous positive pressure within alveoli encourages the return of interstitial oedema into the pulmonary vasculature. Bilevel NIV may also be an effective treatment for pulmonary oedema (Mehta *et al.*, 1997), although the British Thoracic Society (2002) guidelines recommend using CPAP first. Bilevel ventilators can deliver CPAP by setting the same pressures for IPAP and EPAP.

Weaning

With chronic respiratory problems, sudden withdrawal of ventilatory support is likely to result in recurrence of respiratory distress. Therefore, patients often need to be weaned off NIV. Oxygenation can and should (British Thoracic Society, 2002) be monitored continuously using pulse oximetry, remembering to compare saturation readings against haemoglobin levels (see Chapter 29). However, hypoventilation results in hypercapnia, and monitoring carbon dioxide is more problematic. Hypoxia may also cause confusion, drowsiness or other deteriorations in mental state, and compensatory tachycardia.

Carbon dioxide is more problematic to assess. Visual observations can indicate poor ventilation volume if the respiratory rate is very slow or very fast, or chest wall (or accessory muscle) movement is shallow. Carbon dioxide has traditionally been measured by taking a sample of arterial blood (see Chapter 30). This is painful, invasive, and may cause haemorrhage or other vascular damage. However, it remains the 'gold standard' by which other means of assessment are evaluated.

In health, capnography (measuring carbon dioxide in expired air) correlates closely with arterial carbon dioxide levels: $PaCO_2$ (arterial) and $PECO_2$ (capnograph) are usually within less than $1\,kPa$ (Capovilla *et al.*, 2000), but increased pathological dead space, which usually occurs with chronic respiratory disease, reduces $PECO_2$ while increasing $PaCO_2$ (Drew *et al.*, 1998).

Transcutaneous gas measurement is widely used in neonates. Rithalia *et al.* (1992) suggested that it is a reliable means of monitoring, and is potentially under-used in adults. However, adults have more subcutaneous tissue than neonates, so accuracy should logically be reduced. Transcutaneous gas measurement has not been widely used or studied in adults.

Capillary blood gas can be measured, obtaining samples in a similar way to capillary blood glucose measurement. Dar *et al.* (1995) suggest that capillary samples are comparable with arterial, but Sauty *et al.* (1996) and Thompson *et al.* (1999) found that they were not. All three studies used small sample sizes, so reliability of capillary samples remains debatable.

Kramer *et al.* (1995) recommend weaning criteria of:

- Respiratory rate <24
- Heart rate <110
- pH >7.35
- SpO_2 $>90\%$ on 4 litres of oxygen.

However, with severe COPD the normal respiratory rate may exceed 24, and normal SaO_2 may be below 90%. Assessing comfort and mental state is potentially subjective, so although each of these signs may indicate respiratory distress, they do need to be individualised.

Implications for practice

- NIV should be a first line treatment for type 2 respiratory failure
- A respiratory acidosis causing blood pH of 7.25–7.35 is an indication for NIV
- CPAP can support ventilation, but bilevel NIV is more comfortable for the patient, and so better tolerated, provides more benefits, and creates fewer problems
- Patients receiving NIV should be closely monitored and observed, which necessitates sufficient numbers of staff with sufficient knowledge and skills of using NIV to care safely for the patient.

Summary

Ventilatory (type 2) respiratory failure may need ventilatory support. In acute care, CPAP or bilevel NIV is usually used to provide ventilatory support. Because bilevel NIV has more advantages and fewer problems, it is replacing CPAP. In acute health care, NIV is mainly used to support patients with type 2 respiratory failure, but CPAP (more so than bilevel NIV) can resolve pulmonary oedema. Bilevel ventilators can deliver CPAP by setting IPAP and EPAP at the same level.

Clinical scenario

Jack Adams, aged 74, is admitted with an acute exacerbation of COPD. On arrival in A&E he was breathless and cyanosed. Arterial blood gas analysis showed pH 7.27, PaO_2 7.2, $PaCO_2$ 8.3 kPa. Bilevel NIV is commenced, and he is transferred to the medical assessment ward for further observation.

1   List the nursing observations that should be made. Identify which observations should be continuous, and suggest an initial frequency for observations that will be intermittent.

2   Identify problems that Mr Adams is likely to, or may, experience as a result of NIV. Suggest ways these problems could be resolved or minimised.

3   After 2 days of NIV support and other medical treatments, Mr Adams' condition improves sufficiently to consider removing ventilatory support. Make a list of criteria that you would use before removing or to wean off NIV. Identify the rationales for these criteria. Analyse the evidence on which these are based, and how reliable you consider that evidence to be.

Bibliography

Key reading

The British Thoracic Society (2002) guidelines are the single most important resource for all UK staff using NIV. In addition to the journal source in the reference list, these are viewable through the BTS website: brit-thoracic.org.uk.

Lightowler *et al.* (2003) provides the Cochrane review meta-analysis.

Further reading

Useful introductions to NIV from the nursing literature include Perkins and Shortall (2000), Preston (2001).

Chapter 19

Intrapleural chest drains

Philip Woodrow

Contents

Learning outcomes

After reading this chapter you will be able to:

- Understand the benefits and problems of intrapleural chest drains
- Identify the evidence (or lack of evidence) underpinning practice in your own clinical area
- Identify nursing care of patients with chest drains.

Fundamental knowledge

Anatomy of the pleura.

Introduction

Chest drains can be used to drain any abnormal collection of fluid from the thoracic cavity. As there are two main organs in the chest (the heart and lungs), chest drains are almost always used to treat problems with either of these organs. Cardiac drains are widely used following cardiac surgery, but the focus of this chapter is on chest drains used to treat pulmonary problems.

Intrapleural chest drains, more often just called 'chest drains', are used to treat pneumothorax, and pleural effusion (see Chapter 15). Although chest drains have been used for over a century, there is surprisingly little research-based evidence. Most literature remains largely anecdotal (Godden and Hiley, 1998) and is often based on rituals and dated ideas, providing limited evidence for practice (Charnock and Evans, 2001). Research into potentially dangerous practices would be unethical, yet many aspects of chest drain management are based on tradition, leaving many unanswered questions for practice. Nurses are expected to provide the highest quality of evidence-based care that they can reasonably achieve. This chapter reviews current nursing management of chest drains, but practice may develop once more extensive research-based evidence becomes available. While this chapter focuses on management of chest drains, care of patients should include meeting all their needs. For example, the problems that necessitate chest drainage will usually cause patients to be breathless and hypoxic, so their respiratory function (rate, depth, saturations) should be closely monitored, and they will often need supplementary oxygen both before and following insertion of the chest drain.

Physiology

Breathing uses negative pressure. As the diaphragm, intercostal and (sometimes) clavicular muscles move outward, intrathoracic space is increased, making intrathoracic pressure negative in relation to atmospheric (air) pressure. The parietal pleura is attached to tissues surrounding the lungs, so is drawn outward on inspiration. A small amount (about 50 ml) of fluid between the pleura creates sufficient surface tension to draw the visceral (or pulmonary) pleura outward, expanding lung volume and so drawing air from the atmosphere into alveoli.

In health intrapleural pressure remains slightly negative, ranging from minus 2 to minus 6 cmH$_2$O (Hough, 2001). This constant negative pressure helps to keep alveoli patent and prevents atelectasis (Marieb, 2004). If intrapleural pressure equalises with intrapulmonary or atmospheric pressure, the pleura collapse (Hyde *et al.*, 1997), resulting in loss of lung volume and, usually, respiratory distress.

Pneumothorax

A pneumothorax is a collection of gas or air in the pleural space, which may be caused by trauma or be spontaneous (see Chapter 15). Equalisation of pressure across the pleura causes lung collapse, but the pneumothorax remains simple as long as pressure can equalise. If any tension is created between the two sides of the hole, the pneumothorax acts as a one-way valve, drawing more air or fluid into the space with each breath, which cannot escape on expiration (Gallon, 1998). This creates positive (instead of negative) pressure within the thorax (Norman and Cook, 2000), resulting in a life-threatening emergency requiring urgent treatment (Mallett and Dougherty, 2000).

A tension pneumothorax needs urgent removal of the air or blood. If the pneumothorax is small (<20 per cent of the lung) it may be removed through needle aspiration, but larger pneumothoraces necessitate insertion of a chest drain. The chest drain will enable air to escape, so turning a tension pneumothorax into a simple pneumothorax (Norman and Cook, 2000).

Chest drains

Chest drains are inserted to remove air or fluid, so traditionally have a large diameter: 28–40 French Gauge (FG) or larger to drain blood and fluids, 16–24 FG for air (Mallett and Dougherty, 2000). Although larger drains are likely to cause more pain, small drains were traditionally thought to be prone to becoming occluded. Recently 'pig-tail' drains have been introduced, using a 14 FG catheter, which makes them more secure and so enables patients to remain mobile (Miller, 1999).

Drains inserted high in the pleural space (second to fourth intercostal spaces; apical) remove air, while drains inserted lower (fifth or sixth intercostal space; basal) remove fluid (Mallett and Dougherty, 2000).

The end of the drain is inserted into water, so creating a siphon that draws fluid or air to the lower level. Chest drain bottles should therefore be kept below the patient's chest level to prevent the contents of the bottle being siphoned back into the pleura. Water in the drainage bottle creates an underwater seal drain (UWSD), which prevents air returning into the pleural space. A second tube leading out of the collection chamber will either remain open to air or be connected to low suction.

Loops in the drainage tubing can cause air pockets, reducing or preventing further flow (Kam *et al.*, 1993; Charnock and Evans, 2001).

If moving the bottle above the patient's chest level is unavoidable (e.g. during transfer), tubing should be temporarily clamped (Kam *et al.*, 1993). While healthcare staff are usually aware of this danger, Gallon (1998) warns that some patients have placed their chest-drain bottles on lockers to make room for their visitors. Therefore patients with chest drains should also be told why they should never raise the bottle up to their chest level.

The water level in the bottle affects the amount of suction exerted within the pleural space (Carroll, 2000). Most manufacturers mark the level for water, the recommended volume typically being 500 ml or less.

Suction

If the pneumothorax creates a large air leak into the pleural cavity, suction is usually needed to ensure that drainage exceeds the air leak (O'Hanlon-Nichols,

1996; Gallon, 1998). Suction pressures cited in the literature usually vary between minus 10 and minus 20 cmH$_2$O (1–2.5 kPa). Some (e.g. Bar-El *et al.*, 2001) extend the range to minus 40 cmH$_2$O, but such negative pressures may damage the delicate pleural tissue.

Tubing

Drainage relies on a siphon, so tubing must be airtight to prevent atmospheric air being siphoned into the pleura. Graham (1996) warns that an inadequately tied drain 'will' fall out. Godden and Hiley (1998) advise taping connections, although they warn that tape will mask any disconnection. Should the system become disconnected, the pneumothorax will re-collapse, so the drain should be clamped or occluded. Where clamps are not immediately available, Gallon (1998) suggests using a finger, while O'Hanlon-Nichols (1996) recommends petroleum gauze. Neither is ideal, but as a 'first aid' measure either may prove life-saving until help arrives.

Changing bottles

There is no consensus about whether bottles should be changed as indicated, daily or when full (Godden and Hiley, 1998). Practice is increasingly to change the bottle only when full (O'Hanlon-Nichols, 1996; McMahon-Parkes, 1997), remembering that bacteria may enter once closed circuits are broken (Godden and Hiley, 1998).

Dressings

Dressings over the site should be as airtight as possible, securing the drain firmly to the patient both for comfort and to prevent disconnection. A wide waterproof tape, such as sleek or a bio-occlusive dressing (preferably transparent so the insertion site can be seen), is needed to fix and seal the drain into the patient. Some dressings can be very irritating to skin. Patient allergies must be considered and, should they occur, be recorded.

Pain management

If deep breaths and coughs cause pain, a natural response is to breathe shallowly and minimise coughing, both of which increase the risk of chest infection (Gray, 2001). Good pain control is therefore an important part of chest drain management (Miller and Harvey, 1993; Carroll, 2002). Patients' needs will vary, and should be individually assessed, using any available services such as acute pain teams; Fox *et al.* (1999) suggest using patient-controlled analgesia (PCA), while Carroll (2002) suggests using either PCA or epidural analgesia. Inflammation often occurs around the site of the chest drain, so anti-inflammatory drugs are also useful (Gray, 2001).

Observations

In addition to 'basic' respiratory observations, such as rate and depth of breathing and oxygen saturation, nurses should observe whether chest drains are:

- Swinging (between inspiration and expiration)
- Bubbling (on expiration)
- Draining.

If audible sucking is heard at the insertion site, the drain has probably become displaced (Gallon, 1998).

Without suction, *swinging* should be visible, as intrapleural pressure changes between inspiration and expiration. The swing will vary depending on the depth of breathing. Loss of swinging indicates blockage (Gallon, 1998). Suction creates a constant negative pressure, and so drains on suction will not swing.

If no air is in the pleural space, *bubbling* should not be seen. Therefore, basal drains or drains for pleural effusions may not always bubble. Otherwise, cessation of bubbling indicates either that all air has been removed or that the tube has become blocked (e.g. with a blood clot, lung tissue or fat). If bubbling ceases, ask the patient to cough (Gallon, 1998), which may dislodge any occlusion. Normally, chest drains will not be removed until 24 hours after bubbling has ceased (Miller and Harvey, 1993). If drains are on suction, excessive turbulence indicates excessive negative pressure (Bar-El *et al.*, 2001).

Although there will almost always be enough blood *draining* to stain the water in the bottle, the volume will only significantly increase if fluid is drained. The water level should therefore be marked with the time and date during each shift (if possible), so the volume of drainage can be assessed. Drainage may be blood, plasma or pus (or any combination of these), so its colour and type should be noted.

If initial drainage is excessive (more than 1 litre in the first 30 minutes) the drain should be clamped, as rapid drainage is both painful and may cause fatal pulmonary oedema (Kam *et al.*, 1993; Hall and Jones, 1997), as loss of protein causes hydrostatic shifts of fluid into interstitial spaces.

Oxygen

Although oxygen may be needed because patients are hypoxic, Gallon (1998) also reports that high concentration oxygen is sometimes used to increase the absorption of air from the pleural cavity. This practice is, however, rare and questionable.

Mobility

Immobility can provoke many problems, including:

- Muscle wasting
- Deep vein thromboses
- Chest infection.

Early mobilisation reduces mortality (Martinson *et al.*, 2001), so, like all other patients, those with chest drains should be encouraged to mobilise. Chest-drain bottles are now made of durable plastic, so can be safely carried provided patients are taught:

- Never to raise the bottle up to their chest level
- To keep the water level reasonably horizontal
- Always to keep the end of the drain below the water level.

Milking (stripping)

The once common practices of 'milking' drains with fingers or 'stripping' them with roller clamps to encourage drainage towards the bottle are dangerous. Milking can generate pressures in excess of $100\,cmH_2O$, while stripping can generate more than $400\,cmH_2O$ (Kam *et al.*, 1993), which could draw pleural tissue into the drain (Mallett and Dougherty, 2000). To prevent dangerous practice, roller clamps should not be stocked. Milking does not improve patency, although it does increase the drainage volume (Charnock and Evans, 2001), so should not be routinely done (Mallett and Dougherty, 2000). However, blockage, especially from blood clots, may necessitate milking (Godden and Hiley, 1998), using finger movements to dislodge and move clots down the tube.

Clamping

The traditional practice of clamping drains whenever patients were moved was dangerous, as clamping can convert a simple pneumothorax into a life-threatening tension pneumothorax (Hyde *et al.*, 1997). Drains should only be clamped:

- If they become disconnected (Mallett and Dougherty, 2000)
- When moving the drain above the patient is unavoidable (Gallon, 1998)
- When changing bottles
- If there is excessive drainage (see above).

Pneumothoraces may recur following removal of the drain (Gupta, 2001); Gallon (1998) suggests that first-time pneumothoraces recur in 30 per cent of young people and 50 per cent of older people, with higher recurrence rates (70 per cent in young people) in the case of second pneumothoraces. Many authors (e.g. McMahon-Parkes, 1997; Gupta, 2001) recommend clamping drains for up to 24 hours before removal. Should pneumothoraces recur, removing clamps is preferable to inserting a new drain. Gallon (1998) does not recommend this practice, although does not give a reason.

To ensure sealing of the often rigid tubing of chest drains, two clamps should be used, one clamped from the left and the other from the right (O'Hanlon-Nichols, 1996). Clamps should remain in place for the minimum time necessary (Gallon, 1998). If the patient shows signs of respiratory distress (e.g. dyspnoea, cyanosis), clamps should be released immediately (O'Hanlon-Nichols, 1996).

Removing chest drains

Once pneumothoraces have healed, drains are normally removed, although this is a medical rather than a nursing decision. O'Hanlon-Nichols' (1996) suggestion of removing drains when drainage falls below 75 ml per day is dubious. Removal is painful (Owens and Gould, 1997; Gray, 2001), so patients should be given analgesia. Gallon (1998) recommends Entonox.

Removal often needs (and is safest with) two people, preferably one being a doctor who can reinsert a drain if necessary. Traditionally, purse-string sutures were inserted around the sites; this enabled the second person to tighten the suture as soon as the first person had removed the drain. Smaller ('pig-tail') drains are now usually used, often without sutures. In practice, wounds often still need sutures.

Usual practice is to ask patients to hold their breath out (end expiration) while the drain is removed (Godden and Hiley, 1998; Gallon, 1998), or to use the Valsalva manoeuvre (breathing out against a closed glottis, like straining at stool) (McMahon-Parkes, 1997), which again ensures breath is held at the end of expiration. Both ensure that intrapleural pressure is equal to or above intrapulmonary pressure. Bell *et al.* (2001) found similar rates of recurrent pneumothoraces with end-inspiration and end-expiration removal. Although physiologically illogical, they concluded that both were therefore equally safe.

Following removal, lung re-expansion should be checked with a chest X-ray. Close respiratory observations should be maintained for 24 hours (O'Hanlon-Nichols, 1996).

Implications for practice

- If suction is used, limit negative pressures to between minus 10 and minus 20 cmH$_2$O
- Unless there is some over-riding indication, bottles should only be changed when full
- Patients with chest drains usually need strong analgesics, and usually also benefit from anti-inflammatory medicines
- Dressings should be secure and airtight
- Observe for swinging, bubbling, draining
- Listen for air leaks at the insertion site
- Tubing should be examined at least each shift for patency
- Patients should be encouraged to mobilise, having been taught how to manage their drain bottle safely
- Routine milking is not recommended
- Clamping drains is not recommended, except for very brief times during an emergency, to change the bottle, or to move the bottle over the patient
- Roller-clamps should not be kept in stock
- During removal, give additional analgesia (e.g. Entonox).

Summary

Intrapleural chest drains are a useful medical solution to a large (>20 per cent) pneumothorax. However, much nursing and medical practice is based on tradition rather than reliable evidence. Sound research is needed into almost all aspects of management. However, in the absence of adequate evidence, nurses are still expected to deliver care.

Clinical scenario

Mrs Marion Janes has been admitted following a road traffic accident. She is very breathless, with oxygen saturation of 83% on 60% oxygen. Chest X-ray reveals a large pneumothorax, which needs both apical and chest drain insertion. She has been given a bolus of intravenous morphine, which is currently keeping her pain under control.

1   With the help of colleagues from work, list the items that will be needed for insertion of a chest drain.

2   You are asked to assist the doctor inserting the drain. Identify what is expected of you, both by the doctor and to care safely for your patient.

3   Devise a plan of care to manage Mrs Janes' chest drain for the first 12 hours following insertion.

Bibliography

Key reading

Sound nursing reviews are provided by Godden and Hiley (1998) and Charnock and Evans (2001).

Further reading

Miller and Harvey (1993) remains the most widely-followed medical review of chest drains. Pain management is reviewed by Gray (2001).

Chapter 20

Acute coronary syndromes

Noirin Egan

Contents

Learning outcomes

After reading this chapter you will be able to:

- Recognise the priorities of managing acute ST segment elevation myocardial infarction (STEMI) and its common complications
- Appreciate the critical nature of other acute coronary syndromes and their management.

Fundamental knowledge

Anatomy and physiology of the heart, basic ECG interpretation, clotting cascade.

Introduction

Coronary heart disease (CHD) is the single most common cause of death in the United Kingdom today (DOH, 2000b). Those affected by the disease face many challenges that profoundly impact on quality of life, future employment and personal relationships. In an attempt to reduce the morbidity associated with the disease, the National Service Framework for CHD has established clear and measurable standards for its prevention and management.

Recently, the term acute coronary syndrome (ACS) has been used as an umbrella term to describe three main clinical presentations:

1   Unstable angina
2   Non-ST segment elevation myocardial infarction (NSTEMI), which replaces the more traditional terms Non-Q-wave or sub-endocardial MI
3   Acute ST segment elevation myocardial infarction (STEMI).

(Jones, 2003)

The latter term, which refers to a full thickness infarction, is commonly referred to in the clinical setting as 'Barn door infarct'.

The management of STEMI is well documented and clearly defined (DOH, 2000b). Time-dependent interventions implicit in its management highlight a critical situation and hence the need for specialist care right from the outset.

Patients with STEMI should be admitted swiftly to the coronary care unit (CCU). Pressure for beds may mean that patients with other acute coronary syndromes may overflow into less acute areas, such as general medical wards. Some of these patients will be considered to be 'high risk', and will require close monitoring by nursing staff.

This chapter will focus upon STEMI: the pathophysiological processes leading up to it and its critical management within the first 12 hours. Potential complications will be highlighted. Other acute coronary syndromes will then be discussed, as they may require a critical care focus

Pathophysiological processes

Recent advances in treatment options for ACS have developed out of an increased awareness of the pathophysiology of the disease process. It is now known that the pathological process for STEMI is potentially similar to that of other acute coronary syndromes (Figure 20.1; Weston, 1996; Maynard et al., 2000).

The extent of occlusion will depend on its site and duration, as well as the presence of collateral circulation. With unstable angina there is temporary vascular occlusion by a platelet-rich thrombus overlying the atherosclerotic plaque (Jones, 2003).

NSTEMI is associated with more persistent occlusion accompanied by vasoconstriction; however, the distal myocardial territory is usually supplied by a collateral blood supply. If occlusion occurs for more than 20 minutes necrosis will develop, but it may not involve the full thickness of the muscle (Jones, 2003).

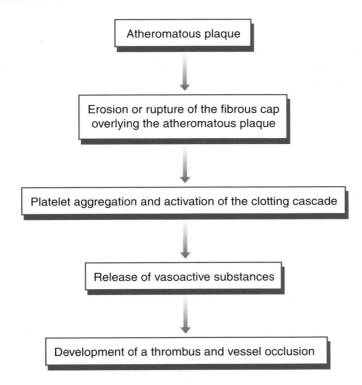

Figure 20.1 The pathophysiological process

In contrast, STEMI results in a fixed and persistent thrombus which restricts myocardial perfusion and causes transmural necrosis (Doering, 1999; Dracup and Cannon, 1999). This thrombus differs in that it is bound by fibrin strands (Jones, 2003).

With STEMI, the wave front of myocardial necrosis begins within minutes of this event and progresses from sub-endocardium to epicardial surface, the outcome being a full thickness area of infarction. Speed is required in an attempt to reverse this pathological process. At present, thrombolysis is the gold standard to be achieved.

Acute ST segment elevation myocardial infarction (STEMI)

Clinical features

- Pain is usually retrosternal in nature, and may radiate to the neck and arms and sometimes to the back.
- Pain is often associated with nausea/and or vomiting
- Sweating can be attributed to the release of toxins from the injured myocardial cells and an increase in autonomic activation (Nolan *et al.*, 1998)

- Blood pressure and heart rate are slightly increased
- If severe myocardial damage has already occurred there may be profound hypotension and arrhythmias may be a feature
- Shortness of breath is usually an indicaton of the extent of myocardial damage.

Management

A patient presenting with symptoms of STEMI is a priority. Initial assessment will be aimed at establishing a diagnosis, assessing haemodynamic function determining suitability for reperfusion therapy and, most importantly, relieving symptoms.

Diagnosis of acute myocardial infarction (STEMI) is based on the following criteria:

- 1 mm of ST segment elevation in standard leads
- 2 mm of elevation in one or more of chest leads
- New left-bundle branch block.

(DOH, 2000b)

Priorities in care include ECG, cannulation, pain relief and establishment of cardiac and vital sign monitoring. The diagnosis of STEMI involves critical decision-making and a clear defined pathway of management.

Pain control

Pain relief is the first priority as uncontrolled pain can cause an increase in sympathetic stimulation, which in turns leads to an increase in myocardial oxygen consumption. This can further aggravate ischaemia, and can increase the threshold for cardiac arrhythmias.

Intravenous diamorphine, a potent analgesia, is given with an anti-emetic (e.g. maxolon). Unrelieved pain may require the administration of a beta-blocker by slow intravenous injection. Beta-blockers can dramatically reduce myocardial oxygen demand and prevent myocardial rupture. By controlling the infarction, left ventricular function may be preserved. Intravenous nitrates will also improve the blood flow to the ischaemic myocardium. Blood pressure should be monitored to detect hypotension.

Supplemental oxygen is an important aspect of management of STEMI, even when oxygen saturation levels are normal (oxygen delivery to the cardiomyocytes is optimised). This may help to limit the degree of ischaemia. Initially, the monitoring of vital signs as frequently as every 15 minutes may be indicated to detect hypotension and cardiac dysrhythmias. This helps to monitor the response to treatment. Monitoring of patients' respiratory rate and oxygen saturations may indicate whether left ventricular failure (LVF) is an associated feature.

The importance of reassuring the patient throughout the critical aspect of care cannot be understated. Anxiety is a major feature, and may cause further ischaemia if not acknowledged and managed. Reassurance can be given by the calm and confident manner with which care is managed. In some areas, coronary care nurses visit the patient in the accident and emergency department to facilitate this.

Many hospitals have fast-tracking procedures to ensure there is little delay in admission to a coronary care unit or other appropriate critical care area.

Thrombolysis

Thrombolysis has now become a major aspect of the management of STEMI. The early survival advantages produced by the administration of thrombolysis and aspirin in the second International Study on Infarct Survival (ISIS 2) have been reported to be maintained for at least 10 years when antiplatelet therapy such as aspirin is continued (Baigent *et al.*, 1998). Aspirin 300 mg is a first-line drug, as it inhibits thrombus formation. It is given in conjunction with thrombolysis.

The aim of thrombolytic therapy is to restore patency in the occluded vessel, thereby reperfusing the myocardium under threat of necrosis. Its mode of action is through the process of lysis. Clot lysis is initiated by activating plasminogen to form plasmin, which in turn degrades the fibrin threads that bind the clot together.

Streptokinase, although rarely used today because of its potential to evoke an antigen antibody response, has revolutionised the management of STEMI. It has been superceded by more synthetic and expensive agents.

Tissue plasminogen activator (t-PA) is another common agent used, and works by activating plasminogen to plasmin, thereby producing lysis of the thrombus. The benefit is that it does not evoke an antigen antibody response and is more specific in its mode of action.

As with the use of all thrombolytic agents, the patient's suitability for administration needs to be assessed carefully and quickly. The risks and benefits of the drug need to be explained to the patient and informed consent obtained. The commencement of thrombolytic therapy requires speed, hence the motto 'Time is muscle'.

Dysrhythmias that occur during thrombolysis can be multiple and varied. They are associated with reperfusion of the infracted area. A surge of oxygen-rich blood can cause electrolyte imbalance and microhaemorrhage (Nieman and Smith, 1999). The circulation may be compromised, but this is usually short lived and is managed by temporarily stopping the infusion and by resuscitative measures where appropriate.

Nurse-led thrombolysis (Bloe, 2001) involves the nurse making a diagnosis (of uncomplicated MI), determining the suitability for thrombolysis, and referring the patient to medical staff who will make the final decision. Success is measured by a 'door to needle time' of less than 20 minutes (DOH, 2000b).

Evidence of successful reperfusion following thrombolytic therapy is provided by:

- Relief of pain
- The return of ST segments to baseline
- The presence of reperfusion arrhythmias.

(Albarran and Kapeluch 2000)

An ECG recorded at 90 minutes will be required to determine this.

Patients with diabetes or those who have a random blood sugar greater than 11 mmol/l will require the administration of a sliding scale of insulin to maintain glycaemic control. Glucose is a major energy source for the ischaemic myocardium, and insulin enhances its uptake (Bennett, 2001). The Digami Study has demonstrated a reduction in 1-year mortality in patients managed according to this protocol (Mamberg *et al.*, 1995).

Complications of acute myocardial infarction

Acute left ventricular failure

Acute left ventricular failure and pulmonary oedema are common complications following STEMI, and are primarily caused by extensive infarction of the left ventricular wall.

Both complications are characterised by sudden acute onset of breathlessness, tachycardia and hypotension. Certain compensatory mechanisms occur in an effort to maintain cardiac output. This can be explained by the principles of pre-load and after-load. Pre-load is the filling phase of the cardiac cycle, and refers to the passive stretching of the myofibrils. According to Starling's Law, cardiac output and the force of contraction are directly related to the amount the muscle fibres stretch during contraction. Pre-load is therefore determined by the blood volume in the ventricle at the end of diastole, and is influenced by the venous return to the heart and the ability of the heart to fill.

After-load is also an important concept, and relates to the resistance to left ventricular emptying and an increase in systemic vascular resistance. Extensive damage to the left ventricle causes a reduction in the ability of the myofibrils to stretch. The heart thus compensates by increasing the heart rate in an effort to maintain cardiac output; this further increases the systemic vascular resistance (SVR), and a vicious cycle begins. When left ventricular emptying is restricted, back-flow to the pulmonary capillaries causes the lungs to become oedematous; the patient therefore becomes breathless and hypoxic. This constitutes an acute emergency situation.

The priorities of management are as follows:

- Sit patient in an upright position (dependent upon blood pressure)
- Give a high flow rate of oxygen
- Administer diamorphine 2.5 mg IV. Diamorphine not only has a sedative effect but also causes venodilation, which in turn decreases venous return and affects pre-load (this reduces the workload of the heart)
- Give maxolon 10 mg IV
- Give frusemide (loop diuretic) IV. This also causes venodilation, reducing the

circulating volume through diuresis. This may be ineffective if the patient is profoundly hypotensive, as there may be insufficient renal flow to achieve this. The use of inotropes to improve blood pressure may be indicated, but they have to be used very cautiously as they may induce further tachy-arrhythmias

■ If the blood pressure allows it, the use of nitrates IV in the acute situation can reduce pre-load and after-load through its biphasic action of venous and arterial dilation

■ The use of non-invasive ventilation such as continuous positive airway pressure (CPAP) is now common in such acute situations. It facilitates more efficient oxygen delivery in the pulmonary capillaries and reduces pre-load by decreasing venous return (see Chapter 18).

Patients who develop acute heart failure in the early stages of STEMI have a worse long-term prognosis (Nolan *et al.*, 1998). Left ventricular remodelling, which can begin in the early stages, leads to a downward spiral of events that involve stretching and thinning of the myocardium, dilatation, compensatory hypertrophy, tachycardia and exacerbated ischaemia (Doering, 1999). Certain drugs such as ACE inhibitors has been shown to prevent this occurrence, and should be started very soon after the initial event in order to prevent the longer-term occurrence of chronic heart failure.

Dysrhythmias

In the acute phase of STEMI, dysrhythmias will primarily be due to a combination of electrolyte imbalance and ischaemia. In the presence of ischaemia, hypoxia precipitates anaerobic metabolism, which leads to a state of acidosis.

Acidosis causes increased stimulation of the sympathetic nervous system and an increase in the automaticity of the myocytes by the release of catecholamines. As a result the resting membrane potential of the cell is decreased, and this results in an increased rate and frequency of depolarisation, leading to the development of tachyarrhythmias.

An increased heart rate leads to increased oxygen demands and a decreased diastolic filling pressure, which is in turn detrimental to an already struggling heart. Anterior wall MI often displays such sympathetic effects and tachyarrhythmias are most common with large anterior wall MI. The most serious are ventricular tachycardia (VT) and ventricular fibrillation (VF). Both pulseless VT and VF can rapidly prove fatal unless the patient is defibrillated within 90 seconds. This is an expanded role.

Ischaemia can also increase extracellular potassium and levels of adenosine, causing slowing of the impulses in the conducting system. The parasympathetic nervous system may also be stimulated and can cause suppression of the sinus or atrioventricular node. Slowing of the heart rate often complicates inferior wall MI (IFWMI) accompanying right coronary artery occlusion. The right coronary artery also supplies the conductive tissue, which explains why bradycardia and heart blocks may be more common with IFWMI

Heart blocks that cause the patient's condition to be compromised will require the insertion of a temporary transvenous pacing wire.

Cardiogenic shock

Cardiogenic shock is a serious complication following STEMI, and will usually present within the first 24 hours of infarction. There is an acute and sustained failure of the heart to maintain adequate tissue perfusion, possibly leading lead to multiple organ failure. Hypotension initiates and sustains a vicious cycle of reduced coronary artery perfusion, leading to further ischaemia and infarct extension and thereby, worsening ventricular dysfunction and restarting the cycle.

Lactic acidosis, which occurs as a result of hypoxia to the tissues, further suppresses myocardial contractility and blunts the response to inotropic and other vasopressor agents. A downward spiral of events ensues unless this cycle is interrupted at an early stage (see Chapter 21).

Management of STEMI in the acute phase requires vigilance and skill of those involved. 'Failing to reperfuse' is a term used for patients who exhibit continuing pain with no resolution, or worsening, of ST segment changes after approximately 90 minutes. These patients may need to be rethrombolysed or, preferably, transferred to a specialist unit where rescue percutaneous transluminal angiography (PTCA) with/without stent can be performed. The use of heparin and other antithrombotic agents such as aspirin and Clopidogrel have been found to be beneficial in stabilising the patient's symptoms, but are limited in their performance of reperfusion.

Unstable angina and non-ST segment elevation myocardial infarction

Unstable angina is defined simply as new onset angina (less than 6 months), worsening of symptoms, or pain occurring at rest. Pain may radiate to the jaw or neck. Radiation down the arm or numbness/tingling in the fingertips may be a feature. Patients may describe a 'dull pressure', squeezing, constricting or burning sensation in the chest, back or arms (Lindsay and Templeton, 2002).

The ECG may be normal or have ST segment depression or T wave abnormalities. It is not associated with a rise in cardiac enzymes. NSTEMI presents similarly, but may be accompanied by a marginal enzyme rise. ST segment changes may be similar in nature. Both conditions are associated with an underlying unstable coronary lesion, and are at risk of full-thickness infarction and/or death (Maynard et al., 2000)

Until recently, professional judgment has played a major part in determining the fine line between these conditions; however, the measurement of serum troponin has enabled clearer risk stratification and better management. Troponin is a specific indicator of myocardial necrosis. Patients with NSTEMI will often have positive troponin results, and will require early investigation because of the nature of their unstable lesion.

The management of ACS in recent years has shifted emphasis from relief of ischaemic pain to relieving the ischaemia itself (Schulman and Fessler, 2001). This emphasis has led to the introduction of some potentially risky interventions aimed at restoring blood flow.

New options to improve blood flow to the myocardium, e.g. glycoprotein 11b-111a inhibitors (such as Tirofiban), have revolutionised the management of ACS. Such drugs are now considered to have major impact on stabilising the acute lesion, and are often used to bridge the critical gap between PTCA and stenting.

Implications for practice

■   Nurses caring for patients with ACS play a pivotal role in identifying significant changes in their condition
■   Monitoring for new ECG changes and careful assessment of the nature of chest pain are vital
■   The emphasis of care is also on preventative measures, through pharmacological management and/or health promotion.

Summary

Nurses working in high dependency environments may not experience caring for patients diagnosed with ACS on a regular basis, although existing patients can develop these problems. None the less, they need to be conversant with current approaches to caring for such patients.

Clinical scenario

Mr Taylor is admitted via a fast-track system. He has suffered an anterolateral MI and has received thrombolysis in A&E. He has continuous unresolved pain, and his ECG has failed to show evidence of reperfusion.

1   Identify the priorities of his immediate management on admission.

2   Discuss other possible complications that may ensue.

3   What drugs/interventions may be used to manage a complication of LVF in this instance?

Bibliography

Key reading

Nolan *et al.* (1998) offers a useful overview of caring for patients with AMI.

Suggested reading

National Service Framework for coronary heart disease, at www.doh.gov.uk/nsf/chd.

Chapter 21

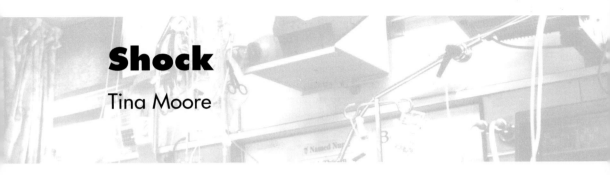

Shock

Tina Moore

Contents

Learning outcomes

After reading this chapter you will be able to:

- Understand the physiological changes during shock
- Recognise the different classifications of shock and the management of each
- Demonstrate knowledge and understanding of how shock affects other organs
- Appreciate the mode of treatment for each type of shock.

Fundamental knowledge

Baroreceptors and chemoreceptors; renin–angiotensin–aldosterone cascade; normal inflammatory response; types of blood cells.

Introduction

Shock is a common complication experienced by many patients. It is crucial that nurses have an understanding of the causes, physiological changes and management of the different types of shock in order for appropriate care to be given.

Definitions of shock fail to recognise its complexity. Hinds and Watson (1999: 1749) state that shock 'is an acute circulatory failure with inadequate or inappropriately distributed tissue perfusion resulting in generalised hypoxia'. Irrespective of the cause of shock, the resultant features will be the same; that is to say, inadequate tissue perfusion and impairment of homeostasis. Whatever the type, it is a life-threatening event requiring aggressive management.

This chapter explains the physiological changes occurring in each stage of shock. Different types of shock are discussed, together with the nursing and medical management.

Stages of shock

Irrespective of the type of shock, there are four identified stages. Each stage is progressive and interrelated. Table 21.1 identifies the physiological changes during each stage. Symptoms may vary depending on the nature of the imbalances.

Table 21.1 Stages of shock

Stage	Pathophysiology
1 Initial stage	Clinical features are not apparent, often unrecognised.
2 Compensatory stage (occurs if the cause persists)	Acute fluid volume loss does not allow for the normal compensatory mechanisms. Many elderly patients and those with chronic diseases may have subtle compensatory responses, which may be overlooked. This stage is designed to preserve cellular function. The responses are first activated by:
	• A fall in circulating blood volume, resulting in decreased cardiac output. If prolonged, baroreceptor reflexes will be initiated, causing stimulation of sympathetic nervous activity. Catecholamines are released, increasing cardiac output and myocardial contractility (stimulating feelings of fear and anxiety with increased ventricular and muscle tremor, sweating and vomiting). Catecholamines also stimulate the liver to convert glycogen to glucose, causing hyperglycaemia. Adrenaline produces an adrenoceptor effect, causing general vasoconstriction, and also increases metabolic rate.

Stage	Pathophysiology
	• Relaxation of bronchial smooth muscles, increased respiratory rate and minute volume improves gaseous exchange. Symptoms include tachypnoea and metabolic acidosis. • Chemoreceptors relay signals to the hypothalamus, stimulating the release of adrenocorticotrophic hormone (ACTH), growth hormone (GH) and antidiuretic hormone (ADH). The combined effect of ACTH and GH increases blood glucose and expands circulating blood volume through sodium and water retention at the renal tubules, resulting in oliguria. • Aldosterone is secreted, aiding the retention of fluid. Increased cortisol production also increases fluid retention and antagonises the effects of insulin, resulting in further hyperglycaemia. Therefore, generalised symptoms include: tachycardia, tachypnoea, hypotension, oliguria, hyperglycaemia, altered level of consciousness, and sweating.
3 Progressive stage	Failure of compensatory mechanisms to restore adequate circulatory volume causes prolonged vasoconstriction, cellular hypoxia and eventual damage. Cellular hypoperfusion and the inability to meet oxygen consumption (VO_2) requirements causes cellular anaerobic metabolism in a worsening acidotic state, and the depletion of adenosine triphosphate (ATP) and failure of the cell membrane sodium–potassium pump. This influx of sodium and water will cause cell swelling, worsening metabolic acidosis. The skin will feel cold and clammy. Capillary refill is poor. Respiratory rate is further reduced. Patients may become restless and confused. Further vasoconstriction makes tissues ischaemic and causes arteriolar vasodilatation as well as dilation of the arterioles, causing pooling of blood in the capillary bed (Hubbard and Mechan, 1997). Together with increased hydrostatic pressure this indicates capillary leakage. The patient may develop hypoxia with hypercapnia. Decompensation processes further aggravate hypovolaemia, with resultant altered cellular metabolism initiating acidosis, cardiac depression, intravascular coagulation, increased capillary permeability and release of toxins.

continued

Table 21.1 continued

Stage	Pathophysiology
4 Refractory stage	Increased vasoactive metabolites released by the damaged cells causes localised vasodilatation of the precapillary sphincters, resulting in hypoperfusion. Histamine released by damaged endothelium increases the permeability of the capillaries, causing proteins to leak into extracellular spaces. Changes resulting from tissue ischaemia can cause disseminated intravascular coagulation. Furthering hypoperfusion, hypercapnia, increased hydrogen ions and bacteraemia will lead to multiple organ failure.

Time out 21.1

1 From your experience, write down the different types of shock that you have seen.
2 How did the clinical features manifest for each patient?
3 Describe the management for each patient.

Classification of shock

Hypovolaemic

Disorders of fluid volume in critically ill patients may be classified as either depletion or expansion disorders, and involve both intracellular and extracellular compartments (Hudak *et al.*, 1998) (see Chapter 35). Hypovolaemic shock develops when the intravascular volume decreases to the point that compensatory mechanisms cannot maintain adequate tissue perfusion and normal cellular function. Inadequate ventricular pre-load is usually manifested by a reduction in circulatory blood volume by 20–25 per cent (Hinds and Watson, 1996).

Causes include:

- Haemorrhage – loss of whole blood. More than 30 per cent of blood loss results in severe shock (Marieb, 2004)
- Plasma loss – increase in capillary permeability leads to a shift of plasma fluid from the vascular space into the interstitial space. This is commonly seen in patients with severe burns
- Third-space fluid shifts – this could occur following trauma or cellular damage, and automatically causes an inflammatory response and vasodilatation. Permeability causes movement of fluids, enabling water, electrolytes and albumin to flow into the interstitial spaces (third space) (Bove, 1994).

Compensatory changes lead to alterations in both regional blood flow and the distribution of fluid between body compartments. Physiological changes include a reduction in venous return to the heart, resulting in a reduction in cardiac output. Persistence causes diversion of blood to vital organs (heart, lung, brain), leading to hypoperfusion of other organs.

Early clinical features include:

■ Dizziness
■ Weakness
■ Nausea, vomiting and anorexia
■ Anxiety/apprehension
■ Hypotension (can appear normal due to the compensatory mechanisms), tachycardia, oliguria.

Severe volume depletion causes:

■ Dehydration – dry mucous membranes, dry furred tongue, sunken eyeballs, acute weight loss
■ Cardiovascular changes – decreased central venous pressure (CVP), decreased cardiac output (CO), rapid/thready pulse, decreased mean arterial pressure (MAP), decreased pulmonary artery pressure (PAP), increased systemic vascular resistance (SVR)
■ Decreased oxygen saturation
■ Disorientation/confusion.

Severe blood loss causes bradycardia. However, with more haemorrhaging the heart rate rises again (Ganong, 2003). Bradycardia may be due to unmasking of vagally mediated depressor reflexes, whose response is possibly a way of stopping the bleeding (Ganong, 2003).

Diagnostic tests for hypovolaemic shock are listed in Box 21.1.

Box 21.1   Diagnostic tests for hypovolaemic shock

■ Blood urea nitrogen levels (BUN) (elevated)
■ Serum electrolyte imbalances (variable, depending on fluid loss type)
■ ABG may reveal metabolic acidosis (occurring in diabetes ketoacidosis or gastro-intestinal loss)
■ Serum osmolality is variable depending on the type of fluid loss and the body's ability to compensate thirst with ADH (greater than 295 mOsm/l)
■ Haemoglobin – low (haemorrhage)
■ Urine osmolality – high, via laboratory specimen.

Management

Immediate restoration of effective circulating blood volume (by optimising the pre-load) and correction of acid–base and electrolyte disturbances is a priority. The aim of a mean arterial pressure of 80 mmHg is considered sufficient (Hinds and Watson, 1999). Fluid resuscitation is both complex and controversial. Whole blood is usually administered in the case of haemorrhage. The use of colloids and crystalloids is non-consensual. Previous systemic reviews have suggested that colloids are no more effective than crystalloids in reducing mortality (Schierhout and Roberts, 1998). The debate regarding whether crystalloid or colloid is the most appropriate to increase volume is ongoing. Crystalloids are free from direct side effects and are rapidly distributed across the intravascular and interstitial spaces. However, two to four times more volume is required than with colloid, and therefore pulmonary oedema may occur. Albumin should be administered with caution, as it is believed to have anticoagulant properties (Soni, 1995).

Fluid balance and vital signs need to be closely monitored (including CVP). Blood products and other colloid solutions are used to assist in acute blood loss. Inotropic support may be indicated if volume replacement attempts fail.

Cardiogenic

Cardiogenic shock results from a loss of critical contraction of the heart (Hudak et al., 1998), causing a reduction in cardiac output and reduced circulatory perfusion.

It is usually caused by myocardial infarction (15–20 per cent), and carries a mortality of 80 per cent. Other causes include tamponade, mitral regurgitation, pulmonary embolism and cardiac dysrhythmias. In addition to the clinical features, signs of myocardial failure (increased central venous pressure, pulmonary oedema and dyspnoea) occur.

Physical assessment and analysis of haemodynamic function (blood pressure and pulse) is required. As a sphygmomanometer reading can be unreliable, more advanced monitoring devices should be used (e.g. Dynamap®). In addition to hypotension, hyperglycaemia, hypernatraemia, hypocalcaemia and dysrhythmias (hypo/hyperkalaemia) may occur (see Chapter 35).

Management

The goals are to correct reversible problems, prevent further ischaemia and improve tissue perfusion.

An inotropic agent (dobutamine) may be used as it improves the contractility of uninjured myocardium and increases cardiac output. By stimulating the adrenergic receptors, vasopressors (e.g. adrenaline) cause vasoconstriction, increasing blood pressure to an adequate mean level (80 mmHg, depending upon the patient's norm). If left ventricular failure is present, diuretics are administered to decrease the pre-load to improve stroke volume and cardiac output. Due to cardiovascular and respiratory symptoms, patients may need to be positioned at a

45° angle. Oxygen therapy is required (this also helps to reduce cardiac pain). Pain control via diamorphine may be indicated. If the patient is overly anxious, sedatives may help to conserve energy.

Correction of electrolyte imbalances and presenting acidosis via sodium bicarbonate 50 ml IV (usually when pH is less than 7.2) is required.

Neurogenic

Causes of neurogenic shock include traumatised or diseased brain stem, spinal cord injury, and some anaesthetic drugs. Neurogenic shock occurs as the result of the loss of sympathetic nerve activity from the brain's vasomotor centre (Adam and Osborne, 1997). With the vasoconstrictor tone being interrupted, the autonomic nervous system controls systemic vascular resistance (SVR). Hence SVR is decreased, causing massive vasodilatation and profound uncontrolled vagal (sympathetic impulse) stimulation. Bradycardia and hypotension occur.

The cause should be treated, but failure of the autonomic response makes inotropic support ineffective (Woodrow, 2000). Poor circulating blood volume may be compensated with fluid replacement and oxygen support.

Anaphylactic

Anaphylactic shock results from an acute hypersensitive reaction to a substance to which the person has previously been sensitised; hence patients are more likely to have a reaction to a second dosage. The hypersensitivity response occurs on the surface of the mast cells, which are located primarily in the lungs, small blood vessels, and connective tissue. The antigen combines with sensitised antibodies from previous exposure (usually immunoglobulin E (IgE) type). The antigen also attaches to basophils circulating in the blood. The immediate reaction is a release of histamine and other mediators (e.g. kinins and esinophils (Guyton and Hall, 2000)), resulting in massive vasodilatation.

Clinical features usually manifest rapidly (within minutes), and include hypotension and tachycardia; visual changes are noted on the skin, e.g. urticaria. Facial oedema (due to loss of protein-rich fluid in the tissues) may cause laryngeal obstruction (indicated by swelling of the lips and face); this is a life-threatening situation and can be very frightening for both patient and nurse. Bronchospasm can also occur, causing wheezing.

Management

Severe cases will result in laryngeal oedema (causing noisy breathing – stridor). Maintenance of an open airway is critical. Adrenaline should be administered as a first-line drug (Resuscitation Council, 2002); this causes an increase in blood pressure through vasoconstriction, and inhibits the mediators released by the immune response. The recommended dosage is 0.5 ml of 1:1000 (500 mg) intramuscularly, repeated after 5 minutes in the absence of clinical improvement or deterioration. Slow intravenous administration is reserved for those who are in an immediate life-threatening situation, and adrenaline should be diluted at least 1:10000 (never 1:1000) (Resuscitation Council, 2002). It also causes smooth muscle relaxation, and therefore bronchi dilation. Oxygen support is required.

Fluid resuscitation should be initiated if drugs do not reverse the shock status; crystalloids are preferable to colloids (Schierhout and Roberts, 1998). Antihistamines should also be administered to help counteract histamine-mediated vasodilatation. Aminophylline should be given intravenously if bronchospasm persists. This is all done in conjunction with the administration of oxygen, and airway management.

Systemic inflammatory response syndrome

SIRS is the abnormal, generalised inflammatory response reaction occurring in organs remote from initial injury (Dolan, 2003). Controversy of the definition exists; another global consensus is being drawn up at the time of writing.

The presence of two or more of the following is required for diagnosis:

- Temperature greater than 38°C or less than 36°C
- Heart rate greater than 90 bpm
- Respiratory rate greater than 20/min, or $PaCO_2$ less than 4.3 kPa
- Leucocyte count above 12,000 cells/mm³ below 4,000 cells/mm³, or containing over 10 per cent immature neutrophils.

(The American College of Chest Physicians and the Society for Critical Care Medicine, 1992)

Box 21.2 outlines the clinical features.

Box 21.2   Clinical features of SIRS

HOT – fever
- Increased HR and CO
- Increasing cardiac workload
- Increasing myocardial oxygen consumption
- Decreased vascular resistance (impaired tissue perfusion/tissue hypoxia)
- Oedema formation
- Cell damage.

COLD
- Progressive plasma extravasation accelerates hypovolaemia
- Ischaemia increases gut permeability, facilitating translocation of gut bacteria and escalating sepsis
- Local vasoconstrictive mediators unsuccessfully attempt to compensate, making peripheries cold and cyanosed
- Myocardial ischaemia and dysfunction reduce cardiac output.

(Woodrow, 2000)

Management

Oxygen therapy is administered to reverse hypoxaemia. Fluid replacement, usually colloids, is necessary to increase colloid osmotic and perfusion pressures. Inotropes will support myocardial contractility. If infection is present, antibiotics should be prescribed. Nutritional support should be started as early as possible.

Septic

Sepsis is the systemic response to severe infection in the body; its sequence is equal to the generalised inflammatory shock response seen in the progressive stage of illness (Bone *et al.*, 1997).

Sepsis remains life-threatening, and is the most common cause of death in intensive care (Bochud and Calandra, 2003). Management must be instigated quickly. Wiessner *et al.* (1995) suggest that there is a progression via a continuum from SIRS through sepsis and sepsis syndrome to septic shock and death.

The inflammatory response is designed to protect the body from further injury and promote rapid healing. Vasodilatation, increased microvascular permeability, neutrophil activation and adhesion, and enhanced coagulation occur. Histamine, prostaglandin, and bradykinin initiate the vascular response. If regulatory mechanisms fail, uncontrolled systemic inflammation overwhelms the body's normal protective response. Excessive vasodilatation, hypotension and increases in vascular permeability occur (Keen, 2001).

Management

Antibiotic therapy, oxygen supplementation, fluid replacement, inotropes, vaso-pressors sodium bicarbonate (for acidosis), nutritional support, and antipyretic agents are required. Haemofiltration and haemodialysis may be necessary to remove certain circulating cytokines. This treatment will not affect those cytokines that are fixed to cells, and many mediators of sepsis are associated with cells (Clarke, 1997).

Time out 21.2

1 After reading about the different types of shock, identify any similarities in management.
2 What do you think are the fundamental differences in the management of shock?

Organs in shock

Shock can precipitate multiple organ failure.

- Acute lung injury starts early. An increase in permeability of the lung microvasculature occurs. This allows pulmonary oedema to develop, even with low venous pressure. When severe, it can lead to adult respiratory distress syndrome (ARDS). Symptoms/clinical features include severe hypoxaemia (PaO_2 less than 8.0 kPa on 40% inspired oxygen), radiological appearance of bilateral pulmonary infiltrates, reduced lung compliance.
- Acute pre-renal failure (see Chapter 23) may occur as a result of hypoperfusion.
- Interference with glucose and oxygen supply to the brain may lead to agitation, confusion, and coma.
- Liver cell necrosis occurs in shock lasting for more than 10 hours (Gosling, 1995). Hepatic hypoperfusion produces intense angiotensin II release, precipitating vasoconstriction. Symptoms of liver impairment include encephalopathy, jaundice and bleeding problems.

Implications for practice

- Shock necessitates nurses closely monitoring haemodynamic and respiratory function
- Nurses are responsible for monitoring and interpreting patient data for the early detection of shock
- Fluid replacement must be given with great caution, particularly in the older person
- Gut ischaemia increases problems owing to the translocation of gut bacteria; enteral feeding should be encouraged/maintained whenever possible
- Some patients in high dependency care are immunosuppressed, so good infection control is required (Woodrow, 2000)
- Shock can cause prolonged complications, so management should focus on long-term effects; benefits may not be seen for a number of days.

Summary

The nature of shock is complex and controversial. Owing to the severity of the disorder, it is imperative that nurses are well versed in the different types of shock. Through close monitoring of the patient's cardiovascular status, early identification and intervention can help to stop progression, thereby reducing morbidity and mortality.

Clinical scenario

Mr Raymond Robinson, 52 years old, has just returned to England from a holiday in India. Since his return 5 days ago he has suffered from acute diarrhoea and vomiting. He presents in the Accident and Emergency Department complaining of dizziness and excessive thirst.

Clinical examination reveals the following:

B/P   85/50 mmHg
Heart rate   142 bpm sinus tachycardia
Pulse pressure   Low
Respiratory rate   33 bpm
Temperature   37.0°C
Skin   Pale, very dry to touch
Tongue   Dry and furred

He is complaining of general lethargy and dizziness.

1 Identify the type of shock Raymond is suffering from. Give reasons for your answer.

2 With reference to physiological changes, describe your assessment.

3 Formulate an evidence-based plan of care for Raymond.

Bibliography

Key reading

Collins (2000).

Further reading

Hinds and Watson (1999) provides an in-depth discussion on haemodynamic monitoring in shock.

Chapter 22

Haematological disorders: sickle cell anaemia, disseminated intravascular coagulation

Tina Moore

Contents

Learning outcomes

After reading this chapter you will be able to:

- Identify the trigger factors for sickle cell anaemia/causes of disseminated intravascular coagulation (DIC)
- Demonstrate knowledge of the associated symptoms of both disorders

- Understand the related pathophysiological dangers
- Understand your own attitudes towards caring for the patient with sickle cell anaemia
- Devise a plan of care (with rationale) for a patient during sickle cell crisis/DIC.

Fundamental knowledge

Normal physiology of the erythrocyte; complications of blood transfusion; normal physiology of coagulation.

Introduction

Haematology is concerned with circulating blood and blood forming products. The three major functions of the haematopoietic system are the distribution of oxygen and nutrients to all cells of the body; protection of organism from invading microbes and regulation homeostasis. Many disorders manifested by abnormalities of the haematopoietic system are secondary to abnormalities of other organ systems. Two haematological disorders will be discussed in this chapter. *Sickle cell* anaemia and *Disseminated intravascular coagulation (DIC)*; these are described below.

Sickle cell anaemia

Sickle cell anaemia is an inherited blood disorder mainly affecting people of Afro-Caribbean descent, but it can be found in Eastern Mediterranean and Middle Eastern people. Haemoglobin S (HbS) forms long polymers upon deoxygenation. These rod-like polymers change the normally round and pliable red blood cells into stiff cells with a crescent (or sickle) shape. Bundles of these deformed cells act as plugs within the capillaries. This results in a reduction of blood flow, causing localised tissue hypoxia and promoting further sickling. If uncorrected, tissue necrosis and infarction follow, causing severe pain, multisystem organ damage and possibly early death (Tigner, 1998).

Most sickle cell crises last for approximately 5–7 days. Triggers for a crisis can include acute infection (especially viral), stress (both emotional and physiological), dehydration, or external temperature (Tigner, 1998).

Time out 22.1

Think about a patient that you have nursed with acute sickle cell anaemia (if you have not, then consider to the pathophysiology of the disease).

1 List the clinical features in order of priority.
2 Give reasons for your answer.
3 What would patients consider to be the priorities of care that they should receive?

Clinical features

The most common clinical picture during adult life is vaso-occlusive crisis. Pain is considered a major symptom of sickle cell, and is thought to be due to the site and degree of vaso-occlusion. The pain is variable, and can be localised or diffused, constant or intermittent. Some patients suffer from fever and swelling in the joints of the hands or feet. Long bones can also be affected. Occasionally abdominal pain is the major symptom, and this may be associated with distension and rigidity (a picture very similar to an acute abdomen requiring surgery).

The degree of pain is comparable to that experienced in myocardial infarction (Pasero, 1996), yet in patients with sickle cell the complaint of pain is not taken seriously or treated with the same degree of urgency. It is a symptom that is doubted by a significant number of nursing and medical staff (Alleyne and Thomas, 1994). Studies show a relationship between the frequency of painful crises and early death (Pasero, 1996).

Secondary symptoms predominantly result from the pain experienced, and include disablement and fright. Hostility and anger may ensue if nurses are perceived to be slow to respond to or are openly sceptical of the pain reports of the patient.

Sickle cells have a short life span (about 15 days in comparison with 120 days for normal red blood cells), and the increased haemolysis causes chronic anaemia. Patients may also look jaundiced (mainly seen in the conjunctivae). Tachypnoea, hypertension, nausea, vomiting and fever may be accompanying symptoms.

There may be multiple organ involvement, with micro-infarcts affecting the heart, lung, central nervous system and spleen. Urinalysis may indicate haematuria, infection or elevated bilirubin levels (which increase as the sickle cells are destroyed).

Diagnosis

Table 22.1 illustrates the blood profiles of a patient in sickle cell crisis (Hoffbrand et al., 1999).

Table 22.1 Blood profile – sickle cell crisis

Blood profile	Results
Haemoglobin	6–8 g/dl
Reticulocyte count	Elevated
Erythrocytes on peripheral blood film	Sickled
Sickling test	Positive
Haemoglobin electrophoretic pattern	Absence of HbA and a preponderance of HbS

Accurate pain assessment, administration of analgesics and oxygen, and intravenous hydration are the first steps in managing a sickle cell crisis (Gorman, 1999). Where an underlying infection is present, IV antibiotics are administered.

Controlling the patient's pain can pose a challenge to nurses. Continuous intravenous infusion of an appropriate analgesia is usually required, and this may be in the form of morphine. Satisfactory dosages are necessary to ensure that the patient remains mobile, helping to avoid pulmonary atelectasis as a result of diaphragmatic splint. Prescriptions should be written on an individual basis. Over-prescribing of opioids may lead to respiratory depression. When appropriate, patient-controlled analgesia (PCA) should be started. Many healthcare professionals are apprehensive about patients becoming addicted to the analgesia, but at present there is no conclusive evidence demonstrating the link between sickle cell pain and drug addiction. Indeed, under-treating the pain actually encourages such behaviours and predisposes the patient to pseudoaddiction syndrome (Hegarty and Portenoy, 1994), where the patient displays addictive behaviour without being dependent upon a substance. Treatment can sometimes be detrimental to the patient – for example, patients receiving high dosages of narcotics need to be monitored for side effects such as constipation, urinary retention, nausea and vomiting. In addition to pharmacological treatment, alternative methods of pain control should be implemented – for example, aromatherapy, distraction, heat and cold application.

Dehydration not only precipitates a crisis but can also occur during one. Replacement of insensible loss (particularly due to fever) is required. Intravenous hydration with 0.9% saline or 5% glucose in saline should be administered, together with careful monitoring for signs of fluid overload (e.g. tachycardia, hypertension, jugular vein distension and crackles). The aim should be a high fluid intake, of 70 ml/kg over 24 hours (Provan and Henson, 1999). Therefore, an average 70 kg patient would need $70 \, (\text{ml}) \times 70 \, (\text{kg}) = 4,900$; $4,900/24 \, (\text{hours}) = 204 \, \text{ml}$ per hour.

Conflicting evidence exists regarding the use of oxygen therapy. It is suggested that oxygen should be given even in the absence of hypoxaemia (Hoffbrand *et al.*, 1999), as oxygen is an anti-sickling agent. However, Tigner (1998) maintains that oxygen suppresses erythropoietin levels, thus exacerbating the crisis. The effect of suppressing erythropoietin is not immediate, and therefore oxygen therapy is beneficial during the early stages of a crisis. Patients can become acidotic, so regular monitoring of arterial blood gas should be carried out as pulse oximetry readings will provide a falsely high SpO_2, particularly during the sickle cell crisis (see Chapter 29).

In the early stages of the crisis, blood transfusions are of a low priority. At this point many patients have developed chronic haemolytic anaemia and therefore have lower haemoglobin and haematocrit levels. Patients with sickle cell can manage relatively well with low haemoglobin levels (Hoffbrand *et al.*, 1999). If the HbS is 30 per cent or higher, an exchange transfusion of packed red blood cells should be performed, with the aim of reducing the concentration of HbS to less than 30 per cent. This involves removing one unit of blood and transfusing one unit, then repeating the process. Alternatively, this process can be achieved via a plasmapheresis machine (Distenfield and Woermann, 2002). This approach may cause blood to become more viscous and increase the chances of sickling. The same result can be achieved by rapid transfusion, up to 12–14 g/dl (Weatherall, 1999), thus helping to prevent the haematocrit level from becoming too high. This procedure may compromise both cardiac and respiratory functions.

Folate stores are often depleted and will require supplementation (folic acid 5 mg daily). Problems associated with multiple transfusion including iron overload should be considered.

Limb tourniquets should be avoided, as they cause local hypoxia and so may precipitate sickling. Any major procedures are best carried out after an exchange transfusion.

Time out 22.2

1 What are the specific psychological needs of patients in sickle cell crisis?
2 Consider your own values/attitudes towards patients who constantly ask for analgesia and become aggressive in the process.
3 Now consider the situation from the perspectives of the patient and your colleagues.

Patients' familiarity with opiates and specific requests for a particular drug or dosage can be misinterpreted. Many patients with sickle cell pain receive covert or sometimes overt messages from healthcare professionals (including nurses) who believe that the pain is exaggerated and that medication is wanted for non-medical reasons (Pasero, 1996). From the patients' perspective this accusation becomes both humiliating and unprofessional. Nurses need to explore their own beliefs and values and be aware of them.

Patients vary in their coping abilities. Many describe feelings of helplessness regarding the disease, and express concerns about premature death (Gorman, 1999). This may lead to depression. Treatment can be enhanced by approaches that incorporate psychological, social and behavioural components. However, in many British hospitals the focus is exclusively on the physical aspects of pain, ignoring psychological and sociocultural dimensions (Thomas *et al.*, 1998). Empowering the patient to reduce stress through appropriate strategies (see Chapter 3) should help to reduce anxiety and allow time to regain some control over the situation.

Complications

Acute lung infarction (acute lung syndrome) is one of the most common causes of death from sickle cell, and accounts for a large proportion of admissions of these patients. It is demonstrated by deteriorating radiological appearances of the chest, and blood gas analysis showing increasing hypoxia. There is also a fall in packed cell volume and platelet count (Hoffbrand *et al.*, 1999). Some degree of cardiomegaly may be evident, and a variety of flow murmurs may be heard. This situation represents a medical emergency. It is managed by analgesics, respiratory support (oxygen in the first instance), antibiotics and transfusion.

Damage to the kidneys promotes an inability to concentrate urine, resulting in polyuria and nocturnal enuresis. In older patients there is chronic glomerular damage that may lead to chronic renal failure.

Sickling in the liver can lead to liver failure. A combination of the pooling of blood and a drop in haemoglobin can be life-threatening.

There may be periods of transient bone marrow aplasia (aplastic crisis), resulting in a low white cell count and an increased risk of infection.

Cerebrovascular accidents and retinopathy may also occur. Repeated crises may cause permanent damage to the vital organs, precipitating multi-organ failure. The outcome of this is bleak; it is believed that only half of the patients survive beyond the age of 50 years (Platt *et al.*, 1994).

Disseminated intravascular coagulation

DIC is not a disease or a symptom, but a syndrome. Its presence almost always indicates underlying disease. DIC is characterised by systemic intravascular activation of coagulation, leading to widespread deposition of fibrin in the circulation (Levi and Cate, 1999). This means that DIC is a thrombohaemorrhagic disorder, which is usually secondary to an underlying clinical condition. It is very rarely of idiopathic origin.

DIC involves an extremely complex pathophysiological process (Yu *et al.*, 2000). Normally coagulation is a dynamic action, with the balance between clot or thrombus formation and lysis being carefully regulated to provide competent homeostasis.

DIC syndrome results from an inappropriate, excessive and uncontrolled activation of the haemostatic process in which excessive procoagulant is released by the vascular endothelium (see Box 22.1). It is caused by severe stress or exposure to bacterial endotoxins (Cavenagh and Colvin, 1997).

Box 22.1 Abnormal clotting cascade in DIC

Platelets and coagulation factors are activated by a disease stimulus and are rapidly consumed

↓

Thrombin is formed very rapidly, and inherent inhibitors cannot stop the formation of the vast amounts of thrombin generated

↓

The fibrinolytic system lyses fibrin and impairs thrombin formation

↓

Fibrin degradation product (FDP) results from fibrinolysis, changing platelet aggregation and inhibiting fibrin polymerisation

---

The endothelial or tissue injury acts as a trigger for the excessive release of pro-coagulant material. This is usually in the form of cytokines and tissue factors known as interleukin 6. As a result the intravascular formation of fibrin causes thrombic occlusion of small and mid-sized vessels, possibly precipitating organ failure. Severe bleeding complications may result from the consumption and subsequent exhaustion of platelets and coagulation proteins initiated by the ongoing activation of the coagulation process (fibrinolysis). Two proteolytic enzymes, thrombin and plasmin, are activated and circulate systemically. Their balance determines a bleeding or thrombotic tendency. Underlying disease processes profoundly affect bleeding or thrombosis in DIC (Baird, 2001).

Acute DIC is often characterised by profound and unexpected bleeding or clotting. Microcirculation and microcirculatory thrombosis lead to hypoperfusion, infarction and end-organ damage, with the possibility of shock. Massive blood loss may lead to further coagulation factor and platelet depletion, thus aggravating the situation.

In chronic DIC (compensated), subacute bleeding and diffuse thrombosis confined to a specific anatomic location have been associated with aortic aneurysm and giant haemangionomas. Here, the activation of coagulation and fibrinolysis does not occur rapidly enough to exceed the rate of production of clotting factors in inhibitors (Baird, 2001).

Causes

Causes include any factors that result in damage to the endothelium or tissue, thus triggering the accelerated clotting response. Common causes include:

- Gram-negative bacterial sepsis (Cavanagh and Colvin 1997). A common pathogenic feature resulting from severe infection is the generalised inflammatory response, characterised by systemic release of cytokines (Levi et al., 1999).
- Viruses, especially varicella, hepatitis.
- Obstetric damage during delivery/abortion (the placenta and brain are especially rich in thromboplasin). Obstetric complications associated with the activation of blood coagulation include eclampsia, and haemolysis elevated liver enzymes and low platelets (HELLP) syndrome (Ruggenenti et al., 1997)
- Some traumas, including crush injuries. A combination of mechanisms, including release of tissue material in the circulation (fat, phospholipids), haemolysis and endothelial damage, may also be contributing factors to DIC (Roumen et al., 1993)
- Disorders that produce necrosis, e.g. severe burns and trauma, brain tissue destruction.
- Neoplastic disease such as acute leukaemia, metastatic carcinoma (Contrino et al., 1996).
- Other disorders including incompatible blood transfusion, drug reaction, shock, diabetic ketoacidosis, pulmonary embolism, sickle cell anaemia, cardiac arrest, surgical causes.

Clinical features

These will include symptoms of the underlying disorders, in addition to:

■ Microvascular thrombosis, including dyspnoea, haemoptysis (pulmonary infarct may lead to ARDS), confusion/disorientation, renal failure
■ Haemorrhagic (due to excess plasmin formation) bleeding (more commonly epistaxis), generalised bleeding/bruising, persistent bleeding from invasive sites (e.g. venepuncture sites, urethral catheters)
■ A mixture of thrombosis and haemorrhaging in various systems.

The major problem and presenting feature of acute DIC is bleeding (Isbister, 2003). When DIC occurs in acutely ill patients with multi-organ dysfunction, the prognosis is poor.

Time out 22.3

1 Assess the patients within your own clinical practice setting.
2 Identify those patients who you think are susceptible to developing DIC.
3 Give reasons why you think this is so.

Diagnosis

Early recognition and prompt intervention is essential if the patient is to have a chance of survival. In addition to the clinical examination, diagnosis is made on the basis of laboratory findings. The main tests are listed in Table 22.2.

There is no single test to diagnose DIC accurately. As haemostasis is a complex phenomenon, test results may be variable and difficult to interpret. Significant DIC can be present despite normal standard coagulation tests, and some patients may show laboratory features of DIC without any clinical sequence (Isbister, 2003). A combination of a clinical condition that may be complicated by DIC with a number of positive laboratory results will establish the presence of DIC with an acceptable level of certainty (Levi *et al.*, 2000).

Table 22.2 Diagnostic tests for Disseminated Intravascular Coagulation (DIC)

• Platelet count (shows thrombocytopenia)
• Fibrinogen levels (decreased)
• Prothrombin time (likely to be prolonged)
• Partial thromboplastin time (prolonged)
• Fibrinopeptide (elevated)
• Fibrin degradation product (FDP) (detectable in the plasma)
• D-Dimer test (specific fibrinogen breakdown test for DIC) (raised)

Management

Whilst there is general agreement on diagnostic criteria, the management of DIC is controversial and complex. It is controversial in that there is a lack of properly conducted research on this particular topic, mainly in relation to treatment. This may be due to the complexity of the syndrome. However, the principles of management appear to be threefold:

1   Identify and treat the cause
2   Optimise the patient's condition
3   Replace clotting factors as appropriate (Kesteven and Saunders, 1993).

In some cases, the DIC will completely resolve within hours after resolution of the underlying condition. Throughout, measures should be undertaken to support organ function, thus maintaining adequate tissue perfusion and preventing further clinical deterioration.

Thrombic

These patients are prone to developing deep vein thrombosis (DVT); their calves should be regularly checked for signs of inflammation, redness, heat, pain. Blockage to the lower extremities may manifest in cold, mottled-looking limb(s). When the patient is stationary, elevating the legs 15–30° together with limb exercises may help to prevent venous stasis. The patient's respiratory status should be monitored very closely for signs of distress resulting from pulmonary emboli.

Drugs may include antifibrinolytic agents (such as aminocaproic acid and transexamic acid) to inhibit fibrinolysis, vitamin K (phytonadione), and folate. Thrombolytic agents, e.g. streptokinase tissue plasminogen activator (TPA), are not indicated with patients with thrombosis as they may facilitate excessive bleeding. The benefits of using heparin are uncertain, and again it may facilitate bleeding (Provan and Henson, 1999).

Haemorrhagic

Assessment of the patient includes looking for signs of bleeding (internally and externally), which may manifest in bruising. Puncture sites (IV sites etc.) should be inspected regularly for visual signs of blood. Urinalysis should be used to check daily for blood. Invasive blood pressure monitoring may be an alternative for these patients, as it reduces the risk of bleeding under the skin caused by external cuff pressures. Changing the patient's position must also be done with caution. Hygiene (particularly oral) should be given (or the patient educated) with caution.

Blood component replacement, i.e. fresh frozen plasma, cryoprecipitate (for patients with markedly decreased fibrinogen levels), may be prescribed. If indicated, red blood replacement, vitamin K and folate should be given.

Complications

These can be either haemorrhagic or thrombic, and include:

- Lung conditions, especially ARDS, pulmonary emboli and pulmonary hypertension
- Kidney conditions (intrarenal failure)
- Liver failure
- Cerebral conditions (microthrombi may cause confusion or cerebrovascular accidents)
- Hypoxia and anoxia, which may lead to severe striated muscle pain
- Shock and coma
- After fibrinolysis, severe to fatal haemorrhaging of vital organs can occur without warning.

Implications for practice

- Nurses should be open and alert to the needs of the patient with sickle cell anaemia, particularly pain control
- Through clinical supervision and reflective practice, the care of patients during sickle cell crisis and those patients with DIC should improve
- Any critically ill patient has the potential to develop DIC; therefore nurses must carefully monitor patients for unexplained haemorrhaging or interference with normal tissue perfusion
- Early recognition of DIC is essential if the patient is to have a chance of survival
- Strategies must be adopted to try and prevent further injury to the patient, particularly during invasive procedures.

Summary

Sickle cell anaemia and DIC are disorders of the blood which can pose a challenge for nurses. Both are potentially life-threatening. Early detection and administration of treatment is required to enable a reasonably favourable outcome for the patient.

Clinical scenario

Philip Anthony is 35 years old, and has suffered from sickle cell anaemia since his childhood. He is usually admitted to hospital twice a year for treatment of sickle cell crises. This time, on admission he is complaining of severe abdominal pain. The pain ruler score is ten. His pulse is 135 bpm (sinus tachycardia), BP 150/100 mmHg, temperature 38.2°C. His Hb is 5 g/dl, and the sickle cell test is positive.

Philip is very anxious and very vocal in his expression of pain.

1 Identify the priorities for the nursing management during Philip's sickle cell crisis.

2 Discuss the specific care required by Philip during an exchange transfusion. Include the identification of potential problems and evidence with your answer.

3 Evaluate Philip's condition, and suggest health promotion strategies to help reduce the occurrence of another sickle cell crisis.

Bibliography

Further reading

Hoffbrand *et al.* (2001) provides a comprehensive detailed account of haematological disorders.

Tigner (1998) gives information about nursing care.

Chapter 23

Acute renal failure

Sandra Gallacher

Contents

Learning outcomes

After reading this chapter you will be able to:

- Understand the functions of the kidneys and renal system
- Demonstrate knowledge of the causes and effects of acute renal failure
- Use this knowledge to anticipate the appropriate medical and nursing management.

Fundamental knowledge

Structures of the renal system; glomerular filtration.

Introduction

The nature of critical illness predisposes to renal failure. Although the renal system is complex, understanding it can explain many of the symptoms patients present with (Challinor, 1998). This chapter will discuss the common causes of renal failure in the critically ill, and current methods of medical and nursing management.

Anatomy and physiology of the renal system

The renal system has seven main functions that impact on body systems:

1   Urine formation
2   Urine secretion
3   Regulation of body fluids and electrolytes
4   Excretion of metabolic waste products
5   Regulation of acid–base balance
6   Regulation of blood pressure
7   Hormone secretion.

The formation and secretion of urine occurs in the kidneys and consists of three processes:

1   Simple filtration
2   Selective reabsorption
3   Secretion.

Regulation of body fluid and electrolytes

The renal system is able to regulate fluid and electrolyte balance by increasing or restricting the amount of filtrate produced, and by the ability of the renal tubules to absorb or excrete electrolytes and waste products of metabolism (Waugh and Grant, 2001). The end product of this process is urine.

Urine is formed from the blood by a process of filtration followed by selective reabsorption. Filtration occurs under pressure from the glomerulus. The thin vessel walls allow water and other small molecules to pass through, but blood and protein molecules are too large to pass through and are therefore not constituents of urine (Watson, 2000b).

Selective reabsorption occurs in the convoluted tubules, where water, glucose and salts are retained. Healthy individuals will not excrete glucose in urine (Watson, 2000b). Water is reabsorbed in the distal convoluted tubule and this is controlled by the secretion of anti-diuretic hormone (ADH), secreted from the posterior lobe of the pituitary gland (Huether, 1998a). Active secretion also occurs in the tubules. The two most important substances excreted by the renal system are hydrogen and potassium. Although the majority of potassium is reabsorbed, some will be excreted to maintain homeostasis of serum potassium levels

(Barczac, 1998). Metabolites, including chlorine and creatinine, are also excreted in urine (Challinor, 1998).

The efficiency of the renal system is determined principally by the renal blood flow (Walsh, 1997). The kidneys are highly vascular organs, and in adults receive 1,000–1,200 ml of blood per minute. This represents approximately 25 per cent of the cardiac output (Huether, 1998a). There are three mechanisms in place that can protect renal blood flow for a short period of time:

1   The process of auto-regulation can compensate for fluctuations in blood pressure and maintain renal blood flow at a constant pressure of 70–80 mmHg (Weiskittel, 2001). Critically ill patients may suffer periods of hypotension, which adversely affect renal function. If blood pressure falls, the afferent arterioles dilate to maintain blood flow. If blood pressure increases, the afferent arterioles constrict to prevent an increase in glomerular blood flow and filtration pressure (Huether, 1998a). In this way, fluctuations in the glomerular filtration rate are avoided and water and electrolyte balance is maintained (Short and Cumming, 1999). Prolonged or profound hypotension can, however, challenge the efficiency of this mechanism.

2   Renal blood flow is also protected by neural regulation (Huether, 1998a). A decrease in systemic arterial pressure results in an increase in renal sympathetic nerve activity, which responds to the carotid sinus and the baroreceptors of the aortic arch. The result is renal arteriolar vasoconstriction. This leads to a decrease in glomerular filtrate, and less sodium and water are excreted (Challinor, 1998). The retention of sodium and water increases the circulating blood volume and thus the blood pressure.

3   The third protective mechanism is the hormonal response, known as the renin–angiotensin cycle (Donnison and Criswell, 2002). Renin is an enzyme formed in the cells of the juxtaglomerular apparatus, which is a collection of specialised cells at the afferent arteriole (Huether, 1998a). Renin is also stored here. When renin is released, following a fall in blood pressure or sodium concentration, it combines with angiotensinogen to form angiotensin I. This is then converted to angiotensin II by angiotensin converting enzyme (ACE). ACE originates in the capillary endothelial cells of the lung (Challinor, 1998). Angiotensin II is a potent vasoconstrictor. This mechanism can stabilise systemic blood pressure by increasing systemic vasoconstriction and indirectly increasing sodium reabsorption, thereby increasing the circulating volume and increasing systemic vascular resistance (Huether, 1998a). The amount of water and electrolytes excreted by the renal system is also influenced by antidiuretic hormone (ADH). This is secreted from the posterior pituitary gland and increases water permeability along the collecting ducts of the kidney.

Small amounts of potassium are also excreted by the kidneys. Most potassium is reabsorbed to maintain serum potassium levels of 3.5–4.5 mmol/l (Challinor, 1998).

The release of erythropoietin, which stimulates the bone marrow to produce red blood cells, is stimulated by decreased oxygen delivery to the kidneys

(Huether, 1998a). Anaemia from this cause is rare in acute renal failure, but fluid overload can result in low haemoglobin levels. This is known as dilutional anaemia (Schira, 2000).

Time out 23.1

1   Read more about the renal system. Waugh and Grant (2001) provides a useful resource (most anatomy and physiology books would be sufficient).
2   List the actual and potential problems you would anticipate that a patient diagnosed with acute renal failure would experience.

Pathophysiology of acute renal failure

Acute renal failure can be defined as 'a reduction in glomerular filtration, with a resulting inability to excrete nitrogenous waste or maintain an adequate fluid and acid–base balance, occurring over hours or days' (Barry, 1998: 99). It can be the primary reason for admission to hospital, or it can be a complication of critical illness, such as septic shock (Schira, 2000). Acute renal failure is potentially reversible (Challinor, 1998), depending upon the cause. Despite this, mortality remains high in the critically ill patient, at around 60 per cent (Kishen, 2002).

Acute renal failure can be classified as pre-renal, intrarenal or post-renal (Short and Cumming, 1999):

■   *Pre-renal failure* results from a decreased renal blood flow. This causes a reduction in glomerular filtration rate. As there is no structural damage to the kidney, it is usually reversible (Challinor, 1998). Pre-renal failure can therefore result from prolonged hypotension caused by septic shock, cardiogenic shock, volume depletion, burns and haemorrhage (Schira, 2000).
■   *Intrarenal (or intrinsic) renal failure* occurs following damage to the nephrons (Schira, 2000). This damage is commonly caused by ischaemia or nephrotoxicity, which can itself result from delayed or inadequate treatment of pre-renal injury (Bellomo, 2003). Acute tubular necrosis is commonly seen in critically ill patients due to the prolonged ischaemia often seen with sepsis (Seaton-Mills, 1999), although glomerulonephritis and vasculitis can also occur in critically ill patients (Bellomo, 2003).
■   *Post-renal failure* occurs when the ureters are blocked, for example by tumour, enlarged prostate, strictures or calculi (Challinor, 1998).

Management of acute renal failure

Once acute renal failure is diagnosed, it is vital to manage symptoms, such as hyperkalaemia, until renal function returns (Challinor, 1998). Kidney failure may last 10–12 days, with full recovery in 6–12 months. Medical management of renal failure consists of treating symptoms of acute renal failure and supporting renal blood flow and function by maintaining blood pressure (Bellomo, 2003).

In most critical care areas, vulnerable patients will be monitored for increasing blood urea and creatinine levels (Barry, 1998). Creatinine is produced at a constant rate as a product of muscle metabolism (Huether, 1998a). The amount filtered is approximately equal to the amount excreted; therefore an increasing serum creatinine level indicates a reduction in the glomerular filtration rate. It can take several days for the creatinine level to stabilise. This could mean that a patient who has been profoundly hypotensive, although successfully resuscitated, will still experience a rise in creatinine level for several days.

Although the damage to the kidney may have been reduced or reversed by the prompt restoration of renal blood flow, the creatinine may continue to rise. Therefore, it is important to examine other factors to assess the effectiveness of treatment (Huether, 1998a). Serum urea can be used as an indicator of renal function (Walsh, 2002). Urea is produced as a result of protein metabolism and excreted by the kidneys, and an increase in urea can indicate renal failure.

There are other factors that can lead to an increased serum urea. In a patient who is volume-depleted, blood urea nitrogen can rise out of proportion to any change in renal function. Blood urea nitrogen can also be increased by increased metabolism, for example, caused by pyrexia and certain drugs (Woodrow, 2000). A more accurate way of determining renal function is via urine collection, usually for 24 hours (Walsh, 2002). This can provide a figure for the creatinine clearance, which can be applied to the filtration capacity of the kidney. Urine output can also indicate renal failure; however, oliguria does not always occur (Short and Cumming, 1999). Routine urinalysis can also provide evidence of primary renal disease, if proteinuria or haematuria is present. A decreased specific gravity may also indicate acute tubular necrosis (Barry, 1998).

The primary aim of management is prevention (Bellomo, 2003). This is achieved by maintaining the renal blood flow by supporting blood pressure whilst treating the underlying cause. Blood pressure can be supported by volume replacement, usually with blood, blood products or colloids (Barry, 1998). In some cases volume resuscitation will not be sufficient to maintain an adequate blood pressure, and inotropic support may be necessary. Dopamine is an inotropic catecholamine which was frequently used to support renal function in the critically ill (Hoogenberg and Girbes, 1998). Until recently dopamine was thought to improve renal blood flow, but there is little evidence to support this (Bellomo, 2003). The use of 'renal dose' dopamine cannot be supported by evidence (Kishen, 2002).

The use of frusemide has been shown to reduce sodium reabsorption at the tubular level; this reduces the oxygen demand of the tubules, which is felt to be one of the leading causes of acute renal failure (Kishen, 2002). The use of mannitol is also controversial (Donnison and Criswell, 2002). Although urine output can be improved, renal function usually is not. Fluid removal is often of benefit to the hypervolaemic patient (Walsh, 1997).

Nursing management of acute renal failure involves monitoring the effectiveness of medical management and promoting patient comfort and compliance throughout treatments. The nurse is of primary importance in detecting complications and ensuring prompt action. In some areas nurses may receive the blood results, and it is vital that they are aware of the normal values of blood potassium, magnesium, urea and creatinine (see Chapter 35).

Fluid balance charts must be strictly maintained on every patient so that imbalances or oliguria can be detected promptly (Walsh, 1997). Fluid retention or overload can also be detected by monitoring the respiratory rate and depth, and the production of white, frothy sputum, sometimes coloured pink by blood, can indicate pulmonary oedema. A significant increase in the depth and volume of respirations may also indicate a metabolic acidosis, which can develop with renal failure (Walsh, 1997). However, most patients admitted to critical care areas from general wards are dehydrated (Kishen, 2002).

Fluid status can be determined by central venous pressure (CVP) monitoring. CVP can also show a patient's response to the administration of fluid, and thereby assist with the diagnosis of dehydration. Recording weight daily can be misleading in the critically ill, due to the administration of fluid and consequent oedema.

Patients with acute renal failure are also at increased risk of impaired skin integrity. This is caused by a variety of factors, including malnutrition, immobility, infection and oedema, The tongue and oral mucosa are also at risk of damage and infection. This can be due to fluid restrictions, but is exacerbated by the decreased salivary production associated with acute renal failure (Walsh, 1997). Frequent mouth care will be necessary, as ulcerative lesions can develop. This may make patients reluctant to eat due to discomfort or lack of taste, exacerbating the malnourished state associated with renal failure (Bellomo, 2003).

Cardiac function can be affected by potassium retention (irregular pulse), and fluid overload (increased blood pressure) can lead to cardiac failure in susceptible patients (Schira, 2000). In extreme cases, this can lead to fatal cardiac arrhythmias.

Implications for practice

- Critically ill patients are at risk of renal system failure
- Nurses must be educated to deliver safe and effective care for these patients
- Nurses are uniquely placed rapidly to detect changes in renal function and to instigate appropriate interventions.

Summary

The critically ill patient is at risk of developing acute renal failure for a variety of reasons, and it is often prompt detection by nursing staff that allows treatment to be commenced and the condition reversed. The renal system affects other systems in the body, and it is the nurse at the bedside who is best placed to monitor all clinical parameters and promote patient comfort.

Clinical scenario

Mrs Baker is a 75-year-old lady who has been admitted to hospital follow-ing periods of hypotension and shortness of breath on a medical ward. Her blood pressure is stabilised with IV fluids, but she is becoming increasingly breathless. There is no fluid balance chart from the ward, and she states that she has not passed urine for several hours.

1 What action would you take to assess Mrs Baker's renal function?

2 Discuss the type of intervention required to control her symptoms.

3 Devise criteria to suggest successful intervention.

Bibliography

Key reading

Short and Cumming (1999).
Walsh (1997).

Further reading

Weiskittle (2001).

Chapter 24

Upper gastrointestinal bleeds and acute pancreatitis

Philip Woodrow

Contents

Learning outcomes

After reading this chapter you will be able to:

- Understand why patients with upper gastrointestinal bleeds and acute pancreatitis may need urgent treatment
- Recognise and understand the priorities of care, including assessment and observation, involved with gastrointestinal emergencies
- Devise a plan of nursing care for patients admitted with these conditions.

Fundamental knowledge

Anatomy and physiology of the upper gastrointestinal tract; anatomy and physiology of the pancreas.

Introduction

The two most frequent gastrointestinal emergencies are upper gastrointestinal bleeds and pancreatitis.

Pathophysiology is briefly described here, but discussion focuses on nursing interventions. Although underlying causes of these two conditions may be chronic, possibly necessitating later medical or surgical treatments, the rapidity with which these conditions can deteriorate or prove fatal means that identification and prompt and appropriate treatment can improve survival and reduce complications. Once immediate dangers to life have been removed, care and treatment increasingly focuses on causes, underlying problems, and needs.

The gastrointestinal tract is highly vascular, and so susceptible to bleeds. Upper gastrointestinal bleeds are the most common gastrointestinal emergency (British Society of Gastroenterology Endoscopy Committee, 2000). Bleeds in the lower gastrointestinal tract are usually from chronic conditions, so although they can be life-threatening and may require major surgery or aggressive medical treatment, they are less likely to need emergency admission. Lower gastrointestinal bleeds are not discussed in this chapter, but many principles of managing upper tract bleeds apply to lower ones as well, although there is less likelihood of needing urgent resuscitation for the latter. Upper gastrointestinal haemorrhage from oesophageal varices or ulcers (gastric or duodenal) may develop rapidly and can prove fatal.

Pancreatitis may be acute or chronic. Acute pancreatitis usually resolves spontaneously, but one-fifth of mild cases progress into severe acute disease (Uhl *et al.*, 1999). Progression of acute pancreatitis is unpredictable and often rapid.

The potential dangers and urgency surrounding upper gastrointestinal bleeds and acute pancreatitis means that nurses looking after these patients need to be able to detect early signs of deterioration and know what treatments to initiate. Upper gastrointestinal bleeds are often large, obvious and may be immediately life-threatening, but bleeds can be smaller and slower, causing anaemia, but with blood passing down the gastrointestinal tract. As little as 60 ml of blood may cause melaena (Hudak *et al.*, 1998), which may be the first sign of bleeding. Many patients are reluctant to discuss abnormal stools but, if asked whether they have noticed any blood, darkness or other abnormality, may report symptoms. Normal bowel transit time is about 24 hours, with individual variations sometimes extending to several days. Constipation may reduce gut motility further, resulting in signs not appearing in stools until several days after bleeds have begun.

Oesophageal varices

Varices are usually caused by chronic alcoholic liver disease (Giacchino and Houdek, 1998). Cirrhosis obstructs blood flow through the liver, increasing the pressure in veins that flow from the gut to the liver. Increased venous pressure makes them engorged, and some eventually rupture. Collateral circulation relieves venous congestion, but this delays rather than prevents problems. Varices usually form around the lower part of the oesophagus, but can also form in the stomach.

Normal portal pressure is about 5 mmHg, and bleeds often occur once pressure exceeds 12 mmHg (Smith, 2000). When varices rupture, high venous pressure causes a large, often fatal, haemorrhage. Varices develop in about half of patients with cirrhosis (Fallah *et al.*, 2000), with about one-third dying from the initial haemorrhage (Giacchino and Houdek, 1998) and about one-third having severe bleeds (Ghost *et al.*, 2002), of which 30–50 per cent prove fatal (Fallah *et al.*, 2000). Most survivors (70 per cent) rebleed (Sharara, 2001).

Sudden and major haemorrhage usually necessitates:

- Interventions to stop haemorrhage (Sengstarken tube or sclerosing injections)
- Fluid resuscitation
- System support (especially oxygen)
- Replacement of clotting factors.

Balloon tamponade

Various types of tube are marketed to place pressure on oesophageal bleeding points. These tubes are often popularly called Sengstarken tubes (see Figure 24.1), although there are other types. They consist of a large tube which is placed orally through the oesophagus and into the stomach, and usually have two balloons that can then be inflated, one in the oesophagus and one in the stomach, placing direct pressure (tamponade) on bleeding points. There are also usually ports to aspirate both the oesophagus and stomach. Like nasogastric tubes, these are easier to insert if cold (Smith, 2000) and are therefore best stored refrigerated.

Balloon tamponade stops most (70–80 per cent) oesophageal bleeds (Fallah *et al.*, 2000), but half rebleed when the tube is removed (Stanley and Hayes, 1997), so tamponade is an emergency measure to enable other more effective treatments to be instigated (Vargas *et al.*, 1999).

Prolonged pressure may cause ulceration, so use of tamponade is usually limited to 12 hours (Therapondos and Hayes, 2002). Sometimes balloons are periodically deflated or pressure within the balloon is monitored, but both these actions are controversial. Deflation may restart bleeding, and there is little consensus about optimal pressure (Sung, 1997); pressure often needs to exceed capillary pressure to stop bleeding. Traction is sometimes used (Hudak *et al.*, 1998), but this is also controversial.

Blood loss and impaired consciousness normally necessitates nursing these patients in the recovery position. Blood and other fluids in the oesophagus should be removed to prevent aspiration into the lungs. This may be achieved through continuous low suction, or through periodic removal.

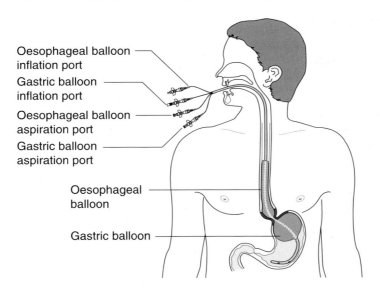

Oesophageal balloon inflation port

Gastric balloon inflation port

Oesophageal balloon aspiration port

Gastric balloon aspiration port

Oesophageal balloon

Gastric balloon

Figure 24.1 **Balloon tamponade ('Sengstarken') tube**

Vasoactive drugs, such as terlipressin, to constrict smooth muscle (Vargas *et al.*, 1999), nitrates, to vasodilate (Sharara, 2001), and beta-blockers, to reduce hypertension (Vargas *et al.*, 1999; Therapondos and Hayes, 2002) may be used to prevent rebleeding, but require close cardiovascular (ECG, BP) monitoring. Other drugs (such as somatostatin and octreotide) have been used, but there is currently insufficient evidence to support this.

Endoscopy

Endoscopy enables bleeding points to be seen and directly treated. The main endoscopic treatments are:

- Injecting sclerosants
- Laser treatment
- Ligation ('banding').

Endoscopy is the most effective way to stop bleeding oesophageal varices, but may take some time to organise and will usually be performed in the endoscopy department.

Sclerosants are usually an alcohol (such as ethanolamine), which is injected into bleeding varices to cause atrophy. Endoscopic sclerotherapy stops most bleeds (90 per cent) (Sharara, 2001), but ligation, which draws varices into the endoscope and then places ligatures (bands) around them, is more effective than sclerotherapy (Gimson *et al.*, 1993) and therefore remains the treatment of choice (Stanley and Hayes, 1997). Laser treatment has largely replaced diathermy.

Shunts

Transjugular intrahepatic portosystemic shunt (TIPPS) uses a catheter to create a fistula between the portal vein and hepatic artery. TIPPS is the best treatment for recurrent bleeds (Vargas *et al.*, 1999) and the treatment of choice if endoscopy fails (Therapondos and Hayes, 2002). Surgery is rarely performed for variceal bleeding.

Ulcers

Ulceration may occur anywhere in the gastrointestinal tract, but ulcers causing acute upper gastrointestinal haemorrhage usually occur in the stomach or duodenum. Most upper gastrointestinal bleeds are caused by peptic ulcers (British Society of Gastroenterology Endoscopy Committee, 2000; Ghost *et al.*, 2002). Hydrochloric acid, secreted by the stomach, is a very strong acid (pH 2). Mucus protects the stomach from acid erosion, but failure of this mucosal barrier exposes the stomach wall to acid. Pancreatic juice, secreted into the duodenum, is strongly alkaline (pH 8), so failure of protective mucus in the duodenum can cause acid erosion above the pancreatic duct or alkali erosion below. A quarter of people with duodenal ulcers develop haemorrhage or other major complications (Shiotani and Graham, 2002).

Failure of the mucosal barrier is particularly associated with non-steroidal anti-inflammatory drugs (NSAIDs) and with the gram-negative bacterium *Helicobacter Pylori*. For people needing long-term anti-inflammatory drugs (e.g. arthritis sufferers) cox-2 inhibitors (e.g. Valdecoxib) cause less risk of gastric ulceration than NSAIDs (Sikes *et al.*, 2002), so the incidence of drug-related ulcers may decline. Most other duodenal ulcers (95 per cent) are associated with *Helicobacter Pylori* (Harris and Misiewicz, 2001). *Helicobacter Pylori* colonisation is widespread, affecting 20–50 per cent of people in industrialised countries (Suerbaum and Michetti, 2002), but infection only causes problems for a minority, making widespread eradication impractical.

Acute illness stimulates a stress response, which increases gastric acid secretion. If patients are eating little, or are nil by mouth, absence of food to reduce gastric acidity together with excessive hydrochloric acid production increases risk of ulceration. Debate about the best prophylaxis for stress ulcers remains inconclusive. Some studies recommend H_2-blockers such as ranitidine (e.g. Cook *et al.*, 1998), while others indicate that this is ineffective (e.g. Messori *et al.*, 2000) or may cause other problems such as obstruction or albumin toxicity (Bradley, 2001). If enteral feeding is possible, even suboptimal amounts for nutrition may prevent gut ulceration (Guzman and Kruse, 2001). Even following gut surgery, early feeding is usually recommended (Lewis *et al.*, 2001).

Complications

Severe haemorrhage usually causes hypovolaemic shock. Even if this does not prove fatal, perfusion failure to other main organs often causes:

- Renal failure (acute tubular necrosis)
- Increased myocardial work, possibly resulting in infarction
- Liver failure, resulting in many complications (see Chapter 26)
- Hypoxaemia (from anaemia).

Complications may progress into multi-organ dysfunction syndrome (MODS), a level 3 illness (see Preface and Chapter 37), which makes survival unlikely.

Neurological complications

Blood in the gut is protein, which may be digested. Protein metabolism produces ammonia, which with impaired liver function may not be metabolised, resulting in neurotoxicity. Toxic ammonia levels increase the blood–brain barrier permeability, leading to encephalopathy, confusion and possible coma.

Therefore, once bleeding has been stabilised, blood should be removed from the gut. This may be through irrigation (e.g. via the gastric port on a Sengstarken tube), through oral laxatives, or through magnesium sulphate enemas. McArdle (1999) recommends aiming for more than one stool each day.

Nursing care

Major gastrointestinal bleeds often need urgent resuscitation, involving:

- Oxygen administration
- Fluids (preferably colloids, with probable need for blood and platelet transfusion)
- Close monitoring, including respiratory rate and depth, heart rate and rhythm, and blood pressure.

Medical help should be summoned urgently. Lying the patient flat and raising the foot of the bed may sustain cerebral circulation until fluids are prescribed. As far as possible, the patient's privacy and dignity should be maintained.

Anything that may provoke bleeding, such as passing nasogastric tubes, should be avoided unless the benefits outweigh the potential risks.

Blood may distress patients and families, so soiled linen should be removed, the patient offered a wash, and the environment cleaned as necessary. The taste of blood can be removed with a drink or mouthwash (including brushing teeth). The patient should be reassured, with information being honest and realistic. Visitors should be informed about what has occurred, warned that their loved one may look and often feel very ill, and that they may see some blood. As distressed visitors might faint, staff should accompany them to the bedside and encourage them to sit down.

Pancreatitis

Pancreatitis is a relatively common and increasing prevalent disease (Larvin, 1999; Palmer *et al.*, 2002), which may be so mild it causes only vague abdominal pain. Very mild cases may not seek medical help or be admitted to hospital, but more severe cases require urgent admission with provision of high dependency (level 2) and sometimes intensive (level 3) care. A minority of people with pancreatitis progress, often rapidly, from appearing relatively well (other than some abdominal pain) to severe acute pancreatitis. Progression is unpredictable, and can occur within a few hours. Therefore, when pancreatitis is suspected or confirmed, nurses should observe and monitor patients closely and frequently as well as providing physical and psychological care.

The pancreas is both an endocrine and an exocrine organ. *Endocrine functions* are production of the hormones glucagon (alpha cells), insulin (beta cells) and somatostatin (delta cells). Although endocrine function may be affected, pancreatitis primarily affects exocrine function. *Exocrine function* is the secretion of digestive enzymes, including amylase, into the duodenum. These powerful pancreatic enzymes are alkaline (pH 8), to neutralise gastric acid. With pancreatitis, the pancreatic or common bile duct is blocked. Uneutralised acid in the duodenum continues to stimulate production of digestive pancreatic enzymes, which eventually rupture the pancreatic duct and begin to autodigest surrounding tissue – mainly the pancreas itself and peri-pancreatic fat. Fistulae may form into surrounding tissues, including the colon. Bacteria entering necrotic tissue usually suppurate. With pancreatitis, serum amylase rises rapidly, often doubling or quadrupling within 2–12 hours (Cole, 2002). Serum lipase is also raised (>110 units/litre) with pancreatitis, while raised alanine aminotransferase (>80 iu/litre) indicates gallstone-induced pancreatitis (Mergener and Baillic, 1998).

Pancreatitis is typically associated with either cholecystitis/biliary disease, where stones or sludge obstruct the common bile duct, or alcoholism, where alcohol atrophies pancreatic ductules, resulting in obstruction. However, only a minority of people with gallstones or chronic alcoholism develop pancreatitis (Fernandez del Castillo, 1993). Biliary causes often occur in women in their fifties (Steinberg and Tenner, 1994; Hale *et al.*, 2000), while alcohol-related pancreatitis typically occurs to men in their forties (Hale *et al.*, 2000). However, pancreatitis may occur at any age and from various other causes, including tumours and scorpion stings (Santamaria, 1997).

Classification

The Atlanta consensus classification is widely used, and should be followed in the UK (Association of Surgeons of Great Britain and Ireland, Association of Upper Gastrointestinal Surgeons of Great Britain and Ireland, British Society of Gastroenterology, and the Pancreatic Society of Great Britain and Ireland, 1998):

- Acute
- Mild acute
- Severe acute
- Acute fluid collection
- Pancreatic necrosis

■ Acute pseudocyst
■ Pancreatic abscess.

People with mild pancreatitis often recover with minimal or no intervention, but should be observed and monitored in case they develop severe pancreatitis. Later complications, such as fluid collection, pseudocysts and abscesses, should also be observed and monitored for, but may occur following discharge.

Pancreatitis may be sterile or become infected, usually from gut bacteria (Uhl *et al.*, 1998). About half of people with severe pancreatitis develop bacterial infections (Steinberg and Tenner, 1994), so infection control should be maintained, and temperature and other signs of infection should be monitored. Uhl *et al.* (1999) suggest that preventing infection is the most promising treatment for pancreatitis. Severe pancreatitis stimulates gross hypermetabolism, so pyrexia (often 38–39°C) may occur without infection.

Complications

Severe pancreatitis can rapidly affect most major organs and systems in the body. The main problems are usually:

■ Pain
■ Cardiovascular failure
■ Respiratory failure
■ Metabolic failure.

(Mergener and Baillic, 1998)

Pain

Most patients with severe pancreatitis experience severe, and rapidly progressing, abdominal pain. Attempting to relieve this pain, they often sit forward, with their knees bent (Banks, 1998). Pain usually causes nausea and (often) vomiting. Half of patients experience pain radiating to their back (Mergener and Baillic, 1998).

Opiates, generally morphine, are usually needed to relieve pain (Banks, 1998). Anti-emetics should also be available.

Cardiovascular failure

Inflammation and stress cause large shifts of fluid from the bloodstream into tissues, causing:

■ Hypovolaemia and shock
■ Ascites
■ Pericardial effusions, often causing dysrhythmias and raised ST segment on ECG
■ Electrolyte imbalances.

Autodigestion can also cause an aneurysm. The pancreas produces a hormone called myocardial depressant factor, which reduces cardiac contractility. Pancreatitis causes excessive production of this, further contributing to hypotension.

Fluid resuscitation should be mainly with colloids (Johnson, 1998), both to sustain blood volume and prevent further tissue oedema. Large volumes of intravenous fluids are often needed (Mergener and Baillic, 1998; Beckingham and Bornman, 2001) to prevent pre-renal failure progressing to acute tubular necrosis (ATN) (Mann *et al.*, 1994). Close monitoring, including continuous ECG, fluid balance and central venous pressure, will usually be needed. Acute tubular necrosis significantly increases mortality and delays recovery (Mann *et al.*, 1994).

Respiratory failure

Breathing may be compromised by

- Pain
- Diaphragmatic splinting from ascites
- Left lower lobe collapse from pleural effusions (Wilson and Imrie, 1991)
- Pleural effusions (Steinberg and Tanner, 1994)
- Pulmonary oedema (Mann *et al.*, 1994).

If the patient is hypoxic, supplementary oxygen should be given (Tham and Collins, 2000). Close and frequent respiratory monitoring should include rate, depth and oxygen saturation. Left lung base collapse can be identified on chest X-ray. Further support, such as non-invasive ventilation, may be needed.

Metabolic failure

Impaired insulin release, insulin antagonism and excessive glucagon release often cause hyperglycaemia (Santamaria, 1997). Aggressive insulin therapy and frequent (possibly hourly) blood glucose monitoring may be needed. Survival from critical illness is improved if blood sugar is maintained between 4.4 and 6.1 mmol/litre (van den Berghe, 2001), although application of this to severe pancreatitis remains presumptive. Many electrolyte imbalances occur, partly from fluid shifts and partly from poor diet or impaired intake. Blood calcium, needed for cardiac conduction, clotting and cell repair, is often low (Mergener and Baillic, 1998; Hale *et al.*, 2000). Biochemistry (urea + electrolytes; glucose) should be checked and stabilised.

Medical treatment

Treating pancreatitis remains problematic. Gallstones may be removed using endoscopic retrograde cholangiopancreatography (ERCP). Various drugs have been trialled and most abandoned, so treatment is largely limited to supporting failing systems and preventing/limiting further complications (Steinberg and Tanner, 1994).

Nursing management

With severe pancreatitis, extensive medical treatments necessitate nursing care being focused largely on administering prescribed drugs and fluids, and monitoring patients' progress, pain assessment and relief. Nurses' knowledge of their patients' social history, together with the close rapport they often build with families, can valuably contribute to diagnosis and treatment. Patients with severe pancreatitis are often able to do little for themselves, so maintaining, as far as possible, normal activities of living (such as hygiene and mouthcare) contributes to the quality of care.

Less severe cases may progress rapidly, so patients should be closely observed and early indications of progression, such as symptoms of shock or deteriorating blood results, reported quickly to medical staff.

Nutrition is needed for recovery. Patients with pancreatitis should be fed enterally if their gut is able to absorb, parenterally if it cannot (Windsor *et al.*, 1998; Wyncoll, 1999).

Implications for practice

- Large bleeds and severe pancreatitis need urgent fluid resuscitation and close haemodynamic monitoring
- Balloon tamponade can quickly stop many variceal bleeds, but is only a temporary measure until endoscopic treatment is available
- When balloon tamponade is removed, many patients rebleed
- Following gastric bleeds, patients should be offered drinks or mouthcare to remove the taste of blood
- Severe pancreatitis causes acute pain, usually needing opiate analgesia and often anti-emetics
- Hyperglycaemia may occur with pancreatitis, while people with gastric bleeding may be malnourished, so blood sugar should be assessed; with pancreatitis, blood sugar may need to be monitored regularly, and insulin infusions may be needed
- Nurses should ensure nutrition is optimised, if possible orally or enterally (gastric or jejunal tubes)
- Blood is a hazardous substance, so acute bleeds may place staff and visitors at risk; patients at risk of severe bleeding should therefore be nursed in an area where risks from blood cross-infection can be minimised.

Summary

Upper gastrointestinal bleeds and pancreatitis often require urgent intervention. Most cases of pancreatitis remain mild, but an unpredictable minority progress rapidly to acute severe pancreatitis, with significant mortality. Medical treatment of severe acute pancreatitis is difficult, and remains largely limited to supporting failing systems. Nursing care focuses on providing relief from pain and nausea, any other care that patients need, and close observation and monitoring so that any deterioration can be reported and treated promptly.

Clinical scenario

Charles Hill, aged 49, is admitted with acute pancreatitis. On arrival he is in obvious pain, despite having been given 10 mg morphine intramuscularly half-an-hour previously. The medical team has prescribed an aggressive fluid regime of Gelofusine® 500 ml over 1 hour, and this was commenced immediately before transfer. The team will review him further within that hour, by which time results from the serum amylase test should be available. He is separated from his wife and gives his next-of-kin as his daughter, whom he describes as 'close', and who manages a care home 'about 50 miles away'.

1   List the immediate priorities of nursing care you would give Mr Hill. Identify your rationales for care.

2   Mr Hill's vital signs are: HR 115 bpm regular, BP 90/60 mmHg, RR 35 per min, temperature 38.5°C. His blood sugar is 24 mmol/l. He is oliguric, having passed 15 ml during the last hour. The medical team has just arrived and Mr Hill is being reviewed. What treatments do you anticipate the team will offer Mr Hill? Include rationales for interventions.

3   The medical team's decisions coincide with your expectations. Devise a plan of care for Mr Hill for the next 12 hours, remembering the possible complications that may occur. Mr Hill's daughter is expected shortly; include information and support that you will offer her.

Bibliography

Key reading

For UK nurses, the UK medical guidelines (Association of Surgeons, 1998) provide the best resource on pancreatitis. Similar guidelines are available in many other countries. Uhl is currently one of the leading European gastroenterologists; his 1998 article provides a useful resource. Other useful medical reviews include Chan and Leung (2002), Baron (1999) and Stanley and Hayes (1997). Although a decade old, Steinberg and Tenner (1994) remains authoritative.

Further reading

Leading specialist medical journals are *Gut* and *Gastroenterology*. A recent valuable addition to nursing journals is *Gastrointestinal Nursing*. Reviews written primarily for medical students and junior doctors appear in various widely accessible medical journals, such as *Medicine* and *Hospital Medicine*. Fewer nursing articles have appeared, but Wright (1998) and McArdle (1999, 2000) provide useful reviews.

Chapter 25

Diabetic emergencies

Tina Moore

Contents

Learning outcomes

After reading this chapter you will be able to:

- Identify the causes of diabetic ketoacidosis, hyperosmolar non-ketotic syndrome (HONK) and hypoglycaemia
- Prioritise nursing assessment and intervention for each diabetic emergency
- Understand the fundamental principles of fluid resuscitation and management in DKA and HONK.

Fundamental knowledge

Blood glucose regulation, acid–base balance, aetiology of diabetes mellitus.

Introduction

A significant number of patients are admitted to the critical care unit (or classified as level 2) following a diabetic emergency. In a number of these instances the patients will be newly diagnosed. Emergencies such as hypoglycaemia are rarely admitted to critical care units, as the condition is easily corrected. Some diabetic emergencies will be very quick in onset, some more insidious, but all could have fatal consequences if not identified quickly and treated appropriately.

There are essentially two types of diabetes: diabetes mellitus and diabetes insipidus. Diabetes insipidus is a disorder where there may be a deficiency of antidiuretic hormone (ADH) or failure of the renal tubules to respond to ADH, resulting in polyuria and potential dehydration and hypovolaemia. Persistent severe diabetes insipidus is rare. Diabetes mellitus is an endocrine problem resulting in disorders of carbohydrate, fat and protein metabolism due to a deficiency in the secretion of insulin. Type 1 diabetes refers to the absence or inadequate production of insulin. Insulin is required to enable the uptake of glucose in the cells. Type 2 diabetes usually occurs in older, often overweight, individuals. It is normally treated through diet, weight control and exercise, sometimes with oral hypoglycaemic medication.

Diabetic ketoacidosis

Diabetic ketoacidosis (DKA) is a common complication of diabetes mellitus (mainly type 1) and results from severe insulin deficiency leading to the disordered metabolism of proteins, carbohydrates and fats. The outcomes of such pathological events are hyperglycaemia, hyperosmolality, ketoacidosis and volume depletion (Lewis, 2000). DKA is the largest single cause of death amongst those with diabetes and aged less than 20 years (Marinac and Mesa, 2000). DKA constitutes an emergency, life-threatening condition, the onset of which usually occurs over the course of hours or sometimes days. Patients suspected of having DKA should be assessed appropriately and quickly by observing for symptoms (such as glycosuria, ketonuria, reduction in blood pressure) in order to confirm diagnosis so that treatment can be started as soon as possible.

Precipitating factors

DKA is common amongst newly diagnosed diabetics. Causative factors include anything that would initiate a physiological stress response (e.g. sepsis). Hypersecretion of glucagons and cortisol results in increasing glucose production. Hence the amount of insulin produced is insufficient to metabolise the glucose. There is also an increase in catecholamines, stimulating a decrease in insulin production (see Chapter 3). Patients may have a history of uncontrolled insulin-dependent diabetes mellitus (type 1). Accidental or deliberate omission of insulin (e.g. patients undergoing surgery) can precipitate DKA.

Clinical features

These can be categorised as general and severe.

General symptoms can be less overt in the older population. This is because some symptoms may be equated to disorders of ageing, and other diseases may mask symptoms (e.g. urinary frequency may be equated to prostatism in men or infection in women). Kussmaul breathing may be mistaken for respiratory problems associated with heart failure or chest infection. The classical symptoms of DKA are listed in Box 25.1.

Box 25.1 Classical symptoms of DKA

- Abdominal pain, usually generalised or epigastric
- Rigid abdomen and irregular bowel sounds
- Polyuria
- Polydipsia
- Nocturia
- Blurring of vision
- Cramps in legs
- Nausea and vomiting.

Some symptoms may imitate gastrointestinal problems, causing diagnosis to be difficult.

Widely accepted criteria for severe DKA include pH <7.3, bicarbonate (HCO_3) <15 mmol/l, blood glucose >14 mmol/l (Keays, 2003). (For information on acid–base balance and metabolic acidosis see Chapter 30) ketonuria (Charalambos *et al.*, 1999.) Diagnostic test findings are listed in Box 25.2.

Box 25.2 Diagnostic test findings – DKA

- Serum glucose level elevated (>14 mmol/l)
- Serum ketone level positive
- Urine ketone level positive
- Serum sodium decreased
- Serum potassium level increased initially then decreased because of the diuresis and reversal of acidosis
- Arterial blood gas reveals metabolic acidosis
- Haemoglobin and haematosis levels elevated because of diuresis and dehydration
- Haemodynamic monitoring pressures below the patient's normal
- Electrocardiogram dysrhythmias from potassium imbalance.

Hyperglycaemia

Osmotic diuresis causes large volumes of water and electrolytes to be lost. Dehydration depletes the intracellular compartment (this is the largest of the body's fluid spaces) and increased serum osmolality causes movement of water out of the cells (see Chapter 35).

In DKA, counter-regulatory hormones, e.g. adrenaline (epinephrine), noradrenaline (norepinephrine), glucagon, cortisol and growth hormones, are released and their catabolic action further exacerbates the hyperglycaemia.

Glycosuria

The renal threshold for glucose of 10 mmol/l is exceeded, and there is up to 200 g of glucose lost per day (Young and Oh, 1997). Glycosuria is also responsible for the loss of water through osmotic diuresis. Compensatory mechanisms, stimulated by hypovolaemia, aid the maintenance of hydration. If the patient is vomiting and therefore unable to replace lost fluids orally, the condition will quickly worsen with acute renal failure potentially occurring. Vomiting will also worsen electrolyte loss and imbalances, especially of potassium, precipitating hypokalaemia and possible cardiac complications. Glycosuria and hyperglycaemia create a favourable medium for the growth of yeast organisms; consequently the patient may complain of pruritis (itching), particularly around the genitalia.

Ketones in the blood and urine

Insulin deficiency prevents the normal utilisation of serum glucose, the outcome of which is cellular starvation, even if there is an abundance of glucose in the blood. The unmet energy requirements of the cells stimulate gluconeogenesis and glycogen conversion in the liver through the release of counter-regulatory hormones. Consequently, the body is forced to break down fat and protein stores to meet energy requirements. The rate of breakdown exceeds the body's ability to use these alternative energy sources. Ketone accumulates in the blood, causing a lowering of the blood pH level, leading to metabolic acidosis. The patient compensates for this acidosis by hyperventilation (Kussmaul respiration).

Kussmaul respiration

Kussmaul respiration results from a low pH that stimulates the respiratory centre, producing an increased rate and depth of breathing (Ganong, 2003). Hyperventilation is the body's attempt to 'blow off' carbon dioxide and compensate for acidosis. The breath smells fruity (acetone).

Dehydration

Glucose exerts a large amount of osmotic pressure in the extracellular fluid and if the glucose concentration rises to excessive values this can cause considerable dehydration (Guyton and Hall, 2000). Some 5–6 litres of free water can be lost (Simpson, 2001). Fluid is also lost via hyperventilation, nausea, vomiting and increased perspiration; combined with decreased oral fluid intake, this leads to dehydration, hypotension and hypovolaemic shock.

Electrolyte imbalances

Low serum concentrations of potassium, phosphate and magnesium can cause cardiac dysrhythmias, including asystole. Hypokalaemia can result from haemo-dilution following fluid resuscitation and inadequate potassium replacement. Initially plasma potassium is decreased. However, as the vascular volumes fall, renal function will be affected. As a result the excretion of potassium will be affected, because this relies on exchange of sodium. If there is a decrease in sodium the exchange will not occur. This will result in serum potassium levels increasing, despite the total body reduction (and cellular level) in potassium levels, sometimes to dangerously high levels (Hudak *et al.*, 1998).

Sodium plasma concentrations are usually normal or slightly low (130–140 mmol/l). Hyponatraemia is caused by the osmotic gradient moving water from the intracellular compartment and diluting extracellular sodium.

Hypophosphataemia can cause muscle weakness, malaise, confusion, respiratory failure and decreased oxygen delivery.

Management

Patients who present in critical care with severe DKA are usually semiconscious with marked hypotension, severe acidosis or electrolyte disturbance. The first 24 hours are critical and require very close monitoring by nurses and medical staff. Managing the patient with severe DKA can be challenging.

The aims of treatment are to correct dehydration and metabolic acidosis. Resuscitation involves fluid and electrolyte replacement in addition to the administration of insulin. In order for treatment to prove successful, the underlying cause should, wherever possible, be treated.

The National Service Framework for Diabetes adopts a proactive approach and advocates health education prior to the development of DKA (thus avoiding this situation); it is, however, unhelpful in its guidance for when such emergencies occur. Local protocols exist within Trusts, and nurses should be familiar with these.

Fluid replacement

The free water deficit in DKA averages 5–6 litres (Simpson, 2001). By rehydrating the patient hyperglycaemia should be reduced (via improving glomerular filtration). Replacement of fluid should take account of the patient's age and degree of dehydration, and issues such as history of cardiac disease (Hand, 2000).

In severe dehydration fluid is lost initially from the intracellular spaces; rehydration using a similar sodium concentration may be used, e.g. hypotonic saline 0.45%.

In the case of hypovolaemic shock, fluid is lost from the intravascular spaces. Fluid replacement is governed by central venous pressure (CVP). Generally, there appears to be a consistent approach to fluid replacement. The choice of fluid is isotonic saline (0.9% saline) administered via rapid infusion in order to restore renal blood flow. Over the first 1–2 hours, 1–2 litres is given (Charalambos et al., 1999), with a total of 6–8 litres over the first 6–8 hours. Hypotonic saline may be used if sodium levels are greater than 160 mmol/l, and then only 1 litre over 8 hours. Plasma expanders may be indicated in some cases if diastolic pressures are less than 100 mmHg. In the case of hypernatraemia, normal saline half strength is used. Fluid can be replaced via colloids. Colloids aid fluid retention in the intravascular space (only one-quarter to one-third of crystalloid will remain in the intravascular space; the remainder enters the interstitial space), depending upon the fluid as well as capillary permeability. Resuscitating the severely hypovolaemic patient with crystalloid fluids only may cause a massive expansion in the intracellular spaces and can result in peripheral, pulmonary or cerebral oedema. When blood glucose levels are less than 15 mmol/l, the infusion fluid should be changed to 5% dextrose (Fleckman, 1993).

Vital signs such as blood pressure, pulse pressures, mean arterial pressures and CVP should be undertaken and closely monitored. ECG rhythm should also be observed for dysrhythmias associated with initial hyperkalaemia (peaked T waves, widening QRS complex; prolonged PR interval; flattened to absent P wave). Hypokalaemia may show depressed ST segments; flat or inverted T waves; or increased ventricular dysrhythmias (refer to Chapter 34).

Attention should be paid to the fluid balance, as impaired renal function (particularly in the older patient) may lead to circulatory overload or prolonged hypotension.

Insulin administration shifts potassium from the extracellular to the intracellular space as glucose enters the cell and restarts the membrane sodium–potassium pump. With rehydration serum potassium can fall further; thus patients are at risk of cardiac dysrhythmias and cardiac arrest. Regular laboratory monitoring of potassium should be performed, with potassium replacement therapy used when indicated.

Insulin replacement

An intravenous infusion using a sliding-scale insulin regime (capillary blood is tested at appropriate intervals and the intravenous infusion of insulin adjusted according to blood glucose levels) helps to lower serum glucose and inhibit ketogenesis, and also begins the reversal process for metabolic acidosis. The infusion should continue until the patient is eating and drinking, and then be substituted with the subcutaneous route.

Serum glucose needs to be analysed (initially 2-hourly) via laboratory rather than a portable glucometer to enable accuracy of results.

Insulin resistance may occur because of the effects of counter-regulatory hormones and acidosis; this may be significant when weaning a patient from the IV route to subcutaneous. Patients may require a 10 per cent increase in their usual insulin dose for several days after the onset of DKA (Page and Hall, 1999). Intravenous infusions of insulin should not be stopped abruptly, as the patient can become totally insulin deficient within 10 minutes; the dosage should be reduced on an hourly basis. Despite normal blood glucose levels, the infusion should not be stopped until the urine is free of ketones (Charalambos *et al.*, 1999); at this stage subcutaneous insulin can be commenced.

Correcting metabolic acidosis

In some critical care units sodium bicarbonate is still used. The role of bicarbonate in treating DKA acidosis remains controversial. Sodium bicarbonate (8.4%) can cause thrombosis of the peripheral veins and excessive sodium load, leading to pulmonary oedema. Wherever possible other treatments should be considered, using bicarbonate only as a last resort together with very close monitoring of the patient, particularly the cardiovascular status. Horne (2001) suggest that acidosis is best corrected by insulin therapy. Arterial blood gas monitoring is also required to establish the degree of metabolic acidosis and evaluate the acid–base balance.

Effective treatment of DKA should reduce or cure abdominal pain within 6–12 hours. If pain persists, another cause is likely. Infection is treated with intravenous antibiotics. A nasogastric tube should be passed in patients who are drowsy or vomiting.

Low doses of heparin should be given to patients at risk of developing deep vein thrombosis. Once the priorities of management and care have been addressed, consideration needs to be given to health promotion.

Complications

- Gastric stasis can lead to acute abdominal distension with copious vomiting and a high risk of aspiration pneumonia. A nasogastric tube should be inserted in order to aspirate stomach contents.
- Salt and water depletion can cause shock and renal insufficiency.
- Over-rapid correction of the biochemical abnormalities can cause hypoglycaemia, hypocalcaemia and hyperkalaemia.
- Respiratory complications/failure present with rapidly progressive shortness of breath, hypoxaemia and bilateral alveolar pulmonary shadowing. The pathophysiology is unclear, but possible links have been made to decreasing osmotic pressures and increased left atrial pressure from excessively rapid fluid replacement (Page and Hall, 1999).
- Mediastinal surgical emphysema (usually affects the chest and neck) can occur in patients with severe acidosis. Symptoms include prolonged hyperventilation and vomiting. Increased alveolar pressure can damage the alveolar walls and allows escape of air into the interstitial lung tissue.

Hyperosmolar non-ketotic syndrome

Hyperosmolar non-ketotic syndrome (HONK) is less common than DKA and occurs mainly in patients over 60 years old presenting with type 2 diabetes mellitus (indicating some insulin production).

HONK is characterised by insulin deficiency (a raised plasma glucose, usually above 30 mmol/l), dehydration, plasma hyperosmolarity and renal impairment. This condition is the second major clinical presentation of uncontrolled diabetes mellitus. In comparison to DKA the onset is more insidious, with clinical features developing gradually (over up to 2 weeks).

Precipitating factors

- Drugs that reduce insulin secretion, such as beta-blockers, thiazide/loop diuretics
- Drugs that increase insulin resistance, such as corticosteroid
- An increase in the osmotic load through feeding (enteral, parental) and excessive IV glucose administration.

Clinical features

Frequently, older patients do not manifest acute clinical symptoms of illness and can become critically ill before the symptoms are recognised. Patients may present with non-specific symptoms, e.g. anorexia, malaise, weakness. Hyperglycaemia is more severe than in DKA, resulting in a significant serum hyperosmolality and pronounced osmotic diuresis. Severe dehydration can occur; patients can lose up to 25 per cent of their body weight, resulting in intracellular dehydration. The blood becomes more viscous and flow is impeded, increasing the risk of thromboemboli. Increased cardiac workload and decreased renal and cerebral blood flow may result in myocardial infarction, renal failure and stroke.

Other features include polydipsia and polyuria, hypotension, tachypnoea with shallow respirations, profound weakness, focal seizures and hypokalaemia. Neurological deficits may be mistaken for senility in the older patient. Some patients may be unconscious or suffer impairment of conscious levels. This is proportional to the severity of hyperosmolality (Young and Oh, 1997).

Although the body's available insulin is insufficient to control blood glucose, it is usually adequate to prevent the formation of ketone bodies, thus avoiding metabolic acidosis.

Diagnostic test findings are listed in Box 25.3.

Box 25.3   Diagnostic test findings – HONK

- Serum glucose level markedly elevated (>14 mmol/l)
- Urine glucose positive
- Serum ketone usually absent
- Urine ketones negative
- Serum sodium elevated, normal or low
- Serum potassium level normal or slightly lowered
- Serum phosphate <1.4 mmol/l
- Serum magnesium <1.5 mmol/l
- Phagocytosis is impaired with serum glucose levels equal to or greater than 200 mg/dl; this can delay wound healing and predispose the patient to infection (Huddleston and Ferguson, 1997).

Management

Treatment is very similar to that for DKA, but patients have a much greater sensitivity to insulin. Insulin is usually administered in low doses via the intravenous route (because of poor tissue perfusion). This condition can sometimes be treated with fluid replacement alone (Horne, 2001). Fluid and electrolyte replacement is via a CVP line, using 0.45–0.9% saline, potassium, sodium, phosphate and magnesium supplements on the basis of laboratory values. Fluid replacement requires flexibility in relation to the patient's level of dehydration/electrolyte imbalances and blood glucose levels.

Time out 25.2

1 Outline the major differences between DKA and HONK.
2 What are the clinical features of hypoglycaemia?
3 Provide a rationale for your answers.

Hypoglycaemia

Hypoglycaemia is the commonest cause of a diabetic emergency, and is usually sudden in onset but correctable. It is an emergency situation in which serum glucose levels fall below 1 mmol/l, and may be caused by a number of factors – for example, missed meal, overdose of insulin, changing insulin therapy/preparations, liver and adrenal insufficiency, and beta-blockers.

If hypoglycaemia is not promptly corrected then irreversible brain damage and myocardial infarction can occur. Prompt reversal of hypoglycaemia occurs with the administration of concentrated glucose. There is the danger of precipitating hyperglycaemia with the administration of too much glucose.

Clinical features

Patients may show altered behaviours, including inappropriate behaviour, withdrawal, irritability, difficulties in motor function (for example walking), and slurred speech that gives the impression of drunkenness. Physiological symptoms include increased heart rate, sweating, and tremor. Patients may even present with epilepsy; in severe cases stupor, seizure and comas are present.

Implications for practice

- Prompt recognition of diabetic emergencies and appropriate intervention is required
- Nurses must conduct a thorough assessment of the patient to aid confirmation of diagnosis
- Maintenance of effective fluid balance is an essential aspect of care
- Caution must be adopted when assessing the older person, as some symptoms may mimic other less acute conditions.

Summary

There are three main diabetic emergencies, all requiring prompt recognition and appropriate intervention. The selected intervention requires the maintenance of fluid and electrolyte balance as well as controlling hyperglycaemia. Once the patient's condition improves, health promotion should begin.

Clinical scenario

Felicity Norris is a 23-year-old who has type 1 diabetes mellitus. She has been diabetic for 8 years and has had several admissions with DKA. Normally her diabetes is controlled with human Insultard 18 units (morning) and 32 units (evening).

On admission she is semiconscious (GCS 15), pulse 140 bpm, B/P 155/65 mmHg, respirations 30/min (Kussmaul respirations) and oxygen saturation 95% (on air).

Test values are pH 7.04, pO_2 18.4, HCO_3 4 mmol/l, pCO_2 2.1, base excess 24.6. Urine indicates ketones +++.

1 From the assessment data, offer a rationale for Felicity's symptoms.

2 Devise a plan of care for the first 6 hours of admission together with criteria for evaluation.

3 Consider the possible causes for Felicity's admission. What health promotion is required to reduce the chances of recurrence?

Bibliography

Key reading

Charalambos *et al.* (1999).

National Service Framework for diabetes, at www.doh.gov.uk/nsf/diabetes.

Further reading

Page and Hall (1999).

Chapter 26

Acute liver failure

Philip Woodrow

Contents

Learning outcomes

After reading this chapter you will be able to:

- Understand the main causes of liver failure
- Recognise the usual symptoms of acute liver failure
- Plan nursing care for patients with acute liver failure.

Fundamental knowledge

Hepatic anatomy and physiology.

Introduction

Some people may be admitted for treatment of liver failure, often caused by alcoholism or viruses, sometimes from intravenous drug abuse; other patients may be admitted for conditions caused or aggravated by underlying liver disease, such as oesophageal varices (see Chapter 24). However, for many critically ill patients liver dysfunction and failure may result from prolonged hypotension, causing progressive damage to, and failure of, hepatocytes.

Symptoms of liver dysfunction are often less obvious than symptoms of respiratory, cardiac or renal failure. Life can be sustained with only 20–40 per cent of normal liver function (Riordan and Williams, 1997), so symptoms of dysfunction only appear once considerable damage has occurred. Focus on other, more obviously symptomatic, failing organs and systems may result in early symptoms being missed. Because the liver has so many functions, effects of liver failure, although slow to appear, are often extensive, affecting most other organs and systems.

After a brief summary of the main liver functions, this chapter identifies likely causes of liver failure and the main symptoms and effects of liver failure that may cause or complicate critical illness. However, the liver has many more functions, and liver disease can cause many more complications, than can be described here, and care should be individualised to meet the needs of each patient. This chapter focuses on acute liver failure, but many aspects identified here apply also to chronic failure. Acute liver failure can progress to chronic failure, which is defined as occurring after 100 days. However, chronic liver failure implies an end-stage disease, fatal unless liver transplantation or artificial support is provided. Acute liver failure is potentially reversible. As with any other organ dysfunction, this is more likely to be achieved if identified early and treated promptly and appropriately.

The functional part of the liver is the lobule. There are 50,000–100,000 lobules, each being hexagonal, with a vein in the centre and an artery and vein at each corner. The arteries supply oxygen, but the corner veins supply nutrients from the gut. The lobule processes these nutrients, which then drain into the central vein, which transports them out of the lobule.

Liver functions

The main liver functions are:

- Bile production and elimination of bilirubin
- Protein, carbohydrate and lipid metabolism (produces cholesterol)
- Heat production
- Regulation of blood glucose and glycogen storage
- Destruction of bacteria absorbed from the gut (specialised macrophages called Kuppfer cells inhabit the liver)
- Production of albumin and other plasma proteins (e.g. globulin, fibrinogen)
- Recycling lactate into bicarbonate (to counter acidosis)
- Storage of minerals and fat-soluble vitamins (A, D, E, K) and minerals (including iron and copper)

- Detoxifying blood, converting ammonia to urea (deammination)
- Metabolism and detoxification of drugs (including alcohol)
- Erythrocyte metabolism, retrieving and storing iron
- Hormone metabolism
- Production of clotting factors
- Production of complements (part of the immune system).

Pathophysiology

Hepatitis (inflammation of liver) may be caused by viruses, drugs (especially paracetamol), chemicals (especially alcohol), and idiopathic (unidentified) causes.

Although hepatocytes regenerate well, the connective tissue between them may generate more rapidly, especially with prolonged inflammation, causing cirrhosis. With cirrhosis (a chronic condition), liver tissue becomes fibrous and progressively dysfunctional. Obstructed blood flow increases pressure in the hepatic portal vein (portal hypertension). Cirrhosis usually progresses to chronic liver failure and cancer.

Classification

At present there is no universally accepted classification for liver failure. *Fulminant hepatic failure* – encephalopathy occurring within 8 weeks of onset of liver disease – remains widely used, but O'Grady's (1999) classification is increasingly popular:

- Hyperacute: encephalopathy develops within 7 days of jaundice appearing
- Acute: encephalopathy develops between 8 and 28 days of jaundice appearing
- Subacute: encephalopathy develops between 4 and 12 weeks of jaundice appearing.

Symptoms

Diversity of liver function means that symptoms of dysfunction can vary greatly. Compared with other main systems, symptoms of dysfunction can often take days, and sometimes weeks, to appear. However, Krumberger (2002) identifies three main signs:

1 Encephalopathy
2 Coagulopathy (e.g. bruising)
3 Jaundice.

Other signs may include:

- Confusion, drowsiness or other changes in neurological state
- Abdominal pain
- Ascites

- Sweet, sickly-smelling breath
- Respiratory failure
- Hypotension
- Infections and sepsis.

Patients' medical and social history may indicate liver disease, although alcoholism or sexually transmitted diseases may be denied or moderated.

Many of these problems can be treated if identified early. Death from liver failure is usually caused by either cerebral oedema progressing to herniation of the brain stem into the spiral column (coning), or overwhelming sepsis (Krumberger, 2002)

Liver function tests

Diversity of liver function creates many biochemical measures. More widely used liver function tests (LFTs) are listed in Table 26.1, together with clotting and albumin (which are sometimes listed separately from LFTs). With liver failure, factors that are produced by the liver (e.g. albumin, clotting factors) are low while factors metabolised by the liver (e.g. bilirubin) are raised. Jaundice, a visible sign of failure, occurs when serum bilirubin levels reach 0.3 mg/dl (Krumberger, 2002).

Albumin is produced, but not stored, in the liver (Nicholson *et al.*, 2000). It has a half-life of about 20 days, so levels start to decline significantly after 10 or more days of liver dysfunction (Beckingham and Ryder, 2001). Starvation, or low-protein diets, may also cause hypoalbuminaemia. Albumin is the main plasma protein, so low serum albumin causes excessive extravasation of plasma, oedema and ascites, hypovolaemia and hypotension. Alanin transferase is raised

Table 26.1 Main liver function tests

Liver function tests (including clotting)	Normal range
Main LFTs:	
Bilirubin	1–20 μmol/litre
Alanine aminotransferase (ALT)	<40 iu/litre
Gamma glutamyl transpeptidase (GGT)	10–48 iu/litre
Alkaline phosphatase (Alk Phos)	<100 iu/litre
Albumin	35–50 g/litre
Other LFTs	
Aspartate aminotransferase (AST)	<40 iu/litre
(Activated) partial thromboplastin time (PTT/APTT)	26–39 seconds or 6 seconds above control
Thrombin time (TT)	15 seconds or 2 seconds above control
Prothrombin time	9.6–12.5 seconds
International normalised ratio (INR)	0.9–1.1
Total protein	60–80 g/litre

with acute and massive hepatic cell necrosis, often before jaundice appears. Gamma glutamyl transferase is raised with all types of liver or biliary tract disease. Alkaline phosphatase usually indicates gallstones, cirrhosis or cancer.

Clotting factors are produced in the liver, so liver failure causes prolonged (activated) partial thromboplastin time (PTT or APTT) and prothrombin time (PT), and an extended international normalised ratio (INR).

Time out 26.1

Using the above table, examine LFT results of patients in your workplace. Where LFTs appear raised, what aspects (if any) of the patient's social or medical history might have caused liver dysfunction? How far has any liver dysfunction contributed to diseases for which they are currently being treated?

Precipitating factors

Paracetamol

Unlike most other countries, paracetamol overdose has long been the main cause of liver failure in the UK. However, 1998 legislation reducing pack sizes and limiting sales has reduced paracetamol-related deaths by one-fifth (Hawton *et al.*, 2001). Metabolism of paracetamol is individual, so small overdoses may prove fatal to some people, while others may survive significantly larger overdoses. Plasma levels above 200 mg/litre after 4 hours or 50 mg/litre after 12 hours usually cause hepatic damage (Weekes, 1997).

Initial symptoms may be limited to nausea, but damage is slow and progressive, peaking 72–96 hours after ingestion. Intravenous acetylcysteine (Parvolex®) or oral methionine given within 10–12 hours of overdose can prevent hepatic failure, and may prevent damage if given within 24 hours (BNF, 2002).

Alcohol

Alcohol causes chronic (rather than acute), liver failure, but alcoholics may be admitted with acute complications, such as gastrointestinal bleeding. Current UK recommendations for daily maximum alcohol intake are 3–4 units/day for men and 2–3 units/day for women. Deaths in the UK from alcohol are increasing (Day, 2002).

Viruses

Many viruses can cause hepatic failure, including varicella, Epstein–Barr and cytomegovirus. Of the many hepatitis viruses, hepatitis A and hepatitis E infections are through ingestion, so tend to be prevalent where sanitation is poor. Infection in the UK is rare (Ryder and Beckingham, 2001). Hepatitis A rarely causes acute liver failure. Hepatitis B, transmitted through blood and other body fluids, is the main cause of acute liver failure (Hawker, 1997). Incidence in the UK is low (Schiodt *et al.*, 1999) with only about 1 per cent of infections progressing to acute liver failure (Jackson and Wendon, 2000), but mortality remains high, with no simple treatment if infected. Hepatitis C is also a blood-borne infection, mainly associated with intravenous drug abuse (Kelly and Skidmore, 2002; Mehta *et al.*, 2002). It may cause early jaundice, but usually causes chronic failure and cancer after a decade or more (Dusheiko, 1999; Simmonds and Smith, 1999). Incidence of hepatitis C is increasing. Hepatitis D is a defective virus, only able to survive in the presence of hepatitis B. Infection is rare and usually self-limiting (Thomas, 1999), but it may accelerate hepatic failure or cause chronic hepatitis. Other hepatitis viruses have been identified, but infection is very rare.

Complications

Neurological

Many toxins that are not cleared in liver failure cause central nervous system complications. Blood ammonia, normally no more than 800–1,000 mcg/ml, can rise to 5,000 mcg/ml (Storer, 1996). Other toxins, such as gamma aminobutyric acid (GABA), increase blood–brain permeability, resulting in encephalopathy (Jackson and Wendon, 2000).

Ammonia, normally metabolised by the liver, is neurotoxic, so with liver failure people may become acutely confused, drowsy or comatose. This often requires skilful psychological support of both patient and relatives, as well as maintaining safety (e.g. preventing aspiration) and providing fundamental aspects of care.

Most people with acute liver failure develop cerebral oedema, with related symptoms:

- Tachypnoea
- Dysconjugate eye movement, dilated pupils and slow pupil reaction to light
- Reversed sleep patterns
- Increased muscle tone, sometimes causing decerebrate posture.

Fitting is, however, rare.

Respiratory

Metabolic acidosis and cerebral oedema may stimulate tachypnoea, drowsiness may compromise the airway, ascites or other abdominal distension may limit diaphragmatic expansion, and hypoalbuminaemia may cause pulmonary oedema. Patients are therefore at risk of hypoxia, ventilatory failure and aspiration. Patients may also have co-existing respiratory disease.

Cardiovascular

Initial compensatory responses may cause tachycardia and hypotension, but hypotension and dysrhythmias often develop later (Shakil *et al.*, 1999). Portal hypertension, and often other factors such as extensive vascular disease, cause central (and jugular) venous pressure to be raised.

Renal

Severe liver failure can cause direct renal damage, but progressive cardiac failure (pre-renal failure) leading to acute tubular necrosis (ATN) is the main cause of renal complications. Uraemia is neurotoxic, so exacerbating acute confusion.

Metabolic

The liver is the main metabolic organ, so liver failure causes extensive complications. These can vary greatly, but often include pyrexia or hypothermia, hypoglycaemia and (metabolic) acidosis.

With severe failure hypoglycaemia can occur rapidly, necessitating monitoring blood sugar every 2–4 hours. Intravenous glucose solutions can increase cerebral oedema (North and Reilly, 1994) so, unless hypoglycaemia is profound, are usually avoided if encephalopathy is suspected.

Infection

The liver produces complements, part of the body's infection control mechanism. It also contains Kuppfer cells, specialised macrophages, to destroy bacteria that transfer across from the gut into the blood. With liver failure, both these defences fail. Most patients with liver failure develop infections – Caraceni and van Thiel (1995) cite rates of 90 per cent within 3 days of hospital admission. Many infections are fungal (Shakil *et al.*, 1999). Minimising infection risks is therefore important, and protective isolation may be needed.

Prognosis

Outcome depends partly on the extent of liver damage, and partly on complications and co-existing diseases. Liver dysfunction from systemic hypotension and poor perfusion causes additional complications to the underlying disease. Severe acute liver failure can be fatal within a few days (Stocklmann *et al.*, 2000).

Implications for practice

- Prolonged hypotension can cause liver dysfunction
- Although signs of liver dysfunction are often less apparent than signs from other dysfunctioning organs, a key sign is jaundice (usually occurring when blood bilirubin exceeds 100 µmol/litre)

- Nurses may detect other signs (such as increasing drowsiness) or receive laboratory results that suggest liver failure; identifying their concerns to medical colleagues may result in earlier and more effective treatment
- Monitoring for hypoglycaemia, which may develop rapidly, is necessary
- Liver dysfunction exposes patients to greater risks of opportunistic infections, so infection control becomes especially important
- If clotting is prolonged, traumatic aspects of nursing care (e.g. wet shaving) should be minimised
- As patients become more drowsy they may need information to be repeated and stated simply
- Causes of liver failure, such as alcoholism or paracetamol overdose, may cause guilt and/or anger among relatives, creating psychological needs for both them and the patient.

Summary

Liver failure may be the cause of admission, but liver dysfunction may develop from prolonged hypotension. Symptoms of liver failure are often less immediately obvious than symptoms from other main organs failing. However, the liver's various functions mean that dysfunction or failure causes many and diverse effects. Early detection can therefore significantly improve outcome.

Clinical scenario

John Sanders, aged 28 years, was staying in a hotel. This morning he was found in a drowsy state. In the ambulance he admitted having taken a paracetamol overdose the previous evening, but would not say how many he had taken. There were two empty 32-tablet packs nearby. He stated that he wished to die, having recently been left by his long-term partner. A stomach washout in A&E produced only a few remains of tablets. He has been transferred quickly to a medical assessment ward, with a parvolex infusion already in progress. He is now less drowsy, with a Glasgow coma score of 11.

John is self-employed. His next of kin, his widowed mother, who lives 250 miles away, has been contacted and is travelling to the hospital by train.

1 From this chapter, and any other sources available, list the nursing priorities immediately following John's arrival in medical assessment.

2 Using this list of priorities, devise a plan for John's immediate nursing care.

3 Paracetamol levels, which were taken in A&E after the washout, are reported as being 200 mg/litre. John has been referred to the regional liver centre, which will review his case in 1 week. Meanwhile, he is to be transferred to a general medical ward once a bed is available. What aspects of physical and psychological care should be highlighted to the ward nurses?

Bibliography

Key reading

Ryder and Beckingham (2001) and Beckingham and Ryder (2001) provide useful medical reviews of acute hepatic failure. Relatively few recent nursing articles have appeared outside specialist journals, but Krumberger (2002) provides a valuable nursing overview of hepatic failure.

Further reading

Specialist medical journals *Gut* and *Gastroenterology* and the specialist nursing journal *Gastrointestinal Nursing* are useful sources for material on this topic. Pratt (2003) provides a useful review of the hepatitis viruses.

Chapter 27

Acute neurological pathologies

Philip Woodrow

Contents

Learning outcomes

After reading this chapter you will be able to:

- Understand the causes of the acute neurological problems described
- Be able to care safely for patients with acute neurological complications
- Plan effective nursing care for patients with these conditions.

Fundamental knowledge

Neurological anatomy (including brain stem, hypothalamus, pituitary gland, formation of cerebro-spinal fluid, myelin, sympathetic and parasympathetic nervous system control, autonomic nervous system).

Introduction

Some patients may be admitted to hospital with neurological problems, but others develop complications when admitted for other pathologies. Even more so than in many pathophysiologies discussed in other chapters, nursing care contributes significantly to recovery from acute neurological disease. Many problems, and so nursing care, are common to many pathologies, so this chapter starts by identifying key problems caused by brain damage, then describes acute neurological conditions seen in many wards and departments of general hospitals including:

- Head injury
- Epilepsy
- Guillain–Barré syndrome
- Spinal cord injury.

Drowsiness and loss of consciousness necessitate a focus on fundamental safety. For example, impaired gag reflexes may expose patients to risks from aspiration, so a clear airway should be maintained by nursing patients in the recovery position. In contrast, conditions affecting peripheral nerves, such as Guillain–Barré syndrome, affect motor, but not cerebral, function.

Key problems caused by cerebral damage

Psychological

As with all highly dependent patients, the less patients are able to do for themselves, the more they rely on nurses to meet their fundamental needs. Relying on nurses to provide fundamental, and often intimate, aspects of care may be psychologically threatening to patients, especially as many of those patients with neurological pathologies are young. Their neurological problem often causes anxiety and frustration, especially as recovery may be protracted. Personality changes may include:

- Reduced inhibition
- Inflexible thinking
- Memory deficits
- Greater irritability.

(O'Neill and Carter, 1998)

Damage to the frontal lobe of the brain is especially likely to cause aggressiveness and loss of inhibition. Neurological problems, especially epilepsy, often bring social stigma (Lanfear, 2002), and sometimes legal restrictions, such as suspension of driving licences. Physical limitations or acute confusion/aggression can make these patients labour-intensive and stressful for nurses. Relatives exposed to aggression or confusion may experience similar stress.

Intracranial pressure

Increased volume in most parts of the body causes distension, tissue and skin stretching to accommodate the increased volume. In contrast, the skull prevents distension, so any increase of intracranial volume increases intracranial pressure. Most of the cranium (an average of 1.4 of its 1.7 litres volume) is filled with brain tissue (Hickey, 1997a), so intracranial bleeding, oedema and tumours compress brain tissue, usually causing neurological symptoms. Some (unhealthy) compensation occurs as pressure displaces the brain stem into the spinal column; once this compensation is exhausted, intracranial pressure rises rapidly and, if unreversed, is usually fatal.

Intracranial pressure (ICP – normally 0–10 mmHg) and cerebral perfusion pressure (CPP – normally 70–100 mmHg (Hickey, 1997a)) can be measured, but measurement is usually confined to ICUs and centres specialising in neurology. The vital (cardiac, respiratory) centres are in the brain stem, so significant and sustained raised intracranial pressure causes abnormal vital signs:

- Abnormal breathing patterns
- Hypertension
- Bradycardia.

These signs ('Cushing's Triad') indicate exhaustion of compensation and likely fatality.

Intracranial pressure can be limited or reduced by:

- Patient comfort (position, analgesia)
- Positions that optimise cerebral drainage (e.g. head tilts of 15-30° (Hudak *et al.*, 1998)), especially ensuring good neck alignment (Odell, 1996); rigid neck collars may impair drainage, so check if they can be removed (Goh and Gupta, 2002)
- Avoiding knee flexion (March *et al.*, 1990)
- Avoiding pressure on any bone flaps if the skull is fractured
- Preventing patients coughing and straining at stool (linctus and laxative drugs may be needed)
- Limiting sensory stimulation – dim lights, quietness (Johnson, 1999).

Discussions about prognosis may cause distress, so should not be made near the bedside (Hickey, 1997a). Friends and family usually provide comfort (Odell, 1996) rather than distress, so visits should be encouraged.

Thermoregulation

In health the hypothalamus regulates body temperature, but cerebral damage may affect hypothalamic function, resulting in pyrexia (Rossi *et al.*, 2001). Pyrexia increases metabolism, consuming more oxygen and nutrients. Loss of peripheral nervous system function may impair thermoregulation by loss of vasoconstriction, shivering, and sweating reflexes. Temperature should therefore initially be assessed frequently. Pyrexia may necessitate antipyretic drugs, such as paracetamol, to provide cerebral protection.

Blood sugar

Blood sugar may be labile, swinging rapidly from hyperglycaemia to hypoglycaemia, so it should initially be monitored frequently. Glucose infusions, such as 5% glucose, should be avoided (Menon, 1999; Eynon and Menon, 2002), as these may increase cerebral oedema.

Nutrition

The brain has few stores of oxygen and nutrition, so relies on almost continuous perfusion. Oxygen is vital; cerebral hypoxia is a major cause of secondary death from head injury. Head injury can increase catabolism by two-fifths (Scott *et al.*, 1998), needing up to 5,000–6,000 calories each day (Hickey, 1997b). Peripheral nervous system diseases, such as Guillain–Barré syndrome, may reduce gut motility. Dietitians should therefore be actively involved in multidisciplinary care. Large-volume feeds may necessitate increasing gut motility with drugs such as metoclopramide. Impaired consciousness may impair the gag reflex, creating dangers of aspiration, so the route for providing nutrition, and the patient's position if enterally fed, should be considered. Inadequate nutrition causes muscle wasting (see Chapter 6), which in trauma patients may delay recovery and discharge.

Diabetes insipidus

Diabetes ('fountain-like') describes the classic symptoms of polydipsia and polyuria. It usually refers to the insulin-lacking disorder of diabetes mellitus, where hyperglycaemia causes osmotic diuresis (polyuria) resulting in hypovolaemia and polydipsia. However, pituitary gland damage may reduce antidiuretic hormone production (see Chapter 35), resulting in reduced renal reabsorption of water (polyuria), and so hypovolaemia and thirst. Urine is dilute but, unlike in diabetes mellitus, glycosuria is absent.

If caused by cerebral oedema or other transitory damage, diabetes insipidus resolves once the cause is removed.

Spasticity

Prolonged immobility can cause severe spasticity (Collin and Daly, 1998), so fundamental care should include active/passive exercises, positioning, and physiotherapy.

Head injury

Every year nearly one and a half million people in the UK suffer head injury (Menon, 1999). Head injuries typically occur in young men (average age 30 (Treadwell *et al.*, 1994)) involved in road traffic accidents (Allen and Ward, 1998) and, to a lesser extent, contact sports such as rugby and boxing (Collin and Daly, 1998). Some injuries are minor, but 150,000 annually necessitate admission to UK hospitals (Treadwell *et al.*, 1994). Recovery from severe injuries may take years, and may remain incomplete; half of people with serious head injury are unable to return to work (Flint, 1999).

Time out 27.1

Reflect on patients you have nursed who had head injuries. What problems and needs were caused by their head injury? List the care and treatments these patients were offered.

Damage at the time of injury is largely irreversible. Following injury, secondary damage from inflammation, including oedema, may cause cerebral ischaemia and hypoxia, and release cytokines. Care for the first 72 hours following injury remains crucial to survival and good recovery (Johnson, 1999).

Trauma often causes multiple injuries, necessitating other support and care. For example, trauma may cause lung contusions, necessitating respiratory support. Because injuries may be extensive some may have been missed during (or developed since) initial assessment, so nurses should actively assess all needs and potential problems of patients with head injury and trauma.

Base-of-skull fractures, which may remain unidentified until X-ray, may result in nasal tubes penetrating the brain, so tubes should be avoided until base-of-skull fractures have been excluded. Base-of-skull fractures may leak cerebrospinal fluid (CSF), which may drain from the nose (rhinorrhoea) or ear (otorrhoea), often forming a yellow ring, or 'halo sign', around bloodstains on linen (Hickey, 1997b).

Epilepsy

Nerve signals rely on a complex balance between excitation and inhibition. Seizures (fitting) occur when there is excessive excitation or insufficient inhibition. Up to 1 in 20 people will have seizures (Lanfear, 2002). Some are known to suffer from epilepsy, and will usually take regular anti-epileptic drugs. Two-fifths of seizures are caused by brain damage from disease or trauma (Lanfear, 2002), such as:

- Head injury
- Raised intracranial pressure (e.g. secondary to liver failure)
- Hypoxia
- Meningitis.

However, epilepsy is unpredictable, and patients with no past medical history of fitting may fit in response to many other factors.

Seizures may be partial (starting in one hemisphere of the brain) or generalised (starting in both hemispheres). Tonic–clonic seizures (formerly called grand mal or convulsions) cause generalised alternation of muscular spasms, often with loss of breathing, clenching of teeth, and single or double incontinence. Seizures may be preceded by an 'aura', which may warn those who have previously experienced fitting. Often their eyes roll upwards. As soon as signs (or in the absence of signs, fitting) occur, patients should be:

■ Placed in the recovery position
■ If in danger from the environment, moved to a safe place (e.g. on the floor, protected by pillows)
■ Provided with privacy and dignity (e.g. by drawing bed screens around the patient)
■ Given an artificial (guedel) airway if possible, but without forcing open clenched teeth.

Seizures usually only last a few minutes (Lanfear, 2002), but they are unpredictable, and may cause aspiration or, if prolonged, hypoxia. Help should be summoned urgently, and 100% oxygen and suction made available. Anti-epileptic drugs may be needed. Nurses should note when the fit began and ended, and which parts of the body were affected.

Seizures can provoke distress in others, so family, friends and observers should be reassured.

Guillain–Barré syndrome

Guillain–Barré syndrome describes two pathologies:

1   Acute inflammatory demyelinating polyneuropathy (AIDP)
2   Acute motor axonal neuropathy (AMAN).

AMAN is more commonly found in China and Japan, whereas AIDP is more common in North America and Europe (Kuwabara *et al.*, 2002). This chapter focuses on AIDP.

Guillain–Barré affects 1.2 per 100,000 of the UK population (Poulter, 1998), making it one of the most common neurological pathologies. Immune dysfunction, usually following minor viral respiratory or gut infections (Seneviratne, 2000; Hudsmith and Menon, 2002), causes ascending demyelination of peripheral nerves (Dawson, 2000), especially motor nerves, resulting in progressive muscle weakness. Sensory nerves are usually unaffected.

Problems experienced by patients often include:

■ Pain, usually severe (Seneviratne, 2000). This is exacerbated by touch (Coakley, 1997) and anxiety, and is usually worse in the evening (Mirski *et al.*, 1995). Opioid analgesia is often needed. Muscle weakness often prevents patients from making themselves comfortable, so patients should be positioned accordingly

■ Respiratory failure, which can be caused by muscle weakness, and may need intensive physiotherapy and sometimes non-invasive ventilation (Vianello *et al.*, 2000)

■ Hypersalivation and loss of gag reflex from autonomic dysfunction, which can create risks of aspiration, requiring oral suction. Facial muscle weakness may cause dribbling

■ Hypotension from widespread peripheral vasodilatation (poor sympathetic tone)

■ Hypertensive episodes, from failure of normal negative feedback opposition to sympathetic stimuli

■ Dysrhythmias, such as sinus tachycardia, bradycardia, asystole (Hund *et al.*, 1993)

■ Sweating from autonomic dysfunction, so nurses should provide frequent washes and changes of clothing for comfort

■ Thrombosis from venous stasis (immobility) and poor perfusion, so patients should have prophylactic subcutaneous anticoagulations and thromboembolytic stockings (Winer, 1994)

■ Limb weakness, necessitating passive exercises to prevent contractures (Winer, 1994) and promote venous return; analgesia cover is often needed for this

■ Incontinence from bladder muscle weakness.

Recovery is unpredictable, relying on regrowth of damaged nerves. It often begins in 2–4 weeks (Skowronski, 2003), but a minority of patients still have significant weakness after 1 year (Seneviratne, 2000). The main treatments are supportive, such as those identified above, but possible medical interventions include plasma exchange (plasmepheresis) and immuno (gamma) globulin intravenously (IgIV), together with support for failing systems.

Spinal injury

Over half of spinal cord injuries affect the cervical spine (Hudak *et al.*, 1998). Higher injuries result in greater loss of function, although injury may be complete or incomplete. Incomplete injury allows some nerve function below the level of injury, so once initial inflammation subsides patients may recover some function during the early weeks following injury. Patients requiring longer-term hospital care are likely to be transferred to spinal injuries units.

The main life-threatening complications of cervical injury are hypotension, bradycardia and spinal shock; and hypoxia and respiratory failure.

(Ball, 2001; Hadley, 2002)

Other complications include:

■ Acute renal failure from hypotension within 48 hours (Hudak *et al.*, 1998)

- Paralytic ileus
- Deep vein thrombosis from venous stasis (Ball, 2001)
- Double incontinence
- Problems with most other systems and functions.

Many patients develop severe pain and spasticity (Burchiel and Hsu, 2001), so nursing care should include pain assessment, analgesia and passive exercises. Patients with cervical spine injury should ideally initially be admitted to ICU (Hadley, 2002), for later transfer either to specialist units or to wards within the hospital.

Injuries of the lower spine cause fewer problems, as most thoracic and abdominal functions remain intact. Thoracic and lumbar injuries will affect the legs (DVTs, immobility) and, until stabilised, patients will still need to be log-rolled to prevent further injury. Lower abdominal organs (bladder and bowels) may still be affected.

Autonomic dysreflexia

This common (Wirtz *et al.*, 1996) complication of spinal injuries above T6 (van Welzen and Carey, 2002), and sometimes as low as T10 (Keely, 1998), occurs at least 4 weeks and more often 6 months following injury.

At rest these patients have excessive parasympathetic stimulation, resulting in underlying bradycardia and hypotension (Naftchi and Richardson, 1997), but on stimulation, absence of inhibitory neurotransmitters (Lee *et al.*, 1995a) cause excessive sympathetic reflex responses (Glasby and Myles, 2000) – life-threatening hypertension and tachycardia (Baxendale and Yeoman, 1997). Severe hypertension causes symptoms such as:

- Blurred vision
- Pounding headaches
- Nasal congestion
- Nausea
- Pupil dilatation
- Profuse sweating and flushing above the lesion
- Pallor below the lesion.

(Halloran, 1995)

A distended bladder (sometimes as little as 200 ml) is the most common cause, with most remaining cases being caused by bowel distension (van Welzen and Carey, 2002). Tight clothing, seams, and other cutaneous, skeletal or visceral stimuli can also cause dysreflexic responses (Halloran, 1995).

Causes should be quickly removed if possible, and hypertension monitored and treated. Once the stimulus for hypertension is removed, antihypertensives may cause profound hypotension. Prophylactic prevention includes monitoring bladder and bowel function, intervening early to prevent distension in patients who have suffered upper spinal injuries.

Implications for practice

- If patients survive to ward admission, most deaths and many disabilities are caused by secondary complications; preventing complications improves survival and reduces morbidity
- Neurological diseases can be particularly frustrating for patients and families; some also bring social stigmatisation and legal restrictions, so psychological and social care and support are especially important
- Skilled nursing care makes a significant contribution to survival and recovery following head injury.

Summary

Patients with neurological conditions may be referred to specialist centres, but many are admitted to and remain in general hospitals. This creates challenges for nurses working in those hospitals. The frustrating nature of many of these conditions, and sometimes their effects on cognition, can make caring for these patients and their families especially stressful. Yet the quality of nursing care is especially important to the outcome of this group of patients. This chapter has discussed some of the more commonly encountered neurological conditions, and nursing interventions, seen in general hospitals.

Clinical scenario

You are making the admission assessment for Tom Walker, 26, who has Guillain–Barré syndrome.

1   List, in order of priority, your main potential concerns and the baseline observations you would undertake.

2   Mr Walker has not previously suffered from this disease, but heard that an acquaintance of his died from it. This makes him very anxious. He and his wife want to know what is likely to happen to him. Write down how you would explain the disease to him.

3   Devise a plan of nursing care for Mr Walker's first few days on your ward.

Bibliography

Key reading

Hickey (1997 – details in 1997a and 1997b) remains the best book on neurological nursing. General medical journals often contain useful articles, such as Seneviratne's (2000) review of Guillain–Barré syndrome. Reviews in general nursing journals are less frequent, but Lanfear's (2002) review of epilepsy is useful.

Further reading

A number of journals are devoted to neurology. Many are medical, but *Neuroscience Nursing* is a useful nursing resource.

Part 3

Monitoring and skills

Chapter 28

Nursing assessment

Sheila O'Sullivan

Contents

Learning outcomes

After reading this chapter you will be able to:

- Understand the role of a comprehensive patient assessment
- Understand the main uses for inspection, palpation, percussion and auscultation
- Describe the advantages and disadvantages of the two main early warning systems.

Fundamental knowledge

Organisation of nursing care, various approaches to performing an assessment of the activities of living, communication approaches used to elicit relevant information from patients about their health problems.

Introduction

There has been a significant change in the role of critical care nurses over the last 10 years to incorporate skills once perceived as being within the remit of the medical profession (Cox and McGrath, 1999). Nurses are now performing more complex assessment to complement technological interventions carried out within critical care units (Field, 1997a). With this comes the requirement to relate normal and abnormal physiology to the observations that are being documented, in order to prioritise patient care. Critical care nurses in the USA, Canada and Australia perform more detailed physical assessment as part of their comprehensive role for patients (Rushforth *et al.*, 1998), and recently education providers in the UK have begun incorporating physical assessment skills into courses for post-registration nurses.

This chapter covers advanced physical assessment for critical care nurses.

Why perform a patient assessment?

Traditionally the role of the doctor was to carry out an assessment to establish a diagnosis, determine the course of treatment or evaluate the effectiveness of interventions.

Nursing assessments determine whether the patient has a problem, establish what impact the condition is having on the patient's independence, and to create a baseline of observations to determine changes in the patient over time (Shah, 1999). These separate assessments by members of the multiprofessional team are now blurring as the holistic care of patients is carried out by the different professionals that make up a critical care team.

Patient assessment

History taking

The goal is to focus on the patient's chief complaint and the events leading up to the current problem (O'Hanlon-Nichols, 1998a). The patient's condition will determine the length and depth of interview. If the patient is unable to talk because of difficulty in breathing, information can be obtained from family members, previous records and any other documentation. Confirm information with the patient using closed questions. It can also be useful to provide the patient with a paper and pen.

For each symptom focus on descriptive characteristics, including:

- Location
- Character
- Quality
- Quantity
- Severity
- Timing (onset, frequency, duration)

- Aggravating or alleviating factors
- Associated symptoms.

(O'Hanlon-Nichols, 1998b)

Past medical history

Discuss each problem separately and gain information regarding how this has changed the patient's life – for example, what is the patient's exercise tolerance in normal health compared to now. Gather information on previous investigations, procedures, illnesses and hospitalisations. For conditions where there may be a familial link, determine which (if any) family members have been diagnosed or treated with this condition.

Allergies

When questioning about allergies, gain information as to the type of allergy and the level of hypersensitivity experienced (e.g. rash, blistering, nausea or full anaphylaxis). Include triggers or diagnosis such as hay fever, asthma, and eczema. Establish how the allergy affects the patient and what has to be done to minimise the symptoms.

Psychosocial history

Ask patients about their home life, activities and key relationships. Find out who the immediate family/friends are, as this information will be required if you need to talk to them about a patient's condition. Has the patients' illness kept them off work? If they have an infectious disease, discuss risk factors or recent travel abroad. Assess their normal level of activity, sleep pattern and appetite.

Current medication

Find out what medications the patient is taking, including any over-the-counter medications like antacids, histamine blockers and analgesia. Discuss whether homeopathic remedies are taken, as these can contribute to symptoms.

Many nurses frequently overlook the value of the health history to get to the 'hands on' aspect of the physical examination (McGrath and Cox, 1998). In order to perform an accurate physical assessment you need to be aware of the full history of the patient's present complaint and long-standing conditions. Without this knowledge pertinent findings cannot become apparent and vital information may be lost during the assessment process

Physical assessment

Once a thorough history has been obtained, the physical examination should confirm and verify the information (Kessenich, 2000). Here, the senses of sight, hearing, touch and smell will be used. The data obtained are then incorporated into a systematic approach for collecting information to complete the picture on the patient's health.

Preparation

Introduce yourself to the patient and inform them of the role you will be playing in their care. It is preferable to obtain the health history of current and previous illnesses when patients are dressed or covered, to maintain their dignity and to minimise anxiety. Remember that they may be worried and possibly frightened, as they will just have been transferred to the critical care unit. Patients may consider the assessment an invasion of privacy, as you will be observing and touching sensitive, private and perhaps painful body areas (Shaw, 1997). Examination requires the patient's consent (Lumley, 2002); therefore give an explanation of what is proposed by briefly explaining what you will be doing, why it is necessary, how long it will take, and why changes in position will be required.

Begin by using A, B, C, D, and E as your assessment process:

- Airway
- Breathing
- Circulation
- Disability (central nervous system)
- Exposure.

Once the initial assessment is completed and the need for advanced life support excluded, the patient will need to be exposed for a thorough top-to-toe assessment. This will include a formal examination of each system to prevent you from missing any critical clues to the patient's condition. This should incorporate a review of the patient's notes, charts, investigations and results that are available (*HELP Booklet*, 2002).

There are four core physical assessment skills:

1 Inspection
2 Palpation
3 Percussion
4 Auscultation.

Inspection

All assessments begin with inspection. Inspection begins from the moment you first meet the patient, and continues throughout the health history and physical assessment. Inspection uses visual skills to gather information on a particular system or the patient as a whole (Rushforth *et al.*, 1998), incorporating vision, hearing and smell to observe for normal conditions and deviations because of disease. Look for obvious and subtle signs, which will then require further investigation during the assessment. As each body system is observed, look for:

- Colour
- Size
- Location

- Movement
- Texture
- Symmetry
- Odour
- Sounds.

Examples include colour of urine with a renal assessment, size of skin redness in patients with sepsis from cellulitis, presence of peripheral and central cyanosis as part of a cardiac assessment, nasal flaring as part of respiratory assessment, and audible wheezing in a patient with severe asthma.

Palpation

Palpation uses touch, with varying degrees of pressure, to assess:

- Texture
- Temperature
- Moisture
- Organ location
- Size
- Swelling
- Vibration
- Pulsation
- Rigidity/spasticity
- Crepitation
- Masses
- Pain.

(Jarvis, 1996)

To palpate accurately and to provide patient comfort, you will need short fingernails and warm hands (Shaw, 1997). Always palpate tender areas last (Epstein *et al.*, 2003). Figure 28.1 illustrates the technique for evaluating posterior chest expansion.

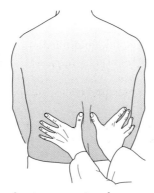

Figure 28.1 Technique for evaluating posterior chest expansion

There are two types of palpation – light and deep. These are illustrated in Figure 28.2 and compared in Table 28.1.

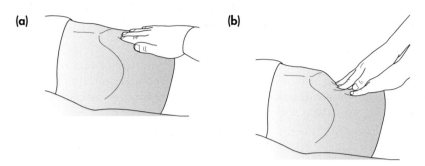

Figure 28.2 (a) Light palpation; (b) two-handed deep palpation

Table 28.1 Comparison of light and deep palpation

	Light palpation	*Deep palpation*
Depress the skin	1.25–2 cm	4–5 cm
Use	Finger pads	One or both hands
Feel for	Surface abnormalities	Internal organs, masses
Assess	Texture, tenderness, temperature, moisture, pulsation, elasticity, superficial organs and superficial masses	Size, shape, tenderness, mobility and symmetry

As each body system is palpated, evaluate the following features:

- Texture (rough or smooth)
- Temperature (warm, hot, cold)
- Motion (still or vibrating)
- Consistency of structures (solid, fluid-filled)
- Moisture (dry, wet, moist).

The areas of the hand used to palpate are:

- The palmar surface of the hand and finger pads to assess size, consistency, texture, fluid, surgical emphysema and the texture of a mass or structure
- The ulnar surface of the hand and fingers to assess vibration
- The dorsal surface of the hands to assess temperature
- The pads of the index and middle fingers to assess pulses.

(Cox and McGrath, 1999)

Percussion

Percussion involves tapping the skin with short, sharp strokes to assess underlying structures. Characteristic sounds aid assessment of size, location and density of underlying organs.

The technique helps to:

- Locate organ borders
- Identify organ shape
- Determine the position
- Determine if an organ is solid or filled with fluid/gas.

(Epstein *et al.*, 2003)

Percussion requires a skilled touch and trained ear to detect slight sound variations. Organs and tissues produce sounds of varying loudness and pitch depending on their density. Each sound is related to the structure underneath. As you percuss, move gradually from areas of resonance to those of dullness and then compare the sounds. You also compare sounds on one side of the body with sounds from the other side (see Table 28.2). Figure 28.3 illustrates percussion over the anterior chest.

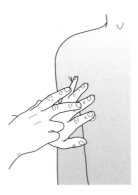

Figure 28.3 **Percussion over the anterior chest**

Table 28.2 Sounds heard during percussion

Sound	Quality of sound	Where it is heard	Source
Tympany	Drumlike	Over enclosed air	Air in bowel and puffed-out cheeks
Resonance	Hollow	Over areas of part air and part solid	Normal lung tissue
Hyper-resonance	Booming	Over air	Pneumothorax, hyperinflated lung
Dullness	Thudlike	Over solid tissue	Liver, heart, pleural effusion
Flatness	Flat	Over dense tissue	Muscle and bone, consolidation (as with atelectasis)

Auscultation

Auscultation is the last step of assessment, and involves listening for sounds produced by the heart, lungs and gastrointestinal tract with a stethoscope pressed firmly against the skin.

The stethoscope should be placed against the patient's skin and not over clothing as this reduces the validity and accuracy of the sounds (O'Neill, 2003).

When auscultating for breath sounds, make comparisons between each lung. Listen to right then left apices, middle zones, bases and axillae. Compare each side and comment upon abnormal breath sounds: fine/coarse crackles, wheeze, bronchial noises, stridor. If present, discuss the location, and where the sound is greater (e.g. R > L). The auscultatory form of vocal fremitus can be monitored by placing your stethoscope on the chest and asking the patient to say 'ninety-nine'. In presence of consolidation, the sound is increased as the transmission is increased through solid tissue and decreased if there is air or fluid between the lungs and chest wall.

When listening for heart sounds, you will be listening for first and second heart sounds, murmurs and any additional heart sounds (Epstein *et al.*, 2003; see Figure 28.4).

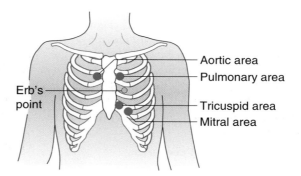

Figure 28.4 **Auscultatory areas for cardiac valves**

When using a stethoscope in clinical practice:

- Provide a quiet environment
- Ensure the area to be auscultated is exposed
- Ensure the ear pieces fit snugly into the ears to ensure good passage of sound down the auditory canal (O'Neill, 2003)
- The tubing should be around 48 cm long; shorter tubing reduces background noise (3M Health Care, 2003)
- Warm the stethoscope head in your hand
- Listen to and try to identify the characteristics of one sound at a time
- Close your eyes to help focus your attention

■ Stretch the stethoscope tubing to improve sound transmission (McGrath and Cox, 1998).

Documentation

Begin documentation with general information, including patient's age, race, sex, and general appearance, communication skills, behaviour, orientation and level of co-operation. Follow that with the patient's complaint, using his or her own words. Then record:

■ Previous medical history
■ Drug history
■ Allergies
■ Family history if relevant.

Use the four physical assessment techniques to obtain information. Complete one body system before proceeding to the next. Depending upon your role, include investigation results and your impression.

Finally, plan the care.

Accuracy

Analyse vital signs together, because two or more abnormal vital signs will provide important clues as to your patient's problem. Take observation measurements at regular intervals, as a series of readings provides more valuable information than a single set. If you obtain an abnormal value, take that vital sign again to ensure it is accurate. It is important to remember that normal readings vary with a patient's age, size and abnormal physiology – which, because of chronic conditions, may be normal for the patient.

Interpret observations and relate them to the patient's condition, but note the following:

■ Always check capillary refill before using pulse oximetry, because if capillary refill is abnormal then pulse oximetry can be inaccurate (O'Hanlon-Nichols, 1997)
■ When using skin turgor to assess for volume depletion, remember that rapid weight loss and advanced age of the patient also lead to decreased turgor (Field, 1997b).

Early warning systems

Patients with the highest mortality in critical care units comprise those admitted from the hospital wards. These patients are often in hospital and seriously ill for some time before admission (Goldhill *et al.*, 1999a). Indeed, in one study 70 per cent of patients had severe physiological abnormalities which were known to medical and nursing staff (Goldhill *et al.*, 1999b).

On admission to these units, patients may be so sick that they die quickly or require a prolonged stay. As a result of these factors, *Comprehensive Critical Care* (DOH, 2000a) recommends the use of an early warning tool to identify which patients are critically ill or deteriorating and to prevent admission or readmission to a critical care unit. Hospital Trusts are using early warning systems to identify at-risk patients through physiological parameters monitored during routine ward observations (Ball, 2002).

Early warning systems are mainly of two types:

1   Those that give an overall score according to the patient's physiology
2   Those that activate a trigger through the patient's physiology.

Systems that give a score according to the patient's physiology have long been used in audit and to evaluate outcomes for groups of patients (Gunning and Rowan, 1999). Scores obtained from scoring systems have been proposed as clinical shorthand; a standard terminology to convey information about a patient. For example, all nurses have used the Glasgow coma scale (GCS) developed by Jennett and Teasdale in 1974 to evaluate neurological responses. This scale helps practitioners to form a quick, objective and easily interpreted judgment of neurological assessment that avoids subjective terminology. However, the GCS may be misleading for some patients that have high cervical injury or hypoxaemia, or are haemodynamically shocked, fitting or post-ictal, as these patients may be unable to move their limbs, or show any responses at all (Dawson, 2000).

The early warning scoring system was developed by Morgan *et al.* (1997) and subsequently adapted by Stenhouse *et al.* (2000) to be used on surgical wards to improve detection of patients developing critical illness. Points are assigned from 0–4, according to disruption of heart rate, blood pressure, urine output, respiratory rate, oxygen saturations, and level of consciousness. The Modified Early Warning Scoring System (MEWS) has been shown to aid the earlier detection of critical illness by scoring all routine observations (Coates *et al.*, 2000; see Table 28.3).

The second early warning system available uses a single observation trigger to alert staff to abnormal physiology (see Table 28.4).

If the patient is not already catheterised, discuss catheterisation; monitor urine output hourly. If oliguria continues for 2 consecutive hours, inform the house officer. If it continues for 4 consecutive hours, call the PERT nurse (Adam, 2002).

The main advantage of these tools is the early identification of the development of critical illness. The key to these early warning systems working is for ward teams to use them on all patients that may go on to develop critical illness. For some patients this will begin the process of referral to a critical care unit.

Table 28.3 Critical care outreach team triggers

Respiratory rate (per min)	<8	>25
Oxygen saturations	<90%	On >35% oxygen
Heart rate (bpm)	<50	>125
Systolic blood pressure (mmHg) Sustained fall in BP (>40 mmHg below normal value)	<90	>200
Conscious level	Sustained alteration in conscious level	
Oliguria (passing <30 ml/hr urine)		

Implications for practice

- Nurses need to have full awareness of the correct method of carrying out a patient assessment
- All nurses need continually to develop their assessment skills as their role progresses from novice to advanced practitioner
- At all times a systematic approach should be used to ensure the full history and assessment/examination are completed methodically.

ummary

This chapter provides a presentation of the key areas and skills required to undertake a patient assessment, including history taking and physical examination, for a patient in a high dependency unit.

Clinical scenario

1 What questions would you ask a patient to elicit information on the descriptive characteristics of their main symptom and the associated problems?

2 Consider how the four physical assessment techniques could assist with the detection of abnormal physiology. Take examples of recent patients you have been involved with.

Bibliography

Key reading

Barrett (2001).

Chapter 29

Pulse oximetry

Tina Moore

Contents

Learning outcomes

After reading this chapter you will be able to:

- Understand the reasons for using pulse oximetry monitoring
- Demonstrate appropriate use of the pulse oximeter within clinical practice
- Interpret the readings within the context of patient care
- Acknowledge the limitations of pulse oximetry and take appropriate action to minimise these.

Fundamental knowledge

Gaseous exchange.

Introduction

Pulse oximeters are now widely used in various healthcare settings. The pulse oximeter measures oxygen saturation by differentiating the light absorbance of reduced and oxygenated haemoglobin during arterial pulsations. Today oximeters are more advanced, and provide a visual digital and waveform display, an audible display of arterial pulsation and heart rate, and have a variety of sensors to accommodate individuals regardless of age, size or weight (Gramlich, 1992).

This chapter discusses the uses of pulse oximetry monitoring within the context of critical care, common limitations are identified and strategies suggested to overcome these.

Time out 29.1

Have you noticed an increase in the use of pulse oximetry to monitor patients within your area of practice? If your answer is yes, what do you think is the reason?

Uses of pulse oximetry

The main function of pulse oximetry is to detect hypoxaemia before it can be detected by sight or before obvious symptoms are displayed. The pulse oximeter provides continuous, non-invasive monitoring of the oxygen saturation in haemoglobin in arterial blood. It is relatively simple to use, and provides immediate results.

This monitoring can be carried out in a variety of settings for a number of patients. These include the following situations:

■ Patients with conditions affecting/potentially affecting respiratory status (e.g. acute cardiac failure with pulmonary oedema, acute asthma)
■ During diagnostic testing for patients with acute problems (e.g. cardiac or respiratory)
■ Monitoring for potential hypoxaemia caused by invasive procedures (e.g. suctioning, exercise testing, cardiac catheterisation, bronchoscopy)
■ Evaluating the effectiveness of oxygen therapy
■ Research studies for sleep apnoea
■ Weaning respiratory support in absence of arterial blood gases.

Pulse oximetry offers continuous monitoring, and changes should be detected almost straight away. It is important to remember that pulse oximetry does not provide all the information in relation to the patient's respiratory and ventilatory status, but can calculate the SpO_2 status and detect hypoxaemia.

As pulse oximeters measure the saturation of arterial oxygen and not ventilation or lung performance (e.g. carbon dioxide levels), they may not provide all the answers required when evaluating the patient's ventilatory status. When indicated, arterial blood gas analysis will be required, as pulse oximeter measurements are not as accurate as arterial blood gas (ABG) testing (see Chapter 30).

How pulse oximetry works

As previously mentioned, pulse oximeters measure arterial blood oxygen saturation (the percentage of haemoglobin filled with oxygen). This is achieved by measuring the absorption of specific wavelengths of light in oxygenated haemoglobin. A probe/sensor (clip-on or adhesive, re-usable or disposable) is placed on a site with an adequate pulsating vascular bed, usually the finger (Figure 29.1). One side of the probe has two light-emitting diodes (LED) that transmit red and infrared light wavelengths through pulsating arterial blood to a photo detector on the other side of the probe. The amplitude of light transmitted is measured by the monitor (Figure 29.2), and depends on:

■ The volume of the arterial pulse
■ The wavelength of light used
■ The oxygen saturation of haemoglobin (Hess and Kacmarek, 1993).

The probe needs to be attached to body parts that are well perfused (where possible).

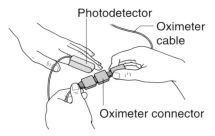

Figure 29.1 **Pulse oximeter probe**

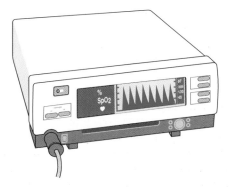

Figure 29.2 **Pulse oximeter monitor**

Oxygen saturation

SaO_2 is the abbreviation for saturation of arterial oxygen, SpO_2 is the abbreviation for saturation of peripheral oxygen, and is the value of haemoglobin oxygen saturation as recorded on a pulse oximeter. A saturation of 95 per cent means that 95 per cent of the total amount of haemoglobin in the blood contains oxygen molecules. However, not all patients with the same SpO_2 levels actually have the same amount of oxygen in their blood. Consider two patients, both of whose saturations are 90 per cent but one has a Hb of 6 g/dl and the other of 12 g/dl. The second patient has double the amount of haemoglobin and hence the potential for more oxygen molecules. Therefore, interpretation of the SpO_2 should be carried out within the context of the whole patient profile.

SpO_2 between 95 and 100 per cent is generally considered to be the normal range. A result below 90 per cent needs to be noted, as this could indicate life-threatening conditions (e.g. respiratory failure). However, it is important to interpret results based on as much information about the patient as is possible, because normal values vary. When monitoring a patient with pulse oximetry, a baseline should be established and accuracy of readings confirmed by ABG analysis.

If the patient demonstrates a decrease in SpO_2, assess his or her status to determine if intervention is necessary (it could be that the problem is mechanical, i.e. the machine and not the patient). Some treatments result in a decrease in SpO_2 levels, e.g. suctioning. If the cause of the decreasing SpO_2 cannot be found, then the patient's lungs should be auscultated for signs that can indicate fluid or consolidation (see Chapter 14). This is to rule out any condition that could decrease arterial oxygenation. ABG analysis may be indicated to determine the underlying cause of the change in SpO_2 levels.

Increasing SpO_2 levels generally indicates an improvement in oxygenation.

Where to place the probe

Manufacturers' guidelines on where to place the probe need to be followed (as different devices are designed for different parts of the body). The probe should be placed on an area that is well perfused. This may be difficult, particularly with the critically ill patient. A finger probe is usually the best with an adult patient, but alternative routes include the toe (Mattice, 1998) and earlobe.

The probe should be moved at least 4-hourly, to prevent pressure sores or thermal damage (Medical Device Agency, 2001).

Time out 29.2

Reflect on situations where you have used pulse oximetry monitoring.

1   What was the rationale for its use?
2   What limitations did you identify in this method of monitoring?
3   How were these limitations overcome?

Limitations of use

Despite the many uses of pulse oximetry, there are a number of limitations/factors that influence the accuracy of both technological and physiological readings.

Jensen *et al.* (1998) found that during severe or rapid desaturations, physiological extremes such as hypotension and hypothermia may cause the failure of the pulse oximeter to record the true SpO_2 accurately. Nevertheless, they acknowledge that the most important criterion for the use of pulse oximetery is that it gives a warning of dangerous levels of oxygen saturation and changes in pulse rate.

If clinical signs do not give cause for concern, power sources need to be checked. Again, it is important for the nurse to follow the manufacturer's guidelines on using the pulse oximeter.

Table 29.1 offers a quick guide regarding how to deal with problems in the use of oximetry.

Other factors that may influence the reading include:

1 Intravenous dyes used in cardiac output studies, which tint the blood and gives a lower level reading. Clarification should be sought from the appropriate department in relation to:

■ the type of dye affecting pulse oximetry readings
■ how long the dye is likely to affect the readings
■ in what way the readings will be affected

2 High levels of carboxyhaemoglobin in patients who smoke (falsely elevated readings)
3 High serum bilirubin level (falsely low reading)

The issue of pigmented skin's influence on pulse oximetry readings is a debatable one. Some studies indicate that deeply pigmented skin does in fact influence the signal quality and accuracy of SpO_2 (Gramlich, 1992), whereas others disagree (Bothma *et al.*, 1996).

Table 29.1 Dealing with problems in the use of oximetry

Cause of interference	Appropriate intervention
There is considerable debate as to whether nail varnish actually affects accuracy of readings (Carroll, 1997); Wahr and Tremper (1996) suggest that blue or black nail varnish can cause errors of 3–5 per cent	Remove patient's nail polish; this should be standard practice to enable monitoring of the patient's colour

Table 29.1 continued

Cause of interference	Appropriate intervention
Long fingernails may interfere with the probe being put on lengthwise	Apply the probe across the nail bed instead of lengthwise (Blazys, 1999); move the probe to another area (e.g. earlobe)
Artificial fingernails	Ideally remove them (remember to gain patient's consent, if possible), as they may interfere with readings
Poor perfusion/vasoconstriction, caused by weak pulses, hypotension, and hypothermia will cause a low, intermittent or unavailable reading	Warm patient's extremities with a blanket or a warmer pack (leave for a short time to avoid heat injury)
Sudden movements and restlessness may cause the sensor to become partially dislodged, or cause motion artifact. This will affect the ability of the light to travel from the LED to the photo-detector. Rhythmic movement (e.g. seizures, shivering) may also cause problems	Explain the importance of keeping still; if the patient is unable to, consider moving the probe to the earlobe, where movement least affects the probe
Interference with the transmission of light may be caused by dirt (e.g. dried blood)	Keep the patient's skin and the equipment clean
Bright light shining directly on the sensor probe will interfere with the readings; this includes direct sunlight, fluorescent lights, surgical lamps	Remove the source of light
Optical shunting may occur when the probe is positioned badly, and the light goes directly from the LED to the photo-detector, missing the vascular bed	Check position and reposition if indicated
Abnormal haemoglobins can occur in patients with carbon monoxide poisoning due to smoke inhalation; the sensor cannot differentiate between oxyhaemoglobin and carboxyhaemoglobin, and will therefore provide a false SpO_2 reading	Do not monitor such patients; ABG analysis should be undertaken instead
Severe anaemia (when haemoglobin levels fall to 3 g/dl) may also cause false readings. Mengelkoch et al. (1994), report that the cause of the error due to anaemia is not fully known, but that it may be due to photon scattering and a shift in	

Table 29.1 continued

Cause of interference	Appropriate intervention
red-light wavelength increasing its absorption)	
Equipment malfunction; damaged/poorly positioned probe	Check the signal strength indicator regularly. A dampened waveform could indicate a reduction in arterial flow; a misaligned sensor could also cause this. In this case the probe will need to be repositioned
Dysrhythmias	Test the equipment on yourself or another healthy person. Correlate the pulse reading with the patient's heart rate (if there is a variance it could indicate that not all pulsations are being picked up). Send blood for ABG analysis. A replacement monitor may be indicated
Intermittent blood flow	Check pulse rate and capillary refill time
Non-arterial pulses can be detected, if, for example, the probe is secured too tightly, causing venous pulsation of the finger. Other causes include right-sided heart failure, where venous obstruction may provide a falsely high reading. Venous pulsation confuses pulse oximeters	Check the position and security of the probe; be aware of signs of right-sided heart failure. Rotate/transfer the probe to different sites frequently
Applying a probe too tightly on a finger or toe or placing a probe on oedematous digits may impece venous return and cause venous pulsation	Check the probe regularly for tightness; loosen tape or change position of probe when indicated
Alterations to recordings occur when Dynamap® blood pressure cuff is used on the same limb	The pulse oximeter sensor needs to be placed on a finger on the opposite side, as blood flow to the finger will be cut off whenever the cuff inflates and readings will be inaccurate

Implications for practice

■ Pulse oximetry offers a simple, reliable way to monitor patients continuously
■ The limitations of pulse oximetry must be acknowledged and appropriate strategies used to reduce/eradicate them
■ Nurses should not rely on pulse oximetry alone and should analyse data obtained from respiratory assessment (e.g. hypercapnia, which may occur in patients with COPD)
■ This approach to monitoring should not replace the need for arterial blood gas analysis when indicated
■ Pulse oximetry is inappropriate in patients with carbon monoxide poisoning
■ Positioning the probe on the finger will usually provide the best recordings
■ Caution needs to be exercised when monitoring patients with abnormal haemoglobins (for example anaemia)
■ Pulse oximetry readings must be analysed in the context of the whole person.

(Woodrow, 1999)

Summary

The benefits of pulse oximetry monitoring are greater than its limitations, as many of these limitations can be overcome through appropriate usage/application. However, it must be remembered that there are certain conditions where it is inappropriate/inadvisable to rely on it alone. In this instance, ABG monitoring is desirable.

Clinical scenario

Mr Michael Cormer, a 34-year-old refugee, is admitted to the critical care unit following a 3-week history of acute weight loss, shortness of breath and persistent coughing. On admission he is dyspnoeic, skin colour is pale. He is receiving 35 per cent of oxygen via a facemask.

Assessment data:
Blood pressure   130/90 mmHg
Heart rate   130 – sinus tachycardia
Pyrexia   37.9°C
Respiratory rate   30 per min, very shallow
Oxygen saturation   90%

Following a chest X-ray a diagnosis of bilateral pneumothorax was made. In view of the history and clinical picture the medical staff suspect that Michael has pneumocystis carinii pneumonia (PCP).

1   Identify the reasons for using pulse oximetry monitoring.

2   Devise a plan of care that is required to ensure safe use of this monitoring device.

3   During the shift Michael's condition deteriorates. He becomes severely dyspnoeic; respiratory rate 52 per min, using accessory muscle. Oxygen saturation drops to 80 per cent, heart rate 160 sinus tachycardia. His skin colour is pale and he feels cold and clammy when touched. Evaluate the appropriateness of relying on pulse oximetry readings in Michael's situation.

Bibliography

Key reading

Casey (2001) provides a useful explanation of the physiological process in oxygen transportation, the influencing factors, and the relationship to pulse oximetry.

Further reading

Woodrow (1999) offers a comprehensive overview of pulse oximetry, highlighting benefits and limitations of usage.

Chapter 30

Arterial blood gas analysis

Sandra Gallacher

Contents

Learning outcomes

After reading this chapter you will be able to:

- Understand blood gas exchange
- Recognise common acid–base disorders
- Discuss how these disorders can be corrected
- Apply knowledge of blood gas analysis safely in the clinical area.

Fundamental knowledge

Basic normal acid–base physiology; normal blood gas levels.

Introduction

This chapter will discuss the disorders in acid–base balance most commonly presenting in the critically ill patient. Arterial blood gas analysis is a learned skill that requires knowledge of normal acid–base physiology and experience in interpreting blood gas results (Field, 2000). Although an overview of acid–base physiology will be given, a detailed discussion of the processes involved can be found in the suggested reading list.

Accurate interpretation of blood gas is vital. Nurses providing critical care need to know normal values, and causes and associated treatment of abnormal results.

Acid–base physiology

For normal cell function to occur, a balance between acids and bases should exist (Watson, 2000b). Arterial pH (which reflects the hydrogen ion concentration) is calculated using the partial pressure of carbon dioxide and the plasma bicarbonate level (Abelow, 1998). The pH of blood is a reflection of the acidity or alkalinity of the blood. It is possible to identify a deviation from the normal pH value (7.35–7.45), but it is not possible to identify, alone, whether the deviation is a result of respiratory or metabolic origin (Woodrow, 2000).

Acid–base balance is a complex process that is regulated by several different mechanisms. The benefit of this is that a failure of one mechanism can, in part, be compensated by another (Alspach, 1998). The two major organs that regulate acid–base balance are the lungs and kidney (Abelow, 1998); kidney regulation is referred to as being metabolic, lung regulation as being respiratory. The lungs regulate carbon dioxide and the kidneys regulate bicarbonate, which provides the most effective buffer in the body. In addition, body fluids contain buffers which can help to maintain a normal pH value by stabilising acidic hydrogen ions. Haemoglobin, phosphates and plasma proteins are involved in the process of buffering. Biological processes in cells and tissues can be significantly disrupted with only a slight deviation from the normal acid–base balance, damaging cell membrane permeability and slowing the reaction of enzymes (Huether, 1998b).

Anything that disturbs the normal functioning of the body, such as disease, trauma or shock, can disturb acid–base balance. It is therefore probable that patients requiring critical care will be at risk of developing acid–base imbalance.

Acids are produced by the body as an end product of cellular metabolism (Huether, 1998b). To maintain a normal pH, acid must be neutralised or excreted. Carbonic acid, for example, is dissociated into carbon dioxide and water, and the carbon dioxide is then expelled by the lungs. This respiratory mechanism reacts quickly to acid–base disturbances, resulting in hyperventilation (and a reduced pH). The kidney can maintain acid–base balance by increasing the amount of bicarbonate reabsorbed in the distal tubule (Abelow, 1998). Bicarbonate is consumed by the acids produced by the body's endogenous acid production; therefore normal body activity results in a gradual loss of bicarbonate. The kidney also excretes acids in the form of hydrogen ions (Abelow, 1998), which are excreted in the urine as ammonium salts and hydrogen phosphate (Watson, 2000b).

Arterial blood gases

Arterial blood gas (ABG) analysis is an established method of assessing respiratory and metabolic status in critical care units (Matamis and Papanikolaou, 1998). Whilst it is a standard test, it is important to ensure that the test is necessary. Frequent checking of ABG is a distressing experience for any patient, and nurses can assess respiratory function in other ways (Coombs 2001; see Chapters 14 and 29).

Obtaining a sample for ABG analysis is associated with complications, including pseudoaneurysm of the artery (Nair and Patel, 2002) and iatrogenic anaemia (Merlani *et al.*, 2001). To avoid these, the minimum amount of blood necessary to perform the test should be aspirated (Andrews *et al.*, 1999).

There are two ways of obtaining an arterial blood sample: a 'stab' (obtains a single sample of blood) or an indwelling arterial catheter if frequent sampling is required (Dolan, 2000b). At present the use of arterial catheters is not recommended in general ward areas due to the complications of disconnection and accidental intra-arterial injection (Dolan, 2000b). However, through monitoring the patient closely and good standards of practice this problem should be minimised. To avoid clotting of the sample, it should be heparinised.

The use of pre-prepared syringes is advocated, as too much heparin may distort the carbon dioxide and bicarbonate readings (Abelow, 1998). Blood containing air bubbles may yield falsely low results (Urden and Stacy, 2000) due to air diluting the concentration of gases in the sample. Sedimentation of the sample can affect pH and carbon dioxide results.

The sample should be gently mixed prior to analysis, as a drawn sample will continue to metabolise (Woodrow, 2000). Continual metabolism can lead to increased potassium and carbon dioxide levels, in addition to a fall in pH and oxygen (Abelow, 1998). The sample should be kept in ice. Unless an indwelling arterial catheter is present, nurses do not routinely take arterial blood samples; however, they are required to obtain the results and therefore should understand the principles of arterial blood gas analysis and apply the results to clinical practice. In order to ensure accuracy of interpretation, it is recommended that the same steps of interpretation are applied to each set of results.

Clinical indications for arterial blood gas analysis vary, but the arterial oxygen level is of clinical importance.

■ PaO_2 measures the partial pressure of oxygen in plasma (Woodrow, 2000) and is usually measured in the UK in kilopascals (kPa). Normal values: 11.5–13.5 kPa.
■ Oxygen carried by haemoglobin is not reflected in this value, and is frequently measured by pulse oximetry (Field, 2000). This is referred to as oxygen saturation (SaO_2). It is possible, therefore, for a patient to have a normal SaO_2 and a low PaO_2 simultaneously (Dickson, 1995). This is known

as the oxygen dissociation curve. In order to interpret the clinical significance of the PaO_2, it is necessary to know the amount of oxygen being inspired by the patient at the time the sample was taken.

■ PCO_2 is a measure of the partial pressure of carbon dioxide dissolved in arterial blood plasma. Although the normal range is 4.5–6.0 kPa (Huether, 1998b), it is usual for values outside this range to be accepted as normal for an individual depending on their medical history (Andrews *et al.*, 1999).

■ Bicarbonate (HCO_3) is the component that reflects renal function (Abelow, 1998). A normal range for bicarbonate levels is considered to be 22–26 mEq/l (Coombs, 2001); a bicarbonate below this range indicates metabolic acidosis, and a bicarbonate above this range indicates a metabolic alkalosis. An actual bicarbonate and a standard bicarbonate may be provided, and it is usual to record the standardised result.

■ Base excess is a measurement of the moles of acid or base needed to return 1 l of blood to neutrality (i.e. pH 7.4). Normal base excess is −2 to +2, and a marked deviation from this norm will indicate acidosis or alkalosis. Most blood gas analysers provide a standardisation of base excess, which is known as Standard Base Excess (Woodrow, 2000).

Interpreting ABG results

Interpreting ABG results is a skill that can take time to develop. It is important that critical care nurses are able to interpret ABG results and identify any deterioration in a patient's condition to inform medical staff. By examining each variable in turn, it is possible to monitor a patient's clinical condition and any response to treatment:

■ PH – is it normal? A low pH indicates acidosis, a high pH indicates alkalosis.

■ $PaCO_2$ – is it high? A high $PaCO_2$ could result in a low pH (respiratory acidosis); a low $PaCO_2$ could result in a high pH (respiratory alkalosis); a normal $PaCO_2$ means the cause of the acidosis or alkalosis may be metabolic.

■ Bicarbonate – is it normal? A low bicarbonate indicates a metabolic acidosis; a high bicarbonate indicates a metabolic alkalosis.

ABGs are often required to determine a patient's oxygenation status. The PO_2 should be checked to determine the need for (or effectiveness of) oxygen therapy or respiratory support. By following these steps of interpretation, it is possible to identify acid–base imbalance and identify the cause so that corrective treatment can be commenced promptly.

Metabolic acidosis

Metabolic acidosis is the failure to remove/buffer sufficient hydrogen ions. This may be due to excessive acid production (commonly lactic acid), and occurs with a significant fall in plasma bicarbonate concentration (Abelow, 1998). Causes include:

- Diabetic keto-acidosis associated with starvation and binge alcohol consumption accompanied by vomiting (Abelow, 1998).
- Acute renal failure caused by impaired excretion of acid leading from the kidney (Huether, 1998).
- Gastrointestinal tract problems, especially those associated with the colon (secretes bicarbonate into the gut lumen); severe vomiting and/or diarrhoea; increased fistula drainage.
- Increased acid production – poor tissue perfusion requires cells to move from aerobic respiration to anaerobic respiration, and the by-product of anaerobic respiration is lactic acid (Alspach, 1998). Lactic acidosis is a concern in critical care as the most common clinical cause is circulatory failure, particularly following cardiogenic or septic shock (Abelow, 1998). Other causes of lactic acidosis include severe acute incidences of hypoxaemia, anaemia, and liver dysfunction (its ability to metabolise the acid may be disrupted).
- Ingestion of acids – overdose (e.g. aspirin, methanol).

Clinical features of metabolic acidosis include headache and lethargy (early symptoms), and deep, rapid respirations to aid the excretion of carbon dioxide in an attempt to restore acid–base balance. Severe acidosis can lead to coma and dysrhythmias.

Metabolic alkalosis

Metabolic alkalosis occurs when plasma bicarbonate is increased; this is often caused by an excessive loss of metabolic acids (Abelow, 1998). It is also associated with volume depletion; resultant hypotension initiates the renin–angiotensin cycle, which is a cycle of events to maintain renal blood flow. The presence of angiotensin increases bicarbonate reabsorption. This process is enhanced by adrenergic stimulation (response of the nervous system to hypovolaemia), resulting in bicarbonate reabsorption.

Two factors are associated with metabolic alkalosis:

1   Hypokalaemia, which increases the threshold for bicarbonate reabsorption. Intracellular bicarbonate may leave the cells with the potassium, which causes an intracellular acidosis prompting the renal cells to conserve bicarbonate. Causes include excessive loss of gastric fluid (e.g. vomiting or nasogastric drainage).
2   The use of thiazide or loop diuretics (e.g. frusemide).

Symptoms of metabolic alkalosis are common to volume depletion and electrolyte disorders (Huether, 1998b), and include weakness and muscle cramps. The respiratory system attempts to retain carbon dioxide to normalise the acid–base balance and this leads to slow, shallow respirations. Atrial tachycardia, confusion and convulsions can also occur with metabolic alkalosis.

Respiratory acidosis

Respiratory acidosis results when alveolar ventilation is insufficient to excrete the metabolic production of carbon dioxide (Huether, 1998b) and has many causes, which can be grouped into two categories, pulmonary and non-pulmonary.

1   Causes of non-pulmonary acidosis include drugs, neurological disease and respiratory muscle failure. Many drugs reduce the central drive, affecting the ability of the respiratory centre to respond to changes in arterial carbon dioxide. Morphine and barbiturates are commonly used drugs, but can affect respiratory function in vulnerable individuals (Abelow, 1998). Damage to the neuronal conduction pathway (for breathing) will result in reduced ventilation and respiratory acidosis. This could be caused by spinal cord damage, damage to the phrenic nerves, and any disease that affects neurotransmission (e.g. multiple sclerosis).

2   Acute causes of pulmonary acidosis include pneumonia, asthma, pulmonary embolus or pulmonary oedema. Chronic (compensated) respiratory acidosis is seen in patients with chronic obstructive pulmonary disease (COPD). Carbon dioxide excess is known as hypercapnia. Respiratory acidosis causes a metabolic response to compensate and keep blood pH within normal limits (Field, 2000). This compensation, however, can take several hours or days to develop fully (Huether, 1998b). The kidneys compensensate for the increased $PaCO_2$ by increasing the plasma bicarbonate concentration (usually over 3–5 days).

Respiratory muscle function (severe muscle weakness) can be affected by electrolyte depletion, in particular low potassium or phosphate levels (Abelow, 1998). Although the respiratory rate initially rises, the respiratory centre is able to adapt to the increasing levels of carbon dioxide and respiratory effort gradually becomes depressed (Huether, 1998b).

Symptoms relate to those of the effects of hypercapnia: irritability, disorientation, restlessness, headache (vasodilatation of cerebral vessels), tachycardia, hypotension, dysrhythmias, and hypoventilation.

Respiratory alkalosis

Respiratory alkalosis is caused by an excessive loss of carbon dioxide, and is usually caused by hyperventilation (Abelow, 1998). Hence, hyperventilation and hypocapnia are present. Hyperventilation is stimulated by hypoxaemia resulting from pulmonary disease (Huether, 1998b), acute myocardial infarction, anxiety and early sepsis, to mention a few. Psychological factors (e.g. anxiety) or physical factors (e.g. pain) can cause dyspnoea and hence hyperventilation (Shuldham, 1998).

Arterial hypoxaemia is sensed by the central chemoreceptors in the aortic arch and carotid bodies. The respiratory rate increases to increase PaO_2. This process also results in a lowered $PaCO_2$ (Abelow, 1998).

Causes include anaemia and severe hypotension (Abelow, 1998), resulting in poor tissue perfusion. Haemoglobin is the primary transporter of oxygen in the human body (Dickson, 1995).

Nursing management of indwelling arterial catheters

Local guidelines should always be adhered to, in conjunction with general principles regarding the safe nursing management of indwelling arterial catheters.

Prior to the insertion of an indwelling arterial catheter the collateral circulation should be assessed. Insertion of an arterial catheter is considered an expanded role. The Allen's Test is performed before insertion. This procedure involves compression of the radial and arteries for several seconds until blanching of the skin occurs. When the pressure is released, skin colour should return within 10–14 seconds; this indicates a positive Allen's Test. A negative Allen's Test indicates inadequate circulation, and an alternative site for catheterisation should be found.

Arterial puncture and indwelling arterial catheters are associated with complications, including:

- Haematoma
- Nosocomial bacteraemia
- Numbness
- Sepsis.

Applying pressure to the site of the puncture for 5 minutes following catheter withdrawal and the use of aseptic technique during insertion can reduce these complications. Numbness can indicate nerve damage, and an alternative puncture site should be found. Sepsis can be associated with indwelling arterial catheters, and can be reduced by avoiding sites that indicate the presence of infection (Rogers and Smith, 1998).

Indwelling arterial cannulae reduce the need for arterial puncture. Risks associated with their use include:

- Hypovolaemia (following accidental disconnection)
- Accidental injection of drugs
- Local arterial damage.

Careful nursing management can reduce these risks. The site must be visible at all times (unless the cannula is in the femoral artery), so that disconnection will be detected promptly. Accidental injection can be avoided by clear labelling of the line as arterial. Distinguishing features, such as red bungs instead of white, can also indicate that the line is arterial. Local damage may be indicated by cooling of the limb when the cannula is flushed (Dolan, 2000b). Blanching and cooling of the skin are also common indications.

Implications for clinical practice

- Nurses should understand the safe care of indwelling arterial lines
- Nurses will need to advise colleagues on the correct care of a sample prior to analysis
- Knowledge of AGB analysis is necessary if nurses are to receive results of analysis.

Summary

Critically ill patients may require arterial blood gas analysis. Although nurses may not be required to obtain the sample, receipt of the results will probably be part of their role. Nurses should therefore understand the principles of arterial blood gas analysis, to enable the prompt recognition of abnormal results and appropriate action taken.

Nurses are responsible for caring for patients with indwelling arterial catheters, and need to provide the highest standard of care.

Clinical scenario

Mr Smith is admitted from a surgical ward following episodes of hypotension and oliguria. His respiratory effort is laboured and his respiratory rate has increased, compared to charted observations from the ward.

Arterial blood gas results are pH 7.30, HCO_3 14 mmol.

1 What acid–base disturbance does this sample suggest?

2 What treatment will be necessary to return the results to normal?

3 What nursing interventions could be used to support Mr Smith's breathing?

Bibliography

Key reading

Abelow (1998).

Urden and Stacy (2000).

Further reading

Mallett and Dougherty (2000).

Chapter 31

Suctioning

Tina Moore

Contents

Learning outcomes

After reading this chapter you will be able to:

- Recognise the indications for suctioning
- Understand the correct suctioning procedure
- Appreciate the dangers/complications of suctioning and take appropriate preventative measures.

Fundamental knowledge

Anatomy and physiology of upper and lower airways; gaseous exchange; principles of asepsis.

Suctioning routes

Suctioning can be performed via various routes (Figure 31.1), which are listed in Box 31.2.

Box 31.2   Routes for suctioning

- Oral – for removal of oral secretions
- Oropharyngeal – insertion of a suction catheter through the mouth and pharynx
- Nasopharyngeal – extends from nasal passage and pharynx (Figure 31.2)
- Nasotracheal – insertion of a suction catheter through the nasal passage, pharynx and trachea
- Tracheal – usually occurs through an artificial opening in the trachea
- Endotracheal – through an endotracheal tube
- In specialist areas such as intensive care, closed circuits are used

---

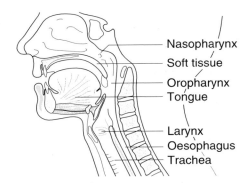

Figure 31.1 **Routes used for suctioning**

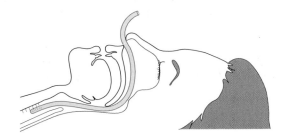

Figure 31.2 **Naso-pharyngeal suctioning device**

Contraindications for nasopharyngeal/nasotracheal suctioning include:

- Nasal bleeding
- Epiglottitis or croup (absolute)
- Acute head, facial or neck injuries
- Bleeding disorders
- Laryngospasm
- Irritable airway
- Upper respiratory tract infection.

(Hilling *et al.*, 1992)

Equipment

Box 31.3 lists the equipment required for suctioning.

Box 31.3   Equipment required for all routes
■ Suction machine (wall-mounted or portable) ■ Suction catheters (a selection of appropriate sizes) ■ Sterile disposable gloves (Ward *et al.*, 1997) ■ Clean disposable gloves (Mallet and Dougherty, 2000) ■ Sterile water for irrigation ■ Sterile lubricant ■ Disposable plastic apron ■ Protective eye wear (not used as standard procedure in some units and is not widely discussed as part of the procedure within the literature) ■ Manual rebreathing bag ■ Sterile disposable container ■ Bactericidal alcohol hand rub ■ Tissues.

Suctioning

Box 31.4 describes the suctioning procedure.

Box 31.4   Suctioning procedure (not oral)
■ Communicate with patient and gain verbal consent (if possible) ■ Explain the procedure to the patient (Mallett and Dougherty, 2000) ■ Check that the suction machine is on (Mallett and Dougherty, 2000) and set it at appropriate suction pressure ■ Calculate appropriate catheter size – for endotracheal and tracheostomy tubes the catheter size should not be larger than one-half of the tube diameter (Wood, 1998) ■ If possible the patient should be sitting upright ■ Wash hands

- Wear a sterile disposable glove on the hand manipulating the catheter (Ward *et al.*, 1997) and a clean disposable glove on the other (Mallett and Dougherty, 2000)
- With the unsterile-gloved hand withdraw catheter from sleeve
- Remove the oxygen supply
- Instilling saline boluses into the airway is dangerous and not recommended (Kinloch, 1999; Akgul and Akyolcu, 2002); instead, a 2-ml saline nebuliser is safer and effective
- Insert the suction catheter via the selected route; do not apply negative pressure on insertion
- On withdrawing the catheter, slowly apply suction pressure (by placing the thumb over the suction port control)
- Withdraw catheter gently; many catheters have holes around their diameters and hence the rotating method is unnecessary
- Monitor patient's oxygen saturation levels and heart rate throughout the procedure for any decrease indicating hypoxaemia
- On completion, wrap catheter around the gloved hand, then pull back glove over soiled catheter and discard safely (Mallett and Dougherty, 2000)
- Rinse connection by dipping its end in the jug of sterile water (Mallett and Dougherty, 2000) and discard other glove
- Wash hands with bactericidal alcohol hand rub
- If further suctioning is required, start the procedure again with another sterile catheter and glove
- Repeat until the airway is clear (auscultate after suctioning), but no more than a total of three suction passes is suggested (Glass and Grap, 1995) in patients without contraindications
- The patient must be allowed to rest between each suction pass
- Reconnect oxygen apparatus as soon as possible
- Evaluate effectiveness by conducting a comprehensive post-suctioning procedure – respiratory assessment (Glass and Grap, 1995)
- Wash hands
- Clean patient's oral cavity
- Document findings
- Allow patient to rest before taking arterial blood for analysis (Hilling *et al.*, 1992)

Frequency of suctioning

Traditionally, critical care units performed this procedure on the patient every 2 hours. Today this practice is seen to be outdated, and the procedure should be performed in response to clinical signs and symptoms rather than on a routine basis (Wainright and Gould, 1996; Blackwood, 1999), reducing the trauma of the experience for the patient and the risk of mucosal damage.

The exact timing to carry out this procedure cannot be identified. However, withholding suctioning until the patient's condition changes may be a dangerous practice. Retained pulmonary secretions become a medium for bacterial growth, with the risk of potential problems including dyspnoea, atelectasis, hypoxaemia and airway obstruction. Therefore, patients require continuous assessment and evaluation by nurses who are deemed to be competent in respiratory care. Particular attention should be given to patients who have chronic obstructive pulmonary disorders (COPD) or those who desaturate very quickly for whatever reason.

If the patient desaturates, Smith (1993) suggests that pre-suctioning oxygen saturation parameters should be returned to before suctioning again. This is achieved by allowing the patient to rest. Supplementary oxygen may also be administered.

Suction catheters

The function of the cough is to alter intrathoracic pressures to aid the mobilisation of secretions (saline can stimulate this). Sometimes a cough is not violent enough to project sections into the oral cavity, only into the trachea, so nurses will need to suction to clear the secretions mobilised.

Suction catheters are available in different sizes; 10–12 FG (French Gauge) are the most commonly used. The size of the suction catheter selected is dependent on the viscosity and volume of secretions – the thicker the secretions and the larger the volume, the greater the bore of the tube (Mallett and Dougherty, 2000). It is also dependent on the size of the artificial airway if intubated. Nevertheless, in order to prevent hypoxia occurring during suction the catheter diameter size should be less than half the tracheal diameter. When calculating the size of a suction catheter for tracheal suctioning, first divide the tracheostomy tube's internal diameter by two. This gives the external diameter of the suction catheter, which should then be multiplied by 3 to obtain the FG size. Therefore, if the tracheostomy tube is size 8, divide this by $2 = 4 \times 3 = 12$ FG. This is difficult to gauge on patients without tracheostomy tubes, and competent clinical judgment is required.

Multiple-eyed catheters cause less damage than the single-eyed catheters. The former dissipate the focus of suction pressure, so it is less like that the mucosa will be sucked into the side holes. Yanker suckers provide the easiest and safest way to remove oral secretions and vomit; however, they are rigid and not as flexible as suction catheters, and may cause trauma of the oral cavity if not used with care.

If the patient is unconscious and unable to cough, it may be necessary to advance the catheter to the carina and then withdraw the catheter 1 cm before suctioning (Dean, 1997; Wood, 1998).

Suction pressure

Negative pressure should be sufficient to clear secretions, although the amount of suction pressure used can affect the amount of secretions removed. Too low a suction pressure can result in inadequate clearance of secretions; if it is too high the suction catheter can adhere to the tracheal wall, causing mucosal damage and atelectasis. With high pressure the suction catheter is more likely to collapse (Czarnik *et al.*, 1991).

Generally, the lowest amount of suction pressure needed to remove secretions should be used. It is suggested that the suction pressure should be between 80 and 120 mmHg (12–17 kPa) (Somerson *et al.*, 1996). Suction pressure should only be applied when removing the catheter; if pressure is applied during insertion, the catheter will adhere to the mucosal wall.

Length of time spent suctioning

Evidence suggests that suction should be applied for no longer than 10 seconds (Mallet and Dougherty, 2000). Do not rely on methods like holding your breath, as this approach does not take into consideration the patient's 'non-healthy' lungs. Indeed, healthy people can hold their breath for up to 25–30 seconds without difficulty. The patient should be encouraged to breath deeply before suctioning, and allowed time to recover between episodes. Always assess the patient's susceptibility to hypoxaemia (sinus bradycardia and hypotension).

At least 2 full minutes of recovery time is needed for adult patients with a closed head injury to return to baseline oxygen saturation values after suctioning (Crosby and Parsons, 1992).

Tracheal suctioning

The presence of a tracheostomy causes cool, dry air to react with the bronchi and lungs, as the trachea is ill-equipped to warm and humidify air (Jackson, 1996b). This results in the drying of secretions, thus making patients susceptible to pulmonary infections and atelectasis. Retention of secretions can be caused by lack of humidification. Systemic dehydration will complicate this further.

Thompson (2000) concludes that the quality of evidence available for tracheal suctioning is lacking in rigorous research design.

Head-injured patients

Caution has to be taken when suctioning patients with head injury. Neuronal viability is threatened due to sudden and acute increases in intracranial pressure (ICP) (Kerr *et al.*, 1997). Hyperventilation can result in hypocapnia, leading to induced cerebral vasoconstriction. This reduces the potential for increased intracranial pressure that occurs during endotracheal suctioning when used longterm (Ropper and Rockoff, 1993).

For these patients, suction passes should be limited to no more than two for each procedure (Rudy *et al.*, 1993). This is because the mean arterial pressure (MAP) increases with each suction pass (Stone, 1991). For patients who have sustained traumatic brain injury, even a moderate increase in ICP will increase cerebral ischaemia and oedema. It is inadvisable to suction patients who have sustained a fractured base of skull, as the suction catheter could accidentally pass through the fracture.

Complications

Suctioning is an important and necessary aspect of care, but may be wrongly viewed as a routine skill. The procedure is full of potential dangers (particularly endotracheal), such as:

- Hypoxaemia due to oxygen desaturation
- Negative pressure removing oxygen from the lungs during withdrawal, which cause dysrhythmias and hypotension
- Contamination of the airway, leading to nonocomial infection
- Cross-infection in the critical care unit if correct procedures are not adhered to (critically ill patients are often immuno-compromised and susceptible to colonisation by the hands of staff during tracheobronchial suctioning)
- Mucosal trauma
- Pneumothorax
- Raised ICP
- Bradycardia and hypotension (Wainright and Gould, 1996), syncope, ventricular irritability, ventricular tachycardia and asystole (Flynn and Bruce, 1993) attributed to mechanical stimulation of the vagus nerve
- Prolonged coughing during the procedure
- Paroxysmal cough caused by stimulation of the tracheal and carinal reflexes, which may in turn affect the venous return and cardiac output and also cause infection (Flynn and Bruce, 1993).

After suctioning

Psychological care

The use of invasive techniques and therapies can result in patients experiencing a feeling of being 'tied down' (Clifford, 1985), thus producing sensations of fear, anxiety and helplessness (Granberg *et al.*, 1996). Ashworth's 1980 classical study provided evidence that nurses' communication with patients in the intensive care unit tends to be task-focused, relatively uninformative, nurse-controlled and associated mainly with physical procedures. Effective communication is a key strategy in preventing anxiety, and explanation of the patient's condition and progress is essential. Therefore, communication between nurses and patients is as vital as it is difficult.

Assessment of sputum

The type, viscosity and amount of secretions should be noted. In the presence of pulmonary disease, infection or dehydration, respiratory secretions may become thick and tenacious, making removal by suctioning difficult. If the patient becomes dehydrated, the mucosal membranes will be drier, mucociliary transport will decrease, and there will be retention of secretions. Therefore, systemic hydration needs to be maintained. If thick and tenacious secretions are linked to dehydration, the patient may need additional fluid replacement or humidification.

If the secretions are loose, copious in amount, pink, frothy and possibly blood-stained, this may indicate fluid overload (pulmonary oedema); yellow/green secretions may be indicative of infection and rusty sputum of pneumonia.

Any deterioration in the patient during suctioning may require termination of the procedure, hyperoxygenation and consequent intervention.

Implications for practice

- Nurses should be competent in assessing the need for performing suctioning
- Suctioning should be performed on the basis of clinical evidence (patient's signs and symptoms)
- Nurses should take particular care when suctioning patients who have additional medical problems (e.g. COPD and head injury)
- Continuous monitoring of the patient for signs of complication during and after the procedure is essential.

Summary

The procedure of suctioning is a necessary part of nursing intervention for the critically ill but should not be viewed as a routine approach. The decision to perform suctioning should be based upon the patient's clinical condition. The correct procedure needs to be adhered to throughout.

Clinical scenario

José Palance, 57 years old, was transferred from the intensive care unit 7 hours ago. Originally admitted with type 2 respiratory failure due to an acute exacerbation of COPD, she has been extubated for 10 hours. She is tachypnoeic, sweating, oxygen saturation 87%. She is coughing but unable to expectorate. Auscultation indicates 'rattling in chest'.

1   What would be your rationale for suctioning?

2   Provide a plan of care for this particular skill, describing the procedure.

3   What criteria would you use to evaluate success?

Bibliography

Key reading

Day *et al.* (2002) provides a relatively comprehensive review of research recommendations
Somerson *et al.* (1996) offers advice to the nurse relating to emergency respiratory care, including suctioning.

Further reading

Day *et al.* (2001) identifies gaps in nurses' knowledge and skill and areas for education.

Chapter 32

Arterial blood pressure monitoring

Philip Woodrow

Contents

Learning outcomes

After reading this chapter you will be able to:

- Understand the significance of mean arterial pressure and pulse pressure
- Recognise causes of inaccurate measurement
- Identify which patients may benefit from invasive intra-arterial monitoring.

Introduction

Although blood pressure and pulse are monitored in most healthcare settings, additional information can be inferred from these observations, and there are potential causes of errors that should be avoided. Some high dependency units may use arterial lines for continuous blood pressure monitoring. This chapter therefore discusses both non-invasive and invasive monitoring of arterial blood pressure.

Arterial blood pressure

Blood pressure, the pressure exerted on vessel walls, is affected by flow and resistance. Flow is created by the stroke volume and the viscosity of blood.

The force of arterial blood flow decreases slightly as the distance from the heart increases, but this decrease is usually more than offset by increased resistance. Resistance is the sum of the arterial wall tone (e.g. increased with atherosclerosis, decreased with dilatation), the vessel size, and the pressure from tissues (e.g. oedema).

Pressure in the ascending aorta is slightly higher than in the brachial artery (the usual site for cuff measurements) or radial artery (the usual site for arterial lines). The difference between brachial and radial artery measurements is clinically insignificant, but elsewhere (e.g. thigh blood pressure cuffs or pedal arterial lines) increased resistance from smaller vessels may make distal measurements up to one-third higher than central pressure (Runciman and Ludbrook, 1996).

Viscosity

The viscosity of blood is determined by its largest components, the blood cells. Of these the largest number are erythrocytes, so viscosity equates with haemoglobin – thus while higher haemoglobin levels increase oxygen-carrying capacity, they also reduce blood flow and hence oxygen delivery. Optimum haemoglobin in critical illness has been much debated, but recent evidence suggests ideal levels of 7–9 g/dl (Herbert *et al.*, 1999).

Fluctuations

The body's circadian rhythm affects blood pressure, the lowest level normally being in the early hours of the morning. Secretion of vasoconstricting hormones such as noradrenaline causes the blood pressure to rise by the time of normal waking (Redón *et al.*, 2001).

Mean arterial pressure

Systolic (maximum) pressure is transient, but perfusion continues throughout the pulse. Therefore, recording the average (mean) pressure across the whole pulse cycle provides a more accurate indication of perfusion. Mean pressure is

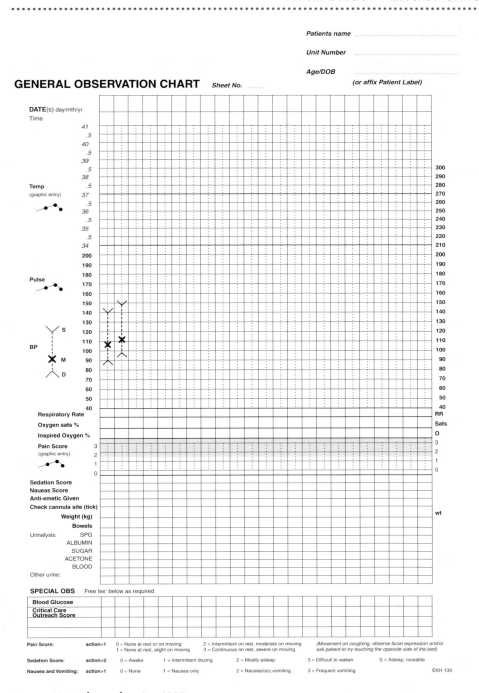

GENERAL OBSERVATION CHART   Sheet No. ....

Patients name ....

Unit Number ....

Age/DOB ....

(or affix Patient Label)

Figure 32.1 Chart, showing MAP

also less affected by artifact and does not alter between different sites (Darovic, 2002b). Mean blood pressure is calculated by most automated blood pressure devices.

Critical illness usually causes poor perfusion, so mean arterial pressure (MAP) should be maintained at least above 70 mmHg if possible, to ensure perfusion to the brain, kidneys and other major organs. The three pressures can be clearly charted by using arrows for systolic and diastolic, and a cross for mean, pressures (see Figure 32.1).

Pulse pressure

Pulse pressure is the pressure created by each pulse, and is measured by subtracting the diastolic from the systolic pressure. For example, blood pressure of 140/90 creates a pulse pressure of 50. Because systolic pressure represents the maximum stretch of the vessel wall, pulse pressure indicates the response (stretch) of the blood vessel to pulse, so wide pulse pressures indicate poor compliance of artery walls (e.g. atherosclerosis) (Campbell, 1997), while narrow pulse pressures indicate hypovolaemia. Wide pulse pressure may be an early indication of risk of chronic heart failure (Haider et al., 2003) or Alzheimer's disease (Qui et al., 2003). Pulse pressure should be assessed against previous readings from the same patient, but taking physiologically 'normal' blood pressure as 120/80, a 'rule of thumb' narrow pulse pressure would be below 30.

Equipment

The speed and reliability (Jones et al., 2003) of readings from automated devices, together with the hazards of mercury, have made sphygmomanometers almost obsolete in clinical practice. However, like any other equipment, automated devices (and sphygmomanometers) are only reliable if maintained and used appropriately. Staff should therefore report equipment that is due for service. Most Trusts check the calibration of automated blood pressure machines once every year, recording on the device when it was last serviced.

Most blood pressure devices automatically inflate cuffs to a pre-set pressure for all patients. This is usually an uncomfortably high pressure for most patients, but can be adjusted. Readers are recommended to try on themselves the devices that they will be using on their patients. If using the timed cycle mode to monitor blood pressure, the benefits of hourly observations (maximum cycle length on most automated devices) should be weighed against any disturbance to sleep patterns – an average sleep cycle is about 90 minutes.

The cuff for measuring arterial blood pressure should be at heart level; being placed lower may give falsely high readings, potentially of up to 10 mmHg (Beevers et al., 2001a).

Although fitted with standard-sized cuffs, larger and smaller cuffs should also be available. The cuff bladder length should be at least 80 per cent of the arm circumference (Beevers et al., 2001a) and its width at least 40 per cent (Bridges and Middleton, 1997). Small cuffs give falsely high readings (Runcimann and Lud-

Table 32.1 Blood pressure cuff size (after Beevers et al., 2001b)

BP cuff size	Cuff width (cm)	Cuff length (cm)	Maximum arm circumference (cm)
Normal adult	12	26	33
Obese adult	12	40	50
Medium-sized child/small adult	10	18	26
Small child	4.0	13	17

brook, 1996), while large cuffs give falsely low readings. Recommended sizes are listed in Table 32.1.

Intra-arterial blood pressure

Direct (invasive) arterial pressure monitoring provides continuous measurement, greater accuracy, and a pulse waveform display. It also gives easy access for blood gas and other blood samples. Because intra-arterial pressures are directly measuring the pressure in the artery, rather than that relayed through flesh between the artery and an external cuff, intra-arterial readings are usually 5–20 mmHg higher (Coad, 1996). Provided the trace looks reliable and there are no other indicators to disbelieve an intra-arterial measurement, it is illogical to check invasive against non-invasive measurements, or to believe cuff rather than intra-arterial pressure.

Arterial blood pressure waveforms (see Figure 32.2) should have sharp and steady upstrokes, caused by steadily increasing pressure as blood is ejected from the left ventricle. Notches on the upstroke (anacrotic notches) are abnormal, indicating resistance to flow (e.g. from aortic stenosis). At the end of ventricular contraction systole is reached, represented by the brief peak on the trace. As aortic pressure falls, the aortic valve closes, causing a brief second surge in pressure – the dicrotic notch. Pressure then falls steadily until diastole is reached. The area under the curve indicates stroke volume, so smaller traces are often seen in heart failure.

A small 'swing' on the baseline over a number of complexes can be caused by breathing, and so is not clinically relevant. Normal breathing reduces blood pressure by 3–10 mmHg (Adam and Osborne, 1997), but deep breaths can cause greater swings. In critical illness, swings greater than 10 mmHg suggest hypovolaemia (Rooke, 1995).

Before reading transduced pressures, transducers should be at heart level and zeroed. Even small differences in height significantly affect blood pressure readings. Zeroing arterial transducers is identical to zeroing central venous ones. With the transducer at heart level, the tap should be opened to both machine and air, but closed to the patient. The instruction to zero is pressed. Once zeroed (a zero will be displayed on the screen, and some monitors state that the procedure is completed) the tap is closed to air, so that it is open to both the machine and the patient. The transducer should be secured at the level at which it has been zeroed.

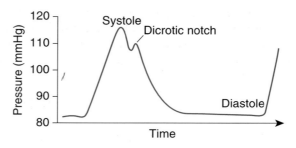

Figure 32.2 **Arterial waveform with dicrotic notch**

Complications of arterial lines

Any invasive device creates complications. While arterial lines provide many benefits, they expose patients to significant risks from:

- Infection
- Occlusion
- Haemorrhage
- Drug error.

Infection risks are similar to those of any in-dwelling vascular devices, but the frequency with which many arterial cannulae are handled (e.g. for blood samples) increases the likelihood of complications. Like any vascular devices, cannulae should be treated aseptically.

Although arteries are smaller than veins, arterial cannulae in clinical use are unlikely to occlude the vessel. However, any synthetic device in blood vessels can cause thrombus formation. The thrombus may directly occlude the vessel, or release an embolus which, propelled by arterial pressure, may wedge in some smaller vessel. Occlusion causes cold and blanched or cyanosed peripheries, so fingers, toes or other tissue beyond the cannulae should be checked frequently. Pressure transducers rely on continuous infusion of heparinised saline in a pressure bag inflated to 300 mmHg. This gives a flow of 3 ml every hour (Hatchett, 2002), which should be enough to prevent thrombus formation without causing other significant complications.

Disconnection of any vascular cannula or infusion can cause haemorrhage, but low blood pressure in veins usually makes bleeds slow. Haemorrhage under arterial pressure is far more rapid, potentially causing fatal exsanguination. Arterial connections must therefore be secure and checked frequently. Whenever possible, arterial line sites should be kept exposed. Setting lower pressure alarm limits within 20 mmHg of diastolic pressure should provide early warning of any disconnection. Critically ill patients often have prolonged bleeding, caused by liver hypofunction, which may cause oozing around the cannula site. If this is significant and cannot reasonably be stopped, the cannula probably needs to be removed.

Arterial lines are intended for pressure measurement and blood sampling; not for drug or fluid infusion. Rapid flow from high arterial pressure can cause toxic concentrations of any drugs given arterially, so arterial lines should be clearly labelled to prevent accidental injection of drugs into the line. Most units place red labels near any connections on arterial lines.

Units of blood pressure

Blood pressure has traditionally been measured in millimetres of mercury (mmHg). Although not a system internationale (SI) unit of measurement, retaining mmHg remained logical as long as mercury sphygmomanometers were used to measure blood pressure. Now this is no longer the case, measurement may change to the SI units of kilopascals (O'Brien, 2001), where 1 kPa = 7.4 mmHg.

Implications for practice

- Arterial BP trends are more significant than absolute figures.
- The mean arterial pressure is the best indicator of perfusion pressure.
- Mean arterial pressure should be maintained above 70 mmHg.
- Pulse pressure is the response of blood vessels to the pulse, and so indicates blood vessel tone and stroke volume; raised pulse pressure indicates cardiovascular disease.

Summary

Blood pressure is a vital sign. Problems with blood pressure (hyper- or hypotension) are, however, symptoms of underlying problems. Nurses caring for highly dependent patients therefore need to consider factors causing abnormal pressure.

In recent years, automated devices have largely replaced sphygmomanometers. This has tended to result in greater accuracy of measurement, and provide useful information about mean arterial pressure. Additional useful information is available through simple calculation of pulse pressure.

Arterial lines can provide useful (and more accurate) continuous blood pressure readings, together with easy availability for arterial blood sampling. However, arterial bleeding can quickly result in massive blood loss, so arterial lines should only be used in areas where patients can be very closely observed, the appropriate equipment is available for continuous monitoring, and staff are skilled in caring for patients with arterial lines.

Clinical scenario

Mr Hugh Barton has been admitted following recent episodes of dizziness. He has a history of hypertension and, despite taking his daily 10 mg of atenolol this morning, his blood pressure is 173/86 and he feels tingling in his fingers. His heart rate is 65 (regular).

1   Comment on this information, identifying what it indicates. Include comments on his systolic, diastolic and pulse pressures.

2   His mean arterial pressure is 115. What does this indicate?

3   An arterial line is inserted into Mr Barton's right radial artery. Devise a care plan to manage Mr Barton's arterial line safely. Include any problems the line may cause him, and strategies to alleviate these problems.

Bibliography

Key reading

Material on blood pressure measurement can be found in most critical care and medical/surgical texts. Darovic's (2000b) text provides a comprehensive review of cardiovascular monitoring. Beevers *et al.* (2001b) provides a valuable medical review of blood pressure measurement, while Lip (2003) offers a useful practical guide for managing hypertension. Staff should read handbooks/manuals for any monitoring equipment used in their workplace.

Further reading

Campbell (1997) provides useful insights into interpreting waveforms from intra-arterial measurement.

Chapter 33

Central venous pressure measurement and cardiac output studies

Philip Woodrow

Contents

Learning outcomes

After reading this chapter you will be able to:

- Read a central venous pressure
- Identify the main causes of high and low central venous pressure measurements
- Apply knowledge of central venous pressure measurement to patient care
- Describe the main options available for cardiac output studies.

Fundamental knowledge

Cardiac physiology.

Introduction

Blood pressure and pulse can easily and reliably be measured in most clinical areas. While these measurements will provide sufficient information to manage most diseases, critical illness may necessitate further monitoring, such as central venous pressure measurement or cardiac output studies.

Blood pressure is the sum of cardiac output and systemic vascular resistance, so:

$$BP = CO \times SVR$$

Cardiac output is the sum of stroke volume and heart rate, so:

$$CO = SV \times HR$$

Combining these formulae:

$$BP = SV \times HR \times SVR$$

Measuring blood pressure may identify a problem, such as hypotension, but the problem may be caused by any (or all three) of these factors, only one of which is easily measurable on most wards. Critical illness provokes acute problems, while critically ill patients often have fewer physical reserves, so early and precise identification can prevent complications such as renal failure from prolonged hypotension.

This chapter focuses on central venous pressure measurement, which will be used in many highly dependent (level 2) patients. However, development of less invasive and more reliable ways to measure cardiac output will lead to these being increasingly used in more clinical areas, so the main cardiac output study measurements are also briefly described.

Central venous pressure measurement

Central lines, or central venous catheters (CVC), are placed in one of the two central veins: the superior or inferior vena cava. Central venous pressure measures the pressure of blood returning to, or filling, the right atrium. This indicates blood volume, vascular tone and cardiac function, and is sometimes referred to as 'filling' pressure, right atrial pressure (RAP) or right ventricular end diastolic pressure (RVEDP).

The majority (about 65 per cent) of the total blood volume is in the veins. In practice, central venous pressure is usually used to assess the blood volume and so guide fluid management. However, central venous pressure will also be affected by:

- Pumps. Blood return to the right atrium is assisted in health by two 'pumps' – the intrathoracic and the skeletal. When breathing in, negative pressure in the thorax draws in whatever it can from outside the thorax. Although this is mainly air into the lungs, it also includes blood from the lower to the upper part of the inferior vena cava. Shallow breathing, or artificial ventilation, therefore reduces blood return to the heart. Muscles contain a rich blood supply. Muscle movement relies on muscular contraction, which squeezes blood out of blood vessels in the muscle. Walking actively increases blood return to the right atrium. Critically ill patients usually mobilise little, so pooling more venous blood in the peripheral vessels. Reduced function of either pump reduces blood return to the right atrium, which reduces central venous pressure.
- Vascular tone. This (and so central venous pressure) may be reduced by vasodilators. Exogenous vasodilating drugs include nitrates (e.g. glyceryl trinitrate, isosorbide mono/dinitrate), but the body also produces endogenous vasodilators, such as nitric oxide, released by ischaemic vascular endothelium. Many critically ill patients have long-standing cardiovascular disease, which may both increase vascular tone and impair right heart function.
- Obstruction to blood flow. This increases central venous pressure, and can be caused by heart failure (especially right-sided failure, such as mitral valve disease); pulmonary congestion (e.g. ARDS, pulmonary hypertension); and increased intrathoracic pressure (e.g. CPAP).

Measurement

Central venous pressure is usually read from the mid-axilla, where lines from the midsternal fourth intercostal space and mid-axilla intersect. In practice, to ensure consistency of the site a small inkmark is usually made on the skin. A few staff may have been taught to measure from the sternal notch. As this will significantly reduce the figures (see below), all staff in one clinical area should measure CVPs from the same point. When receiving patients from elsewhere, staff should check where readings were measured from before comparing them with their own. This chapter assumes measurements are taken from the mid-axilla, but the principles below apply whichever site is used for measurement.

To reflect right atrial pressure, patients should ideally lie supine. However, many breathless patients become distressed in this position, so if they are in a semirecumbent or upright position, the position should be recorded on charts so that future measurements can whenever possible be made in the same position.

Zeroing

'Zeroing' the CVP ensures that the atmospheric pressure at the point of measurement is read as zero. Many high dependency areas measure CVP with monitors that can be electronically zeroed once the transducer (see Figure 33.1) is placed at the right atrial level, with flow from the transducer open to the air but closed to the patient. CVP measurement with water manometers should align the zero on

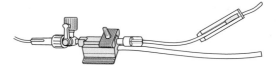

Figure 33.1 **Transduced system**

the scale with the right atrial level; this is usually checked with a spirit level, although commercial light-source devices are also available.

Reading

Digital monitors display a trace and reading once the transducer is closed to air and open to the patient. Provided the scale is sufficiently large, the trace should have a clear waveform (see Figure 33.2), and there will usually be a respiratory 'swing' – the whole trace moving up and down with breathing.

After zeroing, the chamber of a water manometer (see Figure 33.3) should be almost filled with fluid by opening the fluid to the measuring chamber while keeping the tap closed to the patient. Avoid getting the air filter at the top wet – wet filters resist air entry, so giving falsely high readings. The tap should then be turned to stop fluid flow, and the chamber opened to the patient. Gravity makes the fluid level fall until resistance from the patient's central venous pressure matches the pressure of gravity. Slight changes in pressure from the patient's respiratory pattern (usually about 1 cm) make the fluid fall in a 'swinging' pattern, until it oscillates between two figures. Intrathoracic pressure, and so the fluid level in the chamber, falls on inspiration (unless patients are artificially ventilated), so the higher figure of the swing is recorded.

Scale

Central venous pressure may be measured in millimetres of mercury (mmHg) or centimetres of water (cmH_2O). The millimetres of mercury measurement uses the same scale in which arterial and other blood pressure measurements are made, so is used whenever transduced measurement is available. However, mercury is neurotoxic, so manometers have to use water-based fluids, such as 5% glucose or normal saline, which provide readings in centimetres of water. Thus both scales may be used in the same hospital, and sometimes within one clinical area.

Figures are rounded to the nearest whole number, making the two scales

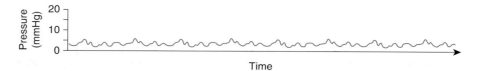

Figure 33.2 **CVP trace**

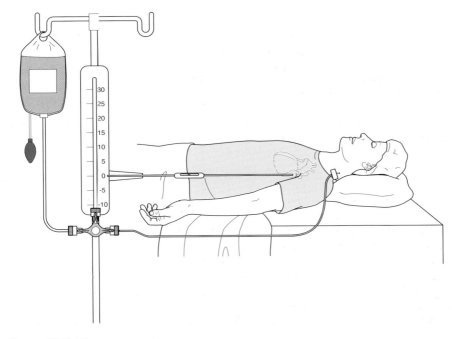

Figure 33.3 **Water manometer**

compatible at low figures; however, with higher figures differences become significant (see Table 33.1).

When receiving patients from other clinical areas it is therefore important to know which scale has been used for CVP measurement.

Pressures

Normal

In health, central venous pressure should be 5–10 mmHg/7–14 cmH$_2$O (mid-axilla) or 0–5 mmHg/0–7 cmH$_2$O (sternal angle) (Henderson, 1997). However, critically ill patients often have abnormally high or low CVPs, with treatment usually aiming to maintain slightly higher than normal CVP to ensure sufficient blood return to the heart. A single central venous pressure measurement has limited significance, but trends show response to treatment and/or disease progression.

Low

A low CVP almost invariably indicates either fluid loss by haemorrhage (e.g. due to trauma or surgery), or excessive diuresis (due to diabetes, diuretics), or poor return (e.g. due to shock).

Table 33.1 Comparison of mmHg and cmH$_2$O pressures

cmH$_2$O	mmHg (exact)	mmHg (rounded)
1	0.74	1
2	1.48	1
3	2.22	2
4	2.96	3
5	3.70	4
6	4.44	4
7	5.18	5
8	5.92	6
9	6.66	7
10	7.40	7
11	8.14	8
12	8.88	9
13	9.62	10
14	10.36	10
15	11.10	11
16	11.84	12
17	12.58	13
18	13.32	13
19	14.06	14
20	14.80	15

mmHg	cmH$_2$O (exact)	cmH$_2$O (rounded)
1	1.36	1
2	2.72	3
3	4.08	4
4	5.44	5
5	6.80	7
6	8.16	8
7	9.52	10
8	10.88	11
9	12.22	12
10	13.60	14
11	14.96	15
12	16.32	16
13	17.68	18
14	19.04	19
15	20.40	20
16	21.76	22
17	23.10	23
18	24.44	24
19	25.82	26
20	27.20	27

High

A high central venous pressure reading may be caused by various factors, including:

- Hypervolaemia (e.g. excessive fluid infusion, renal failure)
- Cardiac failure
- Increased intrathoracic pressure (e.g. from non-invasive ventilation)
- Lumen occlusion/obstruction (e.g. the cannula against the vein wall; thrombus)
- High blood viscosity (rare, but possible following massive blood transfusion)
- Artifact (e.g. viscous drugs/fluids remaining in the line)
- User error (e.g. a wet air filter in water manometers).

The patency of blocked catheters may be restored with urokinase, a thrombolytic agent. With the small doses used to unblock catheters, no complications have been reported (Polderman and Girbes, 2002a)

Cardiac output studies

Central venous pressure measurement provides valuable information about right-sided heart function. In health, ventricular filling and stroke volume are the same on both sides of the heart. However, many critically ill patients have significant heart disease, and so measuring right-sided function may be a poor indication of left-sided function.

Equipment

Pulmonary artery floatation catheters (PAFCs), sometimes called 'Swan–Ganz' catheters (or 'Swans') have largely been replaced by less invasive and non-invasive equipment.

Dopplers, long used to assess peripheral blood flow, have been adapted to measure aortic blood flow, and hence cardiac output. Transtracheal dopplers proved disappointing (Armstrong *et al.*, 1993), but transoesophageal doppler cardiac output studies have been more widely used (Higgins and Singer, 1993).

The capillary blood pressure trace displayed on some pulse oximeters led to the use of *finger blood pressure waveforms* to measure cardiac output. Unfortunately the inaccuracy rate of nearly one-quarter of readings (Hirschl *et al.*, 1997) makes this currently too unreliable to recommend.

Thoracic electrical bioimpedance uses ECG-like electrodes around the neck and thorax to measure differences occurring in aortic flow between systole and diastole. This enables the calculation of cardiac output. High signal-to-noise ratios cause considerable inaccuracy compared with thermodilution measurements (Haller *et al.*, 1995), although Thangathurai *et al.* (1997) consider this mode to be useful.

Peripherally Inserted Continuous Cardiac Output (PiCCO), *lithium-derived cardiac output* (LidCO®) and various other systems measure cardiac studies less invasively than pulmonary artery floatation catheters. However, PiCCO can not be used with any condition where femoral cannulation is contraindicated (e.g. femoral popliteal bypass, severe burns). Lithium-derived cardiac output (LidCO®) uses a central and an arterial line to measure cardiac output and systemic vascular resistance continuously.

Clinical use of PAFCs generated heated debate in the 1980s, advocates considering that they provided valuable diagnostic information whilst opponents considered they exposed patients to unacceptable risks, including increased mortality (Connors *et al.*, 1996). Debate about the value of measuring cardiac output, and the best means to achieve this, may be resolved by the current major UK PACMAN trial. Meanwhile, developments in less- and non-invasive technology are likely to result in increased measurement of cardiac output in various wards and departments.

Information obtained varies between both modes and manufacturers, so readers may find their systems do not give all information below, or may give additional information. If using information not described below, readers should find out what the reading means (from manufacturer's handbooks or company representatives). Normal ranges are given in Table 33.2, but cardiac output studies are usually made when people have heart disease, so abnormal readings will more often be seen in practice. Normal ranges are, however, useful to guide medical management. Indexed figures adjust measurements according to size (body mass index, calculated from weight and height), giving figures that are comparable between patients.

Nurses in most wards therefore have had little or no opportunity to gain the skills needed to make accurate and safe measurements. Until appropriate competence is gained, all measurements taken should therefore be supervised or made by experienced staff.

Cardiac output measurements

Blood pressure is cardiac output multiplied by systemic vascular resistance ($BP = CO \times SVR$). With hypo- or hypertension, either or both of these may be problematic, or compensating for the other. Therefore measuring cardiac output (and thus also deriving systemic vascular resistance) enables treatment for hypotension to target whichever factor causes the problem.

- *Pulmonary artery pressure (PAP).* Pulmonary arteries are more compliant than systemic ones, so have a lower blood pressure. However, severe lung diseases, such as ARDS (see Chapter 15) cause pulmonary hypertension. Pressures above 40 mmHg indicate haemodynamic collapse (Freebairn and Oh, 1997). Low pulmonary artery pressures when CVP is high indicate right heart failure (e.g. mitral valve regurgitation).

- *Pulmonary capillary wedge pressure (PCWP).* Also called pulmonary artery occlusion pressure (PAOP). By inflating a balloon on the tip of a pulmonary

Table 33.2 Normal ranges for cardiac output studies

Cardiac output study	Normal range
Pulmonary artery pressure	
Systolic	5–25 mmHg
Diastolic	5–15 mmHg
Mean	10–20 mmHg
Pulmonary capillary wedge pressure/pulmonary artery occlusion pressure	5–15 mmHg
Stroke volume	60–120 ml
Stroke volume index/stroke index	35–70 ml/beat/m²
Cardiac output (resting)	4–8 l/min
Cardiac index	2.5–4.0 l/min/mm²
Left ventricular stroke volume index	50–60 gm/min/m²
Left cardiac work index	3.4–4.2 kg/min/m²
Right cardiac work index	0.54–0.66 kg/min/m²
Right ventricular stroke work index	7.9–9.7 g/min/m²
Extravascular lung water	5–7 ml/kg
Systemic vascular resistance	900–1,500 dyn/s/cm²
Pulmonary vascular resistance	20–120 dyn/s/cm²
Delivery of oxygen	900–1,100 ml/min
Delivery of oxygen index	520–720 ml/min/m²
Consumption of oxygen	200–290 ml/min
Consumption of oxygen index	100–180 ml/min/m²
Oxygen extraction ratio	0.22–0.30
Shunt fraction	3–5%

'Normal' figures vary slightly between different texts. Where reasonable, rounded figures have been selected.

artery floatation catheter, blood flow through a pulmonary artery can be occluded, or 'wedged'. Measuring pressure beyond that occlusion indicates left atrial, and so left ventricular, function. Occluding blood flow to pulmonary vessels can cause ischaemia, thrombus formation and emboli, so until competent with this skill, staff should be supervised when taking readings.

■ *Stroke volume (SV), stroke volume index (SVI)*. Stroke volume and heart rate determine cardiac output ($SV \times HR = CO$). Many critically ill patients have poor cardiac function, giving a low stroke volume. However, inotropes (e.g. adrenaline) will increase stroke volume, provided filling pressure (CVP, PCWP) is adequate.

■ *Cardiac output (CO), cardiac index (CI)*. Cardiac output is the sum of stroke volume and heart rate, so multiplying the stroke volume by the heart rate, and converting millilitres to litres, provides a calculated cardiac output.

■ *Left ventricular stroke work (LVSW), left ventricular stroke work index (LVSWI), left cardiac work (LCW), left cardiac work index (LCWI)*. In heart failure, assessing the function of each side of the heart can usefully guide treatment. Left-sided function determines systemic stroke volume. So, from mean arterial pressure (MAP) and cardiac output the work of the left myocardium can be calculated. Indexed figures are usually used.

■ *Right cardiac work (RCW), right cardiac work index (RCWI), right ventricular stroke work (RVSW), right ventricular stroke work index (RVSWI).* Right-sided heart function can similarly be calculated. Although often less useful than assessment of left-sided function, right heart failure may need to be treated.

■ *Extravascular lung water (EVLW).* This indicates left heart function. Diseases such as acute respiratory distress syndrome (ARDS) cause excessive accumulation of interstitial fluid in the lungs. Fluid management in such pathologies has generated strong debate, with little evidence to guide practice. The amount of extravascular lung water correlates with mortality (Sakka *et al.*, 2002), so measuring EVLW enables perfusion to be optimised, improving fluid and vasoactive drug therapy (Salukhe and Wyncoll, 2002). The normal extravascular lung water index (EVLW) is 5–7 ml/kg, so (as a rule of thumb) fluid is not usually infused if the EVLW index exceeds 10 ml/kg. This should help to reduce both morbidity and mortality.

■ *Systemic vascular resistance (SVR).* Together with cardiac output, systemic vascular resistance determines blood pressure. It also controls perfusion. So excessive systemic vascular resistance causes hypertension and poor perfusion, while low systemic vascular resistance causes hypotension (shock).

■ *Pulmonary vascular resistance.* Similarly, pulmonary vascular resistance can be calculated. With severe lung disease (e.g. ARDS), this may help guide treatment.

■ *Delivery of oxygen (DO$_2$), delivery of oxygen index (DO$_2$I).* Comparing SvO_2 (from a sample of central venous blood) and SaO_2 enables calculation of oxygen delivery – the ultimate aim of perfusion.

■ *Consumption of oxygen (VO$_2$), consumption of oxygen index (VO$_2$I).* Once oxygen delivery is optimised, calculating oxygen consumption indicates whether tissues can extract sufficient oxygen to meet metabolic needs.

■ *Oxygen extraction ratio (OER/O$_2$ER).* Comparing oxygen delivery to consumption enables calculation of the oxygen extraction ratio, which is expressed as a decimal fraction of 1.0.

■ *Shunt fraction.* 'Shunt' blood is blood that returns to the left atrium with similar gas concentrations to those in blood leaving the right ventricle. In health, unperfused alveoli collapse, and capillaries to unventilated alveoli vasoconstrict. This prevents air entering alveoli or blood entering capillaries where gas exchange cannot occur. However, the inflammatory response that accompanies most critical illnesses prevents the physiological vasoconstriction response, so with severe lung disease considerable shunting of blood occurs. Shunt fraction is expressed as a percentage.

Implications for practice

- Central venous pressure provides a useful indication of blood volume and cardiac function
- Staff measuring CVP should understand how to make accurate and reliable measurements
- Low CVP is usually due to hypovolaemia
- High CVP is usually due either to hypervolaemia or heart failure
- Cardiac output studies can provide useful information to guide therapy, but can be highly invasive or, with some modes, have other significant limitations/complications
- Non-invasive modes are preferable if they are available and reliable
- Trends are more significant than absolute figure
- No observation should be 'routine'; nurses should only perform observations if information may be used, and should consider carefully before delegating tasks to anyone unable to interpret information gained.

Summary

Haemodynamic monitoring provides very useful diagnostic information about critically ill patients. However, invasive modes expose patients to significant infection and other risks, and observation may cause patients stress or inconvenience, so the value of any observation and monitoring equipment should be constantly reassessed and equipment removed when burdens outweigh benefits. Information gained should be evaluated in the context of disease progression and treatments.

For many critically ill patients, monitoring blood pressure and heart rate does provide sufficient information for medical management. Central venous pressure provides a valuable indication of fluid status, although other factors, such as cardiac function, can also significantly affect readings.

Although cardiac output studies are unlikely to be performed on many level 2 patients, this chapter has provided an overview of the main measurements and calculations as a reference point for staff who do see cardiac output studies performed.

Clinical scenario

Mrs Margaret Bowles, aged 68, is admitted to the high dependency unit with shortness of breath. She has long-standing atrial fibrillation and hypertension. Medication on admission includes digoxin, diuretics and anti-hypertensives. On admission, BP is 155/95, heart rate is about 90 (irregular), and respiratory rate is 36, with shallow breaths.

A subclavian central line is inserted. Her CVP is 12 mmHg.

1   What factors might cause Mrs Bowles to have a CVP of 12 mmHg?

2   Devise a self-directed teaching guide for junior colleagues to help them measure CVP accurately. Refer to equipment and systems available at your workplace.

3   Remembering Mrs Bowles' history and current condition, do you think her CVP needs to be reduced or increased? If so, how? If not, at what point would you want her CVP to be treated? Identify likely treatments for both high and low CVP, and discuss these ideas with colleagues.

Bibliography

Key reading

Articles on central venous pressure measurement and central lines appear periodically in the nursing press. Although these vary in quality, Henderson (1997) is the most reliable recent article. Polderman and Girbes (2002a, 2002b) provides a useful recent medical review of problems caused by central lines.

Further reading

Most critical care texts discuss central venous pressure measurement and cardiac output studies. Dillon *et al.* (1997) provides a useful text for interpreting cardiac output studies. Readers should be familiar with handbooks and manuals for equipment used in their workplace.

Chapter 34

Reading electrocardiograms and recognising common dysrhythmias

Philip Woodrow

Contents

Learning outcomes

After reading this chapter you will be able to:

- Understand how normal cardiac conduction relates to the ECG trace for normal sinus rhythm
- Recognise common dysrhythmias

- Recognise the difference between, and implications of, broad and narrow complex tachycardias
- Identify main treatments for dysrhythmias identified in this chapter.

Fundamental knowledge

Cardiac anatomy (including coronary arteries); normal conduction pathways (SA node, AV node, Bundle of His, Branch Bundle, Purkinje Fibres).

Introduction

Level 2 patients may need continuous electrocardiogram (ECG) monitoring or single 12-lead ECGs. This chapter therefore identifies the more frequently seen dysrhythmias, likely causes and main treatments.

Like any skill, reading ECGs takes practice, and can be enhanced considerably beyond the scope of this chapter. This chapter bridges pre-registration introduction to ECGs and advanced study days, texts and courses dedicated to developing this skill. ECG interpretation skills can be developed further through:

- Key texts recommended in this chapter
- Clinical practice, looking at ECGs of patients
- Study days
- Discussion with colleagues.

Familiarity with normal cardiac conduction is presumed. Readers unfamiliar with this should revise normal electrophysiology before proceeding with this chapter.

ECGs represent the three-dimensional electrical activity of cardiac conduction on a two-dimensional graph (see Figure 34.1). The ECG trace can begin on any level, but the height of the complexes represents voltage (1 cm = 1 mv – 2 large squares = 10 small squares) and the length or width of the complexes represents time (1 small square = 0.04 seconds, 1 large square = 0.2 seconds, provided the machine runs at the standard 25 mm/second).

Usually, cardiac muscle contraction follows electrical activity. However, there is one important exception, pulseless electrical activity (PEA), where whatever rhythm is displayed on the ECG does not result in a pulse, and therefore there is little or no cardiac output.

When no electrical activity is recorded, the graph is horizontal (isoelectric). A line upward from the isolelectric line is called a positive deflection, while a line downward is called a negative deflection.

Electrodes

To record the six limb-lead traces, three electrodes are usually used. These three electrodes are normally colour-coded, being placed on the right arm (red), left

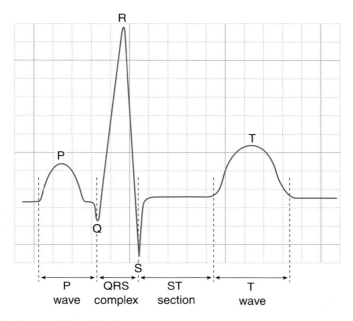

Figure 34.1 **Normal sinus rhythm**

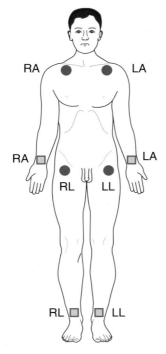

Figure 34.2 **Electrode placement – limb leads**

arm (yellow) and left leg (green) (see Figure 34.2). Placing can be memorised by remembering 'traffic lights'. The electrical 'picture' is unchanged along the limb, so electrodes may be anywhere between the hand/foot and the shoulder/hip. When taking a 12-lead ECG a fourth limb electrode is placed on the right leg (black), which acts as a 'neutral' trace.

The six chest-lead traces each use a single electrode (see Figure 34.3), numbered from the patient's right to left:

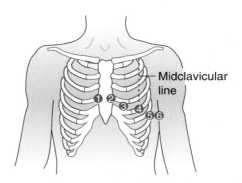

Figure 34.3 **Electrode placement – chest leads**

- C1: 4th intercostal space (right of sternum)
- C2: 4th intercostal space (left of sternum)
- C4: 5th intercostal space, mid-clavicular line
- C6: 5th intercostal space mid axilla
- C3: between C2 and C4
- C5: between C4 and C6.

Although often colour-coded, colours overlap with the limb electrodes, so chest leads are best remembered by the numbers 1–6. Some monitors may record a single (modified) chest lead. This is most often placed on C1, so becoming *modified chest lead 1* (MCL-1).

Reading ECGs

ECGs are mathematically logical, but contain much information in a small graph, so are best deciphered in logical stages, using a framework such as Box 34.1.

When analysing 12-lead ECGs, it is best to start with a single lead. Printouts often contain a single, longer sample of one lead, usually II or C1. In a healthy heart, lead II follows the normal axis cardiac conduction, and so is the most positive. However, people with cardiac disease may have axis deviation. Right axis deviation (relatively rare) makes lead III more positive, while left axis deviation makes lead I more positive.

Begin by looking at the regularity of the rhythm. Using scrap paper, mark two R waves (peaks), then move the paper one or more complexes. The gap between

---

Box 34.1   Reading ECGs

Regularity:
Is the rhythm regular?
If not, is it:

- regularly irregular (is there a pattern?)
- irregularly irregular (no pattern)?

P wave:
Does the P wave appear before the QRS?
Is there one P wave before every QRS?
Is the shape normal?
Is the P wave missing?

PR interval:
Is the PR interval 3–5 small squares?

QRS complex:
Is the QRS positive or negative?
Is the QRS within 3 small squares' width?
Does it look normal?

ST segment:
Does the isoelectric line return between the S and the T?
If not, is it:

- elevated
- depressed?

T wave:
Does the T wave look normal?

Tachycardia (>100 bpm):
Narrow complex (usually with P waves) = atrial (supraventricular)
Wide complex (without P wave) = ventricular

R waves should remain constant. If it is, the rhythm is regular. Regular rhythms can be pathological (e.g. ventricular tachycardia is an arrest situation). If the rhythm is not regular, is it:

- Regularly irregular (is there a pattern?)
- Irregularly irregular (no pattern)?

P wave

The P wave represents atrial depolarisation. This should be followed by ventricular depolarisation, so check: is there a P wave?

Atrial muscle disease can cause abnormal shapes, or total absence of the P wave:

- Does the P wave appear before the QRS?
- Is there one P wave before every QRS?

Atrial muscle mass is small, so voltage (height) is limited. The shape should, however, be a smooth curve above the isoelectric line, so:

- Is the shape normal?

When P waves look abnormal but the QRS looks normal, the dysrhythmia is atrial (supraventricular) in origin – e.g. narrow complex tachycardias.

PR interval

There is no specialised conduction pathway in the atria, so impulses are conducted from one muscle fibre to another. This makes conduction time across the atria relatively slow in proportion to muscle size. Impulses are then normally delayed at the atrioventricular (AV) node, so the PR interval, from the beginning of P wave to the beginning of QRS, should be 3–5 small squares (0.12–0.2 seconds):

- Is the PR interval 3–5 small squares?

Prolonged PR intervals, often from atrioventricular node disease, delay conduction (see First degree block, below).

Q wave

The first negative deflection represents septal depolarisation. Normally, Q waves are either small or absent. A deep (>2 small squares = >0.04 seconds (Sleight, 1999)) Q wave suggests myocardial infarction; however, up to 40 per cent of myocardial infarctions do not cause Q waves (Hudak *et al.*, 1998) (see Chapter 20).

QRS complex

From the atrioventricular node, impulses pass down the Bundle of His, which soon divides into a left and right branch. The left branch bundle further divides into the left anterior hemibranch and the left posterior hemibranch. From these three branches, impulses spread through Purkinje fibres into ventricular muscle cells.

The QRS represents ventricular depolarisation. Although tall (due to the large muscle mass of the ventricles) it is narrow (due to the speed with which the Bundle of His and branch bundles conduct impulses through the muscle). The QRS should be no wider than 3 small squares (0.06–0.12 seconds). Check:

- Is QRS positive or negative?
- Is its width within 3 small squares?
- Does it look normal?

When QRS complexes look abnormal but P waves look normal, the dysrhythmia is ventricular in origin – e.g. wide complex tachycardias.

ST segment

After the QRS, the trace should return rapidly to the isoelectric line:

- Does the isoelectric line return between the S and the T?

Ventricular conduction abnormalities can cause the ST to be depressed or raised. Either effect can have various causes, but elevation typically occurs following myocardial infarction, while depression is often due to either ischaemia or electrolyte (especially potassium) deficiency.
  If not, is it:

- Elevated
- Depressed?

T wave

This represents ventricular repolarisation, and should be a similar shape (only slightly larger) to the P wave. Tall T waves are one of the earliest signs of both myocardial infarction (Channer and Morris, 2002) and hyperkalaemia (Humphreys, 2002).

- Does the T wave look normal?

Artefact

Electrocardiographs will record any electrical activity they detect. All muscle conducts impulses using electrical charges, so skeletal muscle activity, such as shivering, may be recorded on the ECG paper. Similarly, external electrical activity, such as interference from electrical equipment, may be recorded on the graph. On ECGs, any electrical activity that does not originate from cardiac electricity results in artefact. This usually creates constant interference ('fuzz') throughout the trace.

Patient care

ECGs can provide useful diagnostic information whenever there is concern about myocardial function. However, like any observation, ECGs should only be recorded if information will be beneficial for patient care.

Many people fear cardiac disease more than most others, so cardiac investigations may cause stress. The stress response increases endogenous adrenaline (epinephrine) release, which accelerates hypertension and myocardial ischaemia. Therefore, for both psychological and physiological reasons the procedure should be explained.

Continuous ECG monitoring limits mobility, and wires can be dangerous if patients are disorientated and restless. Like any other intervention, the benefits of ECG monitoring should be weighed against their disadvantages.

Dysrhythmias and common treatments

Dysrhythmias are symptoms, and are only treated if they are causing (or likely to cause) problems. Some of the more frequently seen dysrhythmias are identified below, along with more common treatments:

1   Conduction defects:

- bradycardic dysrhythmias – positive chronotropes (e.g. atropine)
- atrial excitability – digoxin
- ventricular conduction excitability – beta-blockers (e.g. esmolol, sotalol, propanolol), calcium antagonists (e.g. amiodarone, verapamil), lignocaine (rhythm stabiliser)

2   Thrombi – anticoagulants
3   Poor cardiac output – positive inotropes (e.g. adrenaline, dobutamine).

If drugs fail, cardioversion or pacing (temporary or permanent) may be used. Oxygen is commonly given.

The appendix to this chapter lists other drugs commonly used to treat dysrhythmias.

Sinus arrhythmia

Some young adults, especially athletes, create sufficient negative pressure when breathing in to stimulate the vagus (parasympathetic) nerve, which reduces the sinoatrial rate so sinus rhythm slows slightly on inspiration, and increases on expiration. Typically, monitored heart rate alternates between two figures, often only about 4 beats per minute (bpm) apart. Sinus arrhythmia (Figure 34.4) is a healthy rhythm and should not be treated.

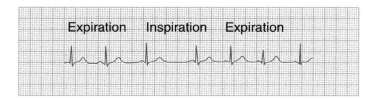

Figure 34.4 Sinus arrhythmia

Sinus bradycardia

This is a sinus rhythm below 60 bpm. If very slow (<40 bpm), positive chronotropes are given to increase the rate. Underlying causes (e.g. hypothermia) should be resolved.

Sinus tachycardia

This is a sinus rhythm above 100 bpm. Tachycardias reduce diastolic time, so reduce myocardial oxygenation at the same time as increasing myocardial oxygen consumption. Very fast rates (especially >140 bpm) usually need to be slowed with drugs such as amiodarone, digoxin, verapamil or beta-blockers. Tachycardia may be caused by abnormal re-entry of impulses into the atria (paroxysmal). Supraventricular tachycardia (SVT) usually implies rates above 160 bpm, requiring urgent treatment.

Ectopics

These are isolated beats from an abnormal pacemaker, with different complexes from the underlying rhythm. Their origin may be atrial, junctional or ventricular.

Atrial impulses will have an abnormal P wave and/or PR interval, but a normal QRS (see Figure 34.5). Junctional impulses will not have a P wave, but will have a normal QRS. Ventricular impulses have either no P wave or an abnormally placed one, with wide and bizarre QRS complexes. If all ventricular ectopics have the same shape, they are from the same focus ('unifocal'). If there are many different shapes, they are from different foci ('multifocal') (see Figure 34.6).

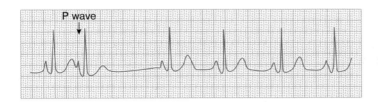

Figure 34.5 **Atrial ectopic**

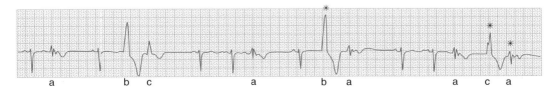

Figure 34.6 **Ventricular ectopics**

Ectopics are called 'premature' if they occur before the expected complex of the underlying rhythm, and 'escape' if the expected complex did not occur, allowing the ectopic focus to initiate the abnormal impulse. So, for example, a premature atrial ectopic (PAE), sometimes called a premature atrial contraction (PAC), is an atrial ectopic occurring before the expected sinus complex. Isolated ectopics are not usually treated, but can be symptomatic of underlying problems (such as hypokalaemia) that require treatment.

Atrial kick

With sinus rhythm, atrial contraction precedes ventricular contraction. This sequence increases ventricular filling prior to ventricular contraction. Almost all rhythms not originating from the sinoatrial node lose this sequential filling, so reducing ventricular stroke volume and cardiac output by up to one-quarter (Huff, 1997).

Atrial fibrillation (AF)

Atrial fibrillation (Figure 34.7) is the commonest dysrhythmia (Lip and Beevers, 1995). Multiple rapid (300 + bpm) but very weak impulses in the atria cause the muscle to 'quiver', resulting in the characteristic wavy baseline to the ECG, and absence of any clear P waves. Only the strongest impulses will be conducted by the atrioventricular node. Strong impulses reach the AV node totally irregularly, making ventricular response irregularly irregular. Ventricular conduction is usually normal, so each QRS complex will look normal.

Atrial fibrillation is usually a chronic condition, and provided it is controlled (<100 bpm) should not prevent people living relatively healthy lives. However, uncontrolled atrial fibrillation usually requires treatment with digoxin or other drugs (e.g. beta blockers). Atrial fibrillation may be reversed by cardioversion.

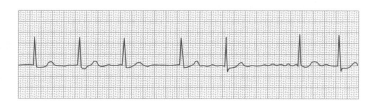

Figure 34.7 Atrial fibrillation

Atrial flutter

This is caused by an ectopic atrial pacemaker firing very rapid impulses (Figure 34.8). P waves are regular but 'saw-toothed'. Ventricular response will be regular, usually with a regular block. Increased conduction can quickly cause life-threatening tachycardias, so atrial flutter usually requires urgent treatment by cardioversion. If cardioversion fails, then drugs may be tried:

- Flecainide
- Calcium antagonists
- Digoxin
- Beta blockers
- Anticoagulants.

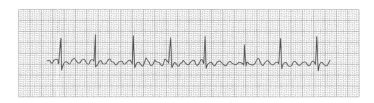

Figure 34.8 **Atrial flutter**

Nodal/junctional rhythm

This is a rhythm originating in or near the atrioventricular node (junction; see Figure 34.9). Rates will usually be 40–60 bpm, which can be tolerated without treatment, although slower rates may require pacing. However, the cause for the atrial block should be investigated and treated.

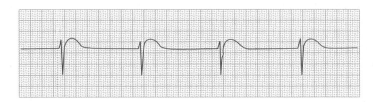

Figure 34.9 **Nodal/junctional rhythm**

Ventricular dysrhythmias

Impulses that originate in ventricular muscle do not use the normal conduction pathway, and so spread from muscle fibre to muscle fibre. This causes prolonged ventricular depolarisation, and so a wide QRS. Any atrial depolarisation is retrograde, following the QRS. P waves are not usually seen, but if they do appear they usually have no relationship to the QRS or are abnormal.

Ventricular dysrhythmias are often life-threatening, requiring urgent treatment. Dysrhythmias and ectopics may be caused by electrolyte imbalances, especially potassium, so provided the rhythm is not immediately life-threatening, potassium and other electrolytes (calcium, magnesium) should be checked if reasonably possible. Mild hyperkalaemia (5.0–6.0 mmol/l) is often treated with enteral calcium resonium, provided the gut is functioning, but higher levels (>6.0 mmol/l) may cause life-threatening dysrhythmias (Humphreys, 2002) and will usually be treated with intravenous insulin and glucose, which transfers serum potassium into cells. Intravenous calcium gluconate/chloride will often also be given to stabilise myocardial conduction.

Hypokalaemia (physiologically <3.5 mmol/l, but <4.0 is often treated with cardiac disease) requires potassium supplements. However, potassium loss largely correlates with urine volumes, so diuresis should also be considered when treating serum potassium levels.

Blocks

A block in conduction pathways causes an abnormal ECG. Four types are discussed here:

1 First degree block (delayed atrioventricular conduction)
2 Second degree block (incomplete heart block)
3 Third degree block (complete heart block)
4 Bundle branch block.

A block in conduction may be caused by infarction, oedema or ischaemia.

Blocks should resolve if oedema or ischaemia can be reversed, but infarction usually results in a permanent block. However, following infarction there will be an ischaemic area around dead myocardium. This ischaemic area will either be reperfused or cause further infarction ('extending').

First degree block (see Figure 34.10) is a delay in atrioventricular conduction, seen on the ECG as a prolonged PR interval and (usually) bradycardia. The atrial node thickens with age, so first degree blocks may be irreversible in some older people. Delayed conduction can also be caused by:

■ Drugs (e.g. digoxin, beta blockers, calcium channel blockers)
■ Acute inferior wall MI
■ Increased vagal tone
■ Hyperkalaemia.

Provided cardiac output and blood pressure remain adequate, first degree blocks are not usually treated, although underlying causes should be reversed if possible. Symptomatic bradycardia may necessitate treatment.

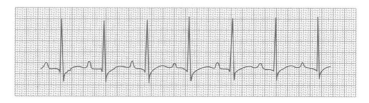

Figure 34.10 **First degree block**

Second degree heart block or incomplete heart block, is where some P waves are conducted and some are not. The block is regular, so there will be a pattern to the ECG (regularly irregular). There are two types of second degree heart block:

■ Type 1 (previously called Wenkebach phenomenon, or sometimes Mobitz type 1) is where the PR progressively lengthens until a P wave remains unconducted (see Figure 34.11).
■ Type 2 (previously called Mobitz, or sometimes Mobitz type 2) is where all conducted impulses are identical, but some P waves will (regularly) not be conducted (see Figure 34.12).

Second degree heart block type 1 occurs more frequently, is usually asymptomatic, and resolves spontaneously. Type 2 is more serious, so more likely to require treatment with:

■ Oxygen
■ Atropine
■ Pacing, if unresponsive.

Third degree heart block (see Figure 34.13) is complete heart block, causing complete dissociation between atrial and ventricular activity. P waves are usually present and regular, but do not initiate the QRS complex (some P waves are often 'lost' in the QRS complex or T wave). The QRS complex originates in ventricular muscle, so is wide and usually very slow (<40 bpm). QRS complexes will usually all appear identical, and be regular. Profound bradycardia usually necessitates urgent pacing. Until pacing can be started, patients should be given 100% oxygen.

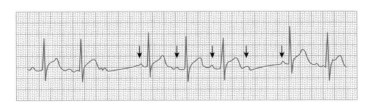

Figure 34.11 Second degree block type 1

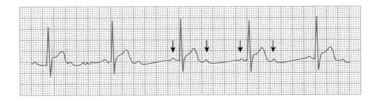

Figure 34.12 Second degree block type 2

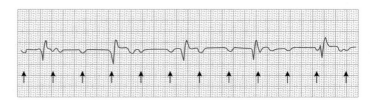

Figure 34.13 **Third degree block**

Bundle branch block (see Figure 34.14) occurs where one of the branches of the bundles of His passes through infarcted, ischaemic or oedematous muscle, and the conduction is completely blocked. Impulses pass through the intact branches, but around the blocked branch(es) by transmission from muscle fibre to muscle fibre. This creates two QRS complexes: a normal complex from the intact branch(es), and a wide ventricular complex from the muscle beyond the blocked branch. These two complexes begin with the same Q wave, creating an M- or W-shaped QRS complex.

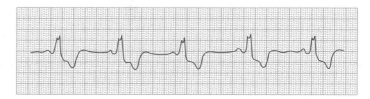

Figure 34.14 **Bundle branch block**

These M/W-shaped complexes can be seen in most limb leads, but to identify whether the block is in the left or right branch bundles look at the chest leads. Left bundle branch blocks (LBBB) have a W in the early chest leads (C1, C2) and an M in the late chest leads (C4–6), while right bundle branch blocks (RBBBs) have an M in the early chest leads (C1, C2) and a W in the late chest leads (C4–6). Bundle branch blocks may be differentiated by the mnemonics MaRRoW and WiLLiaM.

Because the left ventricle supplies the aorta, left bundle branch block is more likely to progress to myocardial infarction and death than is right bundle branch block (Baldasseroni *et al.*, 2002).

Ventricular arrest rhythms

Ventricular tachycardia (VT) (see Figure 34.15) is a regular, but life-threatening rhythm, showing only ventricular (wide) complexes without P waves. Cardiac output and blood pressure will be very poor. Ventricular tachycardia usually rapidly resolves spontaneously, or rapidly progresses to ventricular fibrillation and myocardial infarction. Ventricular tachycardia is an arrest situation, and should be treated according to current resuscitation protocols. Antitachycardic drugs (e.g. amiodarone) may be used. Underlying causes (e.g. hypokalaemia) should be resolved.

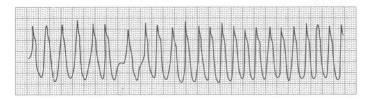

Figure 34.15 **Ventricular tachycardia**

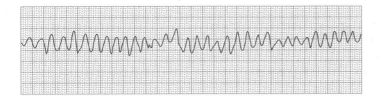

Figure 34.16 **Ventricular fibrillation**

Ventricular fibrillation (VF) (see Figure 34.16) is an irregularly irregular rhythm, with little or no cardiac output. Untreated, it is almost invariably fatal within 2–3 minutes (Guyton and Hall, 2000). It is an arrest situation, and should be treated according to current resuscitation protocols.

Asystole

Also called ventricular standstill, is where there is no cardiac electrical activity, and so the ECG will show only an isoelectric line. It is an arrest situation, and should be treated according to current resuscitation protocols. However, before putting out an arrest call staff should check that electrodes have not become disconnected and the electrode gel has not dried.

Although resuscitation should normally be attempted, few patients survive asystole.

Pulseless electrical activity (PEA)

Previously called electro-mechanical disassociation (EMD), is when there is little or no pulse despite rhythms seen on the ECG monitor (which will usually look abnormal). PEA is an arrest situation, but will be caused by one of the '4Hs and 4Ts':

- Hypoxia
- Hypovolaemia
- Hyper/hypokalaemia and metabolic disorders (e.g. from drug overdose/ intoxication and electrolyte imbalances)
- Hypothermia
- Tension pneumothorax
- Tamponade

■   Toxic/therapeutic disturbances (drug overdose/intoxication)
■   Thrombolytic/mechanical obstruction (e.g. pulmonary embolism, myocardial infarction).

The underlying cause of PEA should therefore be resolved as part of resuscitation.

Implications for practice

■   ECGs are logical, but contain much information is a small graph; to interpret them, nurses should understand normal cardiac electrophysiology and how this is translated onto ECG graph paper. Analyse one lead at a time, using a framework such as in Box 34.1.
■   Reading ECGs is a skill requiring practice, so take every possible opportunity to study ECGs of patients cared for, interpreting information holistically
■   Most dysrhythmias will only be treated if they cause problems
■   Readers should be familiar with current resuscitation protocols (at the time of writing: European Resuscitation Council, 2001), attend annual updates, and have posters of current resuscitation algorithms displayed prominently in clinical areas.

Summary

An ECG presents a two-dimensional graph of the three-dimensional electrical activity created by cardiac conduction. Much information is therefore presented in a relatively small trace. To analyse this information, examine each complex of a single lead, beginning with the P wave. Use a framework such as Box 34.1 to follow through each part of the complex.

The chapter has described how normal electrophysiology is represented in the ECG graph. Understanding this enables interpretation of abnormal rhythms. A summary of the main dysrhythmias and treatments is included, although many other dysrhythmias can occur, so discussion of each dysrhythmia could be considerably extended. This chapter limits depth to present an accessible overview for staff working with level 2 patients. Reading ECGs is a skill that takes practice. With further practice, readers should seek more challenging and advanced texts, as recommended in Further reading.

Exercise

1   Make a list of the main reasons patients having an ECG recorded may be anxious. Identify where a 12-lead ECG may cause more or less anxiety than continuous monitoring. Using this list, what explanations would you normally give to patients before recording their ECG?
2   Find a printout of an ECG from a patient that you have cared for. Cover any printed analysis of the ECG and, using the framework in Box 34.1, analyse the ECG. At the earliest opportunity, discuss your analysis with a nursing or medical colleague skilled in ECG analysis.

3   Reflecting on your experience over the last year, list the dysrhythmias you have seen. What treatments can you remember being used for each dysrhythmia? What dysrhythmias were not actively treated, and why?

Bibliography

Key reading

Readers should know resuscitation protocols (currently, European Resuscitation Council, 2001), and have posters of Resuscitation Council algorithms displayed in their workplace. A number of books and articles are available to help develop ECG skills. Hampton (2003b) and Houghton and Gray (1997) are two useful pocket-sized books describing normal and abnormal rhythms.

Further reading

Readers ready to develop skills beyond this level will find more detail in Hampton (2003a), while Huff (1997) and Hampton (2003c) provide exercises for readers to test and develop interpretation skills.

Appendix: some drugs used to treat dysrhythmias

Drug	Action
Adrenaline (epinephrine)	Alpha and beta agonist: increases heart rate, stroke volume and systemic vascular resistance
Amiodarone	Reverses tachycardia (atrial or ventricular); must be given through a central line
Atropine	Positive chronotrope (increases heart rate)
Calcium chloride/ calcium gluconate	Stabilises cardiac conduction
Captopril	ACE inhibitor; reduces hypertension
Digoxin	Slows and strengthens atrial impulses in atrial fibrillation
Diltiazim	Calcium channel blocker
Disopyramide	Controls ventricular dysrhythmias
Dobutamine	Positive inotrope; beta agonist, so increases stroke volume
Esmolol	Beta blocker
Flecainide	Controls atrial tachycardias
Insulin and glucose	Insulin transports glucose into cell, taking potassium with it
Lignocaine	Controls ventricular dysrhythmias
Losartin	Anti-hypertensive (blocks angiotensin II)
Nifedipine	Calcium channel blocker
Procainamide	Controls ventricular dysrhythmias and atrial tachycardia

Drug	Action
Propanolol	Beta blocker; reduces hypertension
Sotalol	Beta blocker; reduces hypertension
Verapamil	Calcium channel blocker

Chapter 35

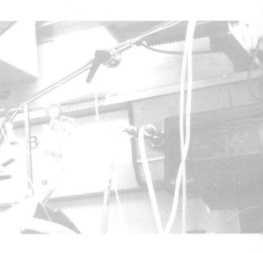

Fluid and electrolyte disturbances

Tina Moore

Contents

Learning outcomes

After reading this chapter you will be able to:

- Outline the homeostatic mechanisms of water and electrolyte balance
- Conduct an appropriate assessment of the patient's fluid and electrolyte status
- Identify appropriate intervention for the prevention and treatment of potential/actual disturbances
- Describe the aetiology of electrolyte disturbances
- Understand the rationale for clinical features of the above.

Fundamental knowledge

Basic knowledge of the functions and homeostatic mechanisms of water and electrolyte balance; sources of water intake and losses; sources of various electrolyte intake and areas of loss; medication affecting water balance.

Introduction

Water is an essential element for all body processes. It is involved in the transportation of substances to and from the cells, the promotion of necessary chemical activity and the maintenance of a physicochemical constancy (important in normal cellular function). The influence of water in the regulation of sodium balance aids the control of blood pressure. Water and electrolyte disturbances generally occur simultaneously. However, to enable clarity of information within this particular chapter fluid and electrolytes will be discussed separately.

Fluid balance

In the 'average' adult male approximately 60–65 per cent of total body weight is water (i.e. 40–45 litres). In the 'average' female (due to higher body fat content) this figure is reduced to 50 per cent (Marieb, 2004). Consequently, obesity also incurs a lower total body weight (water) percentage.

With age, the body increases its fat content and loses a significant amount of muscle mass (muscle holds 40 per cent of total body water). Consequently, the older person is more at risk of becoming dehydrated.

There are two main body fluid compartments:

1 Intracellular fluid (ICF) is contained within the cells and account for approximately 40 per cent of total body weight
2 Extracellular fluid (ECF) surrounds the cells, and is subdivided into two types: interstitial fluid and plasma fluid volumes (20 per cent of the total body weight). Interstitial fluid is water between the cells and outside the blood vessels. The transcellular component (also considered part of interstitial fluid) consists of a collection of biochemically distinct fluids, including cerebrospinal, synovial, pleural, pericardial and peritoneal fluids, and digestive secretions, which are separated from the interstitial compartment by a layer of epithelium (Flanning, 2000). Plasma (intravascular fluid) is contained within the blood vessels and plasma volume.

Normally, the composition and concentration of ECF is altered and modified as the body reacts with its surrounding environment. ICF remains relatively stable. During critical illness there is an alteration in the normal distribution of fluids, namely a depletion of ICF and an increase in ECF.

A third space exists and generally occurs in illness, taking place as a consequence of increased capillary hydrostatic pressure, decreased plasma colloid osmotic pressure or both. It enables movement of fluid (often referred to as transcellular fluid) into body cavities, for example in paralytic ileum (where the fluid pools into the bowel), oedema and effusion.

Maintaining fluid balance

Initially, fluid volume and osmolality are maintained within normal limits by the hypothalamic thirst mechanism, and by several hormones – notably aldosterone, antidiuretic hormone (ADH) and atrial natruiretic peptide, which act on the kidney to regulate urine volume and osmolality. A reduction in plasma osmolality inhibits ADH release, and thus increases the excretion of water. An increase in osmolality stimulates ADH production and increases kidney tubular reabsorption of water.

In normal ageing, the release of ADH appears to be increased in response to a variety of stimuli that can result in the retention of fluid. Aldosterone is an important regulator of fluid volume that is released by the adrenal cortex. The release of aldosterone is stimulated by an increase in potassium levels and decrease in sodium levels. It promotes reabsorption of sodium in the distal tubules in the kidney and from the colon.

Fluid and electrolyte homeostasis is maintained by the cardiovascular, renal, respiratory and gastrointestinal systems, the skin and brain. In illnesses where cardiac volume is insufficient, resulting in renal impairment, selective reabsorption takes place. Sodium is retained and potassium is excreted, maintaining normal osmolality and blood volume. The lungs influence loss of fluid through ventilation.

There are two principle forces that govern the movement of water. *Osmotic pressure* is pressure that must be applied to a solution on one side of a membrane. Sodium and protein are important for the maintenance of osmotic pressure and volume in the ECF compartment. Any changes in sodium concentration will lead to fluid volume changes (water follows sodium). Potassium is the main intracellular cation, and maintains the ICF osmotic pressure. Electrolytes do not move between the cell walls and capillaries as easily as water.

Sodium and potassium concentrations are maintained inside and outside the cells through active transport in the ECF; sodium is pumped out of the cell (keeping intracellular sodium low) and potassium is pumped into the cell (maintaining a high intracellular potassium level). Renal mechanisms aid this distribution, regulating sodium excretion. Despite variations in dietary intake, potassium levels are kept constant. Constancy is achieved by the renal tubular absorption of potassium and the secretion of variable amounts of potassium. When potassium is lost from the body (e.g. in urine), potassium moves out of the cells into the ECF to maintain potassium equilibrium between the ICF and ECF.

In the ECF compartment there is an exchange of water and electrolytes between the interstitial fluid compartment and the intravascular compartment. The principal difference in composition between these compartments is the presence of proteins in the plasma. Proteins cannot pass through the capillary membrane, and therefore function as osmotically active substances holding fluid in the blood vessels. The osmotic pressure exerted by plasma proteins is referred to as oncotic pressure, at approximately 20–30 mmHg. With sodium, the plasma proteins control intravascular volume.

Hydrostatic pressure of blood is the pressure exerted by fluid against the vascular wall. When the osmotic pressure changes in one fluid compartment, water moves across the semipermeable membrane from an area of lesser osmotic pressure to that of greater osmotic pressure until equilibrium is achieved. The volume of blood flowing through the vessels creates hydrostatic pressure, and this driving force causes filtration of fluid through the semipermeable membranes of the capillaries. Water and small electrolyte molecules pass easily; larger colloid substances and protein are held back.

Disturbances to fluid balance

Water balance disorders are manifested by alterations in plasma osmolality (which measures the ability of a fluid to hold water and to draw it through a semipermeable membrane). Normal osmolality is 280–290 mOsm/kg of water, and this provides an environment that is favourable for cellular activity. In disturbances such as dehydration, hyperosmolality occurs.

The osmolality of the ICF compartment must balance that of the ECF compartment in order to maintain a correct and orderly distribution of fluid between the cell and its environment.

Time out 35.1

1 Reflect upon patients you nursed who had developed fluid and/or electrolyte disturbances. How were these disturbances detected (i.e. what symptoms manifested)?
2 What caused the imbalances, and how were they corrected?
3 Think about why monitoring fluid balance is important.

Clinical practice issues

Loss or gain of relatively small amounts of fluid and electrolytes can influence a very delicate balance in an unstable patient. Fluid imbalance is present when regulatory mechanisms are insufficient to compensate for abnormal intake or output of fluid.

Movement of water, electrolytes and albumin occurs into the interstitial spaces. This third space fluid shift leads to localised swelling and lymphatic blockage, causing localised interstitial oedema. A patient might appear hypovolaemic or dehydrated. Fluid has moved into the interstitial spaces, so the total amount of body water may not have changed but just become unequally distributed. These patients can easily become overloaded with fluid replacement. The minimum urine output for critically ill patients should be at least 1 ml/kg per hour or about 1,700 ml, per 24 hours (Gosling, 1999). Hourly monitoring of input, output and overall balance is essential.

Fluid loss – hypovolaemia

Depletion of ECF volume occurs when water loss exceeds water intake over a period of time and the body is in negative fluid balance. A reduction of 5 per cent in body fluids will cause thirst; reduction of 8 per cent results in illness, and a 10 per cent deficit will cause death. Irrespective of the cause of fluid loss, cardiac output will be impaired (diminished pre-load). Presenting problems will reflect the effects of reduced cardiac output, disruption of normal cellular metabolism, and the resulting activation of homeostatic mechanisms to compensate.

Sometimes patients will develop hypovolaemia with fluid overload, e.g. oedema due to increased capillary permeability. Despite clinical signs of shock, positive fluid balance is present. Whilst interstitial overload is present the aim is to expand the vascular space with fluids that will not leak into the interstitial spaces and risk worsening the oedema. Reducing water and sodium intake together with diuretic therapy (optional) should result in a negative balance (Gosling, 1999).

Causes of fluid loss

Fluid loss may be:

- Hyperosmolar due to body water losses. Losses may occur because of food and water deprivation, an increased body or environmental temperature, hyperglycaemia, diuresis in diabetes insipidus, or hyperalimination
- Isosmolar due to loss of fluids and electrolytes (hypotonic dehydration). This may occur because of loss of body fluids containing salt, haemorrhage, burns, peritonitis or surgical intervention
- Hypo-osmolar, where there is solute loss in excess of water excretion (hyper-natraemic dehydration) This type of fluid loss is commonly seen in the critically ill patient. It occurs when a disproportionate amount of free water is retained in the intracellular compartment. It is often associated with diabetic ketoacidosis, disorders causing excessive gastrointestinal loss, and excessive use of diuretics.

Clinical features

General signs of hypovolaemic shock include increased heart rate, thready pulse, reduced blood pressure and CVP, increased SVR, tachypnoea, and a decreased urine output (although this is increased in diabetes insipidus).

Fluid balance results indicate a gross deficit. The patient's skin appears dehydrated (although older patients' skin elasticity is lost, therefore this sign alone will not truly reflect a fluid deficit). The patient's oral cavity, mucous membranes and tongue are dry, while the skin is often cold and clammy. Skin colour changes suggest under-perfusion of tissues, and a reduction in capillary refill is noted. Excessive perspiration accompanies an increased body temperature. Patients may appear apprehensive and restless, and there may be acute weight loss (except when a third space occurs).

Owing to the compensatory mechanisms, the severity of the illness may be misjudged. The older person is particularly vulnerable to hypernatraemic dehydration. Thirst may be present; initially there may be little change in the BP (compensatory responses). In severe cases, mental confusion, hallucinations and a dangerous reduction in renal blood flow may occur.

Diagnostic test results include elevated blood urea nitrogen (BUN) levels; electrolyte disturbances (variable depending upon the type of fluid lost); increased urine specific gravity (the kidney's attempt to conserve water); and increased urine osmolality.

Management

Management is dependent upon treating the known cause. The overall fluid balance should be monitored on an hourly basis initially, and then reduced accordingly. Insensible loss (i.e. fluid loss through respirations, skin and faeces) needs to be estimated; this accounts for approximately 500 ml of water per day. Fluid replacement is given to induce a positive balance. Any infused IV fluids will directly enter the ECF compartment, primarily the vascular space, and will then be distributed into the respective fluid compartments, according to their composition.

The type of fluid replacement will depend upon the type of fluid lost and the severity of the deficit:

- Oral fluids may be encouraged, if tolerated by the patient
- Isotonic saline (0.9%) is appropriate for rapid volume replacement (e.g. in dehydration); it expands ECF only and does not enter ICF
- Hypotonic saline (0.45%) solution is used in the management of patients who have both volume depletion and hypernatraemia or hyperglycaemia (e.g. diabetic ketoacidosis)
- Glucose and water is used to treat a water deficit; it is useful in replacing fluid volume without altering electrolytes (both in ECF and ICF)
- Mixed saline/electrolyte solutions provide additional electrolytes
- Blood and albumin expands the intravascular portion of the ECF only (acute haemorrhage)
- If there is no response in stroke volume to a fluid challenge, then positive inotropic support and vasodilators or vasoconstrictors will be necessary (Adam and Osborne, 1997)
- Low sodium fluid replacement is used in hypernatraemia dehydration (fluid intake of at least 2,500 ml/day unless contraindicated).

If the patient has periodic fluid challenges, then vital signs need to be evaluated. There should also be daily measurement of serum electrolyte balances.

For further information on hypovolaemic shock, see Chapter 21.

Fluid gain – hypervolaemia

Expansion of the ECF is termed hypervolaemia. Iatragenic fluid overload is preventable with appropriate monitoring of treatment.

Causes of fluid gain

Fluid gain may be:

- Hypertonic (more water than sodium is lost or ECF concentration of sodium increases). This can result from increased solutes in the ECF compartment leading to water being drawn out of the cells, or excessive administration of sodium bicarbonate.
- Isotonic (sodium and water are lost in equal proportion). This results from increased fluid and electrolyte gains. Expansion of both ICF and ECF compartments occurs. Excessive infusion of isotonic solutions, congestive heart failure, acute renal failure, nephrotic syndrome, liver cirrhosis can be classified as causes.
- Hypotonic (water intoxication). Here, water moves from the ECF, causing overhydration and swelling of the cells. Possible causes include excessive fluid intake, renal impairment, retention of irrigation fluid, physiological stress (ADH production is affected and increases rapidly, overriding normal regulation). It can result in reduced urine output and osmolality, leading to water retention and hyponatraemia.

Clinical features

Clinical features of overload include increased heart rate (gallop rhythm), BP (unless left-sided heart failure is present), CVP (neck vein distension may be evident) and pulse pressures; delayed capillary filling time; and tachypnoea, dyspnoea and pulmonary oedema may be evident. Lung auscultation reveals crackling, ronchi and wheezes. Urinary output may be increased or decreased, depending on the underlying cause and renal function. Urine osmolality increases in fluid volume deficit (this test reflects the concentrating ability of the kidneys, normal range = 300–1,200 mOsml/l). Diagnostic findings are related to haemodilution.

Gross fluid balance is positive. Signs of systemic overload are apparent; generalised and/or pitting oedema or, objectively, a weight gain is noticeable (rapid gains are generally associated with changes in fluid volume). Skin may be warm, moist and swollen, appearing tight and shiny. Patient's general orientation behaviour may include irritability, and a deteriorating level of consciousness.

Management

The goal of managing this condition is to treat the precipitating problem and return ECF to normal. Patients may require fluid and sodium restrictions; again it is important to monitor fluid balance, as this aids evaluation of treatment and provides an indication of whether the patient's condition is worsening. Care needs to be taken when administering fluid with sizeable amounts of sodium (e.g. 0.9% normal saline); a change in the solution or a slow infusion rate may need to be prescribed. Diuretics may be indicated; loop diuretics (e.g. frusemide) might be indicated in severe hypervolaemia. Patients receiving IV medication need to have it diluted in the minimum amount of solution. Careful monitoring of vital signs (BP, CVP, pulse, respiratory status) should be performed, initially on an hourly basis. In life-threatening hypervolaemia, haemodialysis is indicated.

Time out 35.2

1   Make a list of the electrolytes you can remember.
2   How does a disorder in each affect the patient's physiological functioning?

Electrolyte imbalances

An electrolyte is a substance that develops an electrical charge when dissolved in water – ions are collectively referred to as electrolytes. Electrolytes dissociate into positive and negative ions and are measured by their capacity to combine (mulliquivalents/litre – mEq/l) or by their molecular weight in milligrams (millimole/litre – mmol/l). Electrolytes that develop a positive charge are cations (e.g. sodium, potassium, calcium, magnesium). Electrolytes with a negative charge are anions (e.g. chloride, bicarbonate).

They are a critical component of the ECF and ICF environments. Regulation of electrolyte concentrations depends on a balance between adequate intake of food and drink containing electrolytes and output of electrolytes (in urine, faeces and sweat).

Table 35.1 provides details of various electrolyte imbalances, their causes, features and treatment.

Table 35.1 Electrolyte imbalances

Electrolyte	Disturbance	Causes	Clinical features	Treatment
Potassium • Closely related to reabsorption of sodium and hydrogen ions • Major cation in the ICF compartment; maintains osmotic pressure and volume in this compartment • Essential for transmission and conduction of nerve impulses for the contraction of skeletal, cardiac and smooth muscles • Necessary for movement of glucose into cells Normal values: 3.5–5.5 mmol/l	Hypokalaemia develops when serum potassium levels drop below 3.5 mmol/l	• Reduced potassium intake (anorexia malabsorption and alcoholism) • Excessive loss – diarrhoea and vomiting • Urinary loss via the kidneys, which are responsible for 80% of the body's potassium secretion (Perez, 1995) • Diuretic phase of acute renal failure • Iatrogenic – excessive use of diuretics, prolonged and excessive aspiration of GI tract, IV alkali (e.g. sodium bicarbonate), nephrotoxic drugs (e.g. aminoglycoside antibiotics)	• Usually becomes apparent when levels are below 3.0 mmol/l • Reduces contractility of smooth, skeletal and cardiac muscle; generalised body cramps, cardiac arrhythmias, confusion, disorientation, anorexia, decreased gastric motion, paralytic ileus	• Potassium replacement, oral or IV. May act as irritant IV, therefore frequently inspect the infusion site, monitor the infusion rate carefully; rapid infusions can cause death due to cardiac depression, dysrhythmias or cardiac arrest

Table 35.1 continued

Electrolyte	Disturbance	Causes	Clinical features	Treatment
	Hyperkalaemia	• Increased potassium intake/iatrogenic cause; excessive use of supplements/excessive potassium infusion • Increased supply – hypercatabolic states (e.g. MI, cardiac arrest, massive injury/infection), resulting in wide release of potassium ions from the cells into the ECF • Reduced blood pH – hydrogen ions cross cell membranes into ECF in exchange for potassium ions; cells become potassium depleted but plasma ECF levels increase • Poor excretion due to renal failure • Haemolysis (sickle cell crisis)	• ECG changes – peaked P and T waves, widening of QRS complex • Bradycardia, atrial and ventricular tachycardia • Risk of cardiac arrest (levels – 7.0 mmol) • Respiratory failure • Tingling in extremities • Hypotension	Treatment depends on individual's underlying condition, level and cause of raised potassium • Emergency treatment aimed at counteracting the cardiac effects and shifting extra cellular potassium into the cells – 10 ml 10% calcium gluconate or calcium chloride protects the heart, raises the threshold and prolongs repolarisation; rapidly, but temporarily, reverses adverse effects on the heart • Calcium salts potentiate the effects of digitalis, so should be given with caution to patients already receiving cardiac glycocides; if potassium remains dangerously high, haemodialysis or haemofiltration may need to be considered • Sometimes insulin and glucose, 10 units in 50 ml glucose IV slow bolus or 10 units in 500 ml over 1

Sodium
- Sodium is widely distributed in the body, although most of it is in the extracellular fluid, where it exerts a profound effect on body cells
- Essential for nerve impulses and muscle contractions
- Influences acid–base balance, chloride and potassium levels, maintains osmotic pressure and volume in this compartment

Normal values: 135–145 mmol/l. Serum sodium levels do not necessarily reflect total body sodium, but the relative content of sodium and water in the ECF

Hyponatraemia is the most common imbalance in the acutely ill. Acute hyponatraemia can lead to serious neurological disturbances. When sodium is lost from the body, the osmotic pressure in the ECF is reduced and water then moves into the ICF, leading to overhydration of the cells

A reduced sodium concentration in the ECF results in potassium moving out of the ICF, leading to potassium imbalance as well as a sodium imbalance

- Prolonged restricted dietary sodium intake
- Diarrhoea and vomiting, GI suction, surgery/inappropriate replacement of GI losses (e.g. water without sufficient amounts of sodium)
- Skin – perspiration in fever in high environmental temps, also from the skin surface in burns
- Nephritis, renal tubules do not respond to ADH
- Abuse or overuse of diuretics
- Water gain in CCF, liver cirrhosis, nephrotic syndrome; dilutional hyponatraemia results even though total body sodium may be in excess
- Hyperglycaemia increases tubular flow rates and may promote renal sodium loss in excess of water. Can occur in hypervolaemia – dilution of sodium

- Neurological symptoms include headaches, confusion, coma convulsions (cellular overhydration)
- Muscle cramps, nausea and vomiting, disturbance of fluid volume

- Treatment is dependent on cause and severity of symptoms; if cause is fluid volume deficit, 0.9% sodium chloride will correct both sodium and water deficit
- Fluid volume excess – fluid restriction and occasionally hypertonic 3% or 5% sodium chloride is prescribed

Table 35.1 continued

Electrolyte	Disturbance	Causes	Clinical features	Treatment
	Hypernatraemia develops when, in response to increased ECF osmolality, water moves out of the cells, leading to cellular dehydration Hyperosmolality occurs as a response to hypernatraemia via osmoreceptors in the brain, stimulating ADH and thirst. It is easy for a critically ill patient to develop hypernatraemia, particularly when receiving large amounts of fluid	• Dietary – increased intake or overinfusion of sodium-containing fluids. May cause hypernatraemia in addition to absent thirst response (e.g. in elderly or debilitated states) • GI tract – severe diarrhoea and vomiting • Excessive perspiration in increased body or environmental temperature = excessive water loss • Renal and congestive cardiac failure both involve sodium retention • Reduced water intake/inability to respond to fluid deficit – indeficiency of ADH as a result of diabetes insipidus, pituitary tumours, trauma = brain damage	• Clinical features associated with fluid volume disturbances in excess or deficit • Disturbance of cerebral cell function due to cell dehydration (e.g. irritability) • In severe hypernatraemia, convulsions, drowsiness, lethargy, confusion, coma	• If water loss is the cause, hyperosmolality may be corrected with intravenous replacement of water (e.g. 5% glucose) • If cause is excess fluid, correction of sodium imbalance may be achieved with restricted intake of sodium and with the use of diuretics (e.g. thiazide, which blocks sodium absorption and water reabsorption)

Calcium
- Promotes normal nerve and muscle activity
- Increases contraction of the myocardium
- Maintains normal cellular permeability and promotes blood clotting
- Bone development and healing

Normal values: 2.25–2.75 mmol/l

Hypercalcaemia

- Bone tumours
- Thiazide diuretics
- Renal failure
- Prolonged immobilisation (bone disuse causes increased reabsorption and reduced formation)

Mild elevations usually have few or no symptoms
- Lethargy, headache, nausea, vomiting, thirst, polyuria, loss of muscle tone
- ECG – Q and T wave changes
- Severe elevations may cause coma (older patients are more likely to be symptomatic from moderate elevations)

High volume of IV fluids and diuretics; restricted calcium intake

Hydration is ineffective in patients with kidney failure because diuresis is impossible; therefore, dialysis may be recommended (Bove, 1996)

Hypocalcaemia

- Hypoparathyroidism
- Chronic renal failure
- Vitamin D deficiency
- Increased fluid loss

- Irritability, anxiety, tetany (twitching around the mouth, pins and needles in fingers, laryngeal spasm and convulsions)
- Increased bleeding tendencies
- Possible hypotension
- ECG – Q and T wave changes
- Hyperventilation

Calcium gluconate 10% IV for acute severe cases

Table 35.1 continued

Electrolyte	Disturbance	Causes	Clinical features	Treatment
Phosphate • A vital component in the structure of bone tissue and teeth • Essential in the metabolism of all cells Vital component of adenosine diphosphate and troposphere Normal values: 0.8–1.4 mmol/l	Hyperphosphataemia	• Renal failure • Hyperparathyroidism	• Increased heart rate • Nausea, diarrhoea, muscle weakness	• Treatment is aimed at primary causative condition; phosphate binding antacids, e.g. albumin hydroxide gel
	Hypophosphataemia	• Reduced dietary intake • Impaired absorption • Renal failure	• Lethargy, muscle weakness • Nausea, vomiting • Reduced white blood cell function, haemolytic anaemia	• Treatment: IV phosphate

Magnesium
- A major ICF cation closely related to potassium
- Essential in the function of many enzyme activities
- Has a depressant effect at the neural synapsis; also affects neuromuscular transmission and cardiovascular tone
- Renal function is central to magnesium homeostasis

Normal values: 1.5–2.5 mmol/l

Hypermagnesaemia

- Renal failure
- Excessive magnesium administration

- Bradycardia
- Complete heart block
- Hypotension
- In severe cases, respiratory and cardiac arrest, drowsiness and coma

- Treatment is directed towards promoting urinary output; haemodialysis may be used
- IV fluid replacement and diuretics are used to 'flush out' excessive magnesium
- Calcium chloride via IV infusion (0.5–1 gm) should counteract effects on cardiovascular and nervous systems (Ferrin, 1996)

Hypomagnesaemia
- Common in the critically ill, usually asymptomatic (Noronha and Matuschak, 2002)
- Diarrhoea/vomiting and alcohol abuse
- Increased renal excretion (Ferrin, 1996)

Singularly or combined: three main causes:
- Increased renal losses
- Reduced intestinal absorption
- Compartmental redistribution (Ellin, 1994)

- Muscular weakness/cramps, twitching and tremors
- cardiac arrhythmia – SVT, VT
- Carpopedal spasm (tetany)
- Convulsions and coma in severe cases

- In an emergency, IV route – usually 8–12 mmol/mg over 1–2 min, then 40 mmol/mg over the next 5 hours
- Kidney function should be assessed prior to treatment
- Intramuscular/IV preparation – magnesium sulphate for severely ill 40 mmol/mg day 1, 16–24 mmol/mg on days 2–5 (Noronha and Matuschak, 2002)

Table 35.1 continued

Electrolyte	Disturbance	Causes	Clinical features	Treatment
				• Monitor for signs of magnesium overload, e.g. hypotension
Chloride • Helps maintain ECF osmotic pressure and water balance • Digestion – essential for production of hydrochloric acid Normal values: 95–108 mmol/l	Hyperchloraemia	Possible causes: • Increased retention or intake • Excessive IV sodium chloride • Renal failure • Metabolic acidosis	• Weakness • Lethargy • Deep and rapid respiration	Treatment aimed at treating the cause
	Hypochloraemia	• Increased loss from GI tract • Excessive diuretic use • Excessive perspiration • Metabolic alkalosis • Generally associated with disorders of sodium loss	Those of fluid loss	Chloride replacement

Implications for practice

- Nurses should have in-depth knowledge in this aspect of care
- Prevention, early detection and early treatment should occur
- Elderly and critically ill patients are particularly vulnerable to developing fluid and electrolyte disturbances
- Close monitoring is required, including serum electrolytes.

Summary

Fluid and electrolyte disturbances are common features within clinical practice. All nurses have a fundamental role in the prevention, early detection and treatment of fluid and electrolyte imbalances, yet this is a role that appears to be given a low priority. Failure to recognise and treat fluid and electrolyte disturbances properly, particularly in the critically ill patient, may have fatal consequences. Successful management is dependent upon accurate assessment of the patient. Nurses must have knowledge and understanding of the normal physiological processes of fluid balance in order to deliver safe care. Risks of imbalance must be predicted, detected and evaluated through accurate monitoring and recording of fluid intake and output.

Bibliography

Suggested reading

Edwards (2001).
Flanning (2000).

Part 4

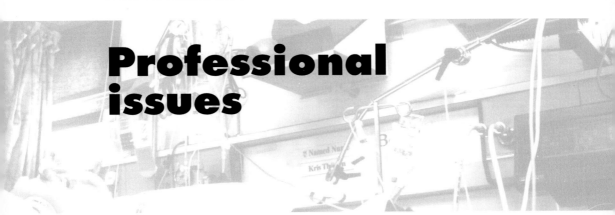

Professional
issues

Chapter 36

Clinical governance

Tina Moore

Contents

Learning outcomes

After reading this chapter you will be able to:

- Define clinical governance
- Appreciate the need for quality improvements within the NHS
- Demonstrate knowledge of the key components of clinical governance
- Discuss implementation strategies with colleagues.

Fundamental knowledge

The meaning of quality; tools used to measure quality.

Introduction

In the past the National Health Service (NHS) in the UK has been driven via an internal market system, which has resulted in a competitive ethos. Consequently, many healthcare professionals felt that the quality of professional care had become subservient to price and quality (Scally and Donaldson, 1998).

Increased publicity, awareness-raising programmes, publication of the Patient's Charter (DOH, 1992) and of the Citizen's Charter (DOH, 1993) have outlined the standards and rights expected from the NHS. This has led to radical changes within health care.

Clinical governance was developed to offer an alternative way of managing the NHS, thus ending the divisive internal market and avoiding the central command and controls system approach characteristic of the NHS for the first 40 years of its evolution. Clinical governance was also a response to addressing the inequalities that existed throughout the country, manifested by a noticeable increase in complaints made by patients and carers about hospital and community services (Wilson and Tingle, 1999).

The principles of clinical governance are designed to help address public concerns originating from well-published cases of poor performance (Scally and Donaldson, 1998), and provides protective mechanisms in avoiding cases like those of Beverley Allitt (a qualified enrolled nurse who was convicted of murdering four children and injuring nine others whilst working on a paediatric unit) and of the Bristol paediatric cardiac consultant whose death rate post-surgery was significantly higher than the national average (*Lancet*, 1998; McSherry and Haddock, 1999).

Its overall aim is to improve the quality of clinical care by creating universality across the NHS. It has been described as the most ambitious quality initiative that has been implemented in the NHS (Scally and Donaldson, 1998).

Meaning of clinical governance

Clinical governance is a complex, integrated care system, the philosophy of which is based on partnership (particularly between patients and healthcare professionals) and innovation, and driven by performance. It is part of a 10-year plan (DOH, 1997). The main principles are efficiency and effectiveness (a value for money ethos), and the needs and rights of the patient are central to all decision-making processes.

It is viewed as a framework through which NHS organisations are accountable for continuously improving the quality of their services and safeguarding high standards. This should be achieved by creating an environment in which excellence in clinical care can continuously flourish (DOH, 1998a) and be disseminated. It thus encourages a proactive rather than a reactive approach.

Clinical governance is described as an umbrella term for everything that helps to maintain and improve high standards of patient care (RCN, 2000). It encompasses a range of quality improvement activities that many healthcare professionals are already involved in, such as risk management, clinical audit and staff development.

It also provides a framework to draw these activities together in a more co-ordinated way. Its implementation is not an option; all healthcare organisations are required to develop local systems for ensuring quality of care, setting standards, and collecting information to demonstrate the quality of their work (DOH, 1998a).

Time out 36.1

1 With reference to your practice area, what mechanisms are in place for patients to receive high-quality care?
2 How is this quality measured?
3 Obtain and read the document on quality (DOH, 1998a)

Quality

Different definitions of quality exist, and this indicates the ambiguous and subjective nature of the concept.

Four areas of quality have been identified (Figure 36.1):

1 Professional performance (technical quality).
2 Resource use (related to efficiency).
3 Risk management (the risk of injury or illness associated with the service provided).
4 Patient satisfaction.

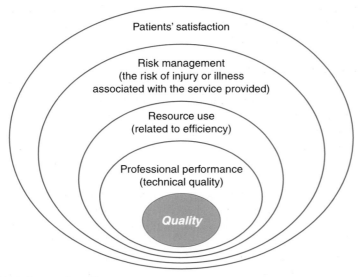

Figure 36.1 **Areas of quality**

(Source: DOH, 1997)

Healthcare organisations have a statutory duty to seek quality improvement. This may prove to be difficult, particularly in the measurement of quality. Healthcare professionals are expected to deliver a high-quality service based upon appropriate evidence. There is therefore a potential conflict between balancing expectations efficiently and effectively, and maintaining quality and standards. For the balance to succeed, there is a need to have strong leadership and the commitment, involvement and co-operation of all clinical staff. Clinical excellence includes the influences of all aspects of care provision.

Time out 36.2

1   Find and read the policies and procedures relating to your practice area.
2   Identify the ones that will potentially enhance quality of care provision.
3   Find out if these policies/procedures are being used in practice.

Themes emerging from clinical governance

Several themes emerge from the literature, all are interrelated (see Figure 36.2).

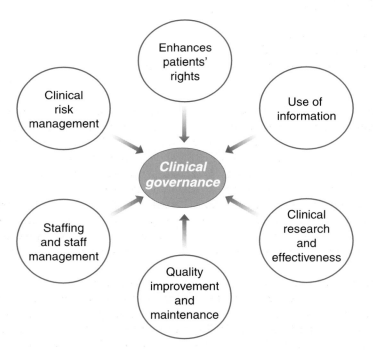

Figure 36.2 **Themes in clinical governance**

Quality audit

The setting of measurable (if possible) local standards could aid in the improvement and maintenance of quality. Clinical audit can be used as a tool for coordinating and promoting action in clinical effectiveness. Previous audit findings should be evaluated, enabling developmental processes.

Clinical research and effectiveness

Nursing is slowly moving away from a reliance on procedures, towards interventions based on rigorous appraisal of evidence (Crinson, 1999). Evidence-based practice occurs through the integration of clinical expertise with the best available external evidence from systematic research. It gives healthcare professionals confidence that their interventions (clinical, educational and managerial) are informed by a current and appropriate knowledge base. Practitioners and guidelines can then be audited and measured against agreed standards at a national or local level (McSherry and Haddock, 1999).

Evidence-based practice is a critical part of clinical governance for achieving clinical effectiveness and quality services to patients. Clinical effectiveness has three distinctive parts:

1   Obtaining evidence
2   Implementing the evidence
3   Evaluating the impact of the changed practice.
                                            (McSherry and Haddock, 1999)

The goal of clinical effectiveness is that nurses will acquire the professional skills and knowledge to practise evidence-based care. Evidenced-based information is available from the Institute for Clinical Excellence. For example, the National Service Framework (NSF) is responsible for issuing recommendations regarding the patterns and levels of service that should be provided for patients (a number for certain clinical disorders have already been developed).

The limitations of the evidence-based practice approach raises the question of what counts as the 'sufficient evidence' required to amend practice. Crinson (1999) questions the sufficiency of a single study, and wonders if a meta-analysis is required where the data from a number of individual studies are pooled and reanalysed.

Patient needs levels are a way of standardising patient dependency categories (see Chapter 37). Research into the effectiveness of early warning systems and their impact on patient outcome (mortality, morbidity and adverse events) has been identified as a future priority for critical care (DOH, 2000c). The development of the nurse consultant and outreach (Chapter 37) has led to a responsibility to be involved in research relating to the critically ill.

Use of information

Clinical governance advocates the move from a restricted culture of blame to one of openness. Guidelines have been provided in the Code of Openness in the NHS (DOH, 1997) outlining the principles of good information-giving. Patients should be actively encouraged to be involved in their care (see Chapter 10) and indeed the running of the NHS.

Changes to the NHS complaints procedure in 1996 reduced the fragmentation and inconsistency of previous arrangements, as well as introducing more openness and lay participation.

The Critical Care Information Advisory Group (CCIAG) has issued guidance relating to information data needs of critical care services (e.g. bed status). This is a multidisciplinary department of health advisory groups, set up as part of the critical care modernisation programme. An information strategy has been developed to improve the quality of patient-based care data. The information required relates to some degree of prediction, which is extremely difficult under any circumstances, but particularly within the critically ill environment.

Nurses working within critical care have a comprehensive network system where they can communicate with each other via local and national networks and national updates. Information relating to various strategic working groups (resulting from comprehensive critical care) (DOH, 2000c) can also be found on the Internet.

Management of staff

Staff development is seen to be the key component in these improvements, through the Continuous Professional Development Standard (NMC, 2002b) (see Chapter 41). Good recruitment, retention and staff development will make a major contribution (Scally and Donaldson, 1998) to quality care provision. This approach requires active participation from staff, who need to examine existing processes critically and with a view to improvement.

The reduction in junior doctors' working hours (DOH, 1998b) and nurses' role expansion (NMC, 2002b; DOH, 1999a) have led to new roles being undertaken by nurses (NHSE, 1996; Doyal et al., 1998). This has created a blurring of the role boundaries between nurse and doctor. As a result, staff need to be managed effectively and efficiently. Managing staff also involves detecting and dealing with good as well as poor performances. In achieving this there is a need to foster an open 'blame-free' culture, and to have 'measurable' factors – e.g. quality indicators (through standards), performance appraisals and reviews, clinical incident reporting, complaints and accolades, and monitoring of sickness and absence. Poorly performing healthcare professionals, including nurses, are not only a risk to patients but also to the organisation they work for. They need to be dealt with fairly and by experienced and highly trained professionals. Equally, the valuing of staff is crucial in order to maintain the motivation and commitment required for the management of change (see Chapter 40).

Education and development are essential to ensure nurses can competently assess and manage patients who are acutely/critically ill. Active educational programmes relating to critical care are in progress in an attempt to address issues that have been neglected in the past.

Competencies relating to critical care are in existence at a local level, and there are plans to make this a national initiative. These competencies will help to address the mismatch between patient dependency and skill mix; and will also help with the identification of professional development for individual nurses.

Clinical risk management

The lifting of Crown immunity in 1995 has led to an increased awareness of the need for risk management. Trusts are now expected to take out a type of insurance (via the Clinical Negligence Scheme for Trusts). To qualify, Trusts need to prove that a clinical risk strategy is in place together with its implementation (policies, procedures, staff development).

Risks attached to the provision of health care need to be minimised. Compliance with statutory regulations (e.g. the Data Protection Act, 1998; Control of Substances; Hazards to Health (COSHH); Medicine Control Agency Approval; Indemnity Insurance etc. have to be proven by the Trusts) (Storey, 2001).

Risk management involves the identification of 'at risk situations' (for patients, practitioners and organisation). These are situations relating to clinical error/ deviations from the 'norm'. Those involved must be helped through guidance, support and development. Thus, rigorous policies and procedures need to be in place, including a comprehensive risk assessment tool. Within critical care, Early Warning Systems are in place to help assess the risk in acutely ill patients (many hospitals have produced a call-out criteria; see Chapter 37).

However, improvement in clinical risk management requires a change in culture (openness and communication) in order that staff are encouraged to report adverse events without fear of being held personally liable. This will take time, if indeed it is at all achievable.

Patient rights

Patient involvement in policies and development of services, reflected in the National Patient Safety Agency (NPSA), allows the public to report concerns. There are areas where examination of the patients' and relatives' 'lived experience' could enhance clinical practice. This is a potential growth area.

Accountability

This relates to every level of care provision, from the individual nurse right up to the Chief Executive of the Trust (see Chapter 41).

Implementation structure

This is described in Box 36.1.

Box 36.1   Implementation structure

New structures to aid in the achievements principles of clinical governance include:

- Nationally agreed standards – National Service Frameworks (NSF).
- A new performance framework with a scorecard of quality effectiveness and efficiency measures.
- NICE (National Institute for Clinical Excellence), which is responsible for producing clinical guidelines for NHS and standard setting, and for the assessment of new treatments, drugs and devices (including guidance on their clinical and cost effectiveness).
- Networking/sharing of good practices.
- CHI (soon to be called the Commission for Health Inspection and Audit) – the Department of Health sets national clinical priorities and CHI is responsible for the monitoring of these standards; it is a government body that is open to public scrutiny, and responsible for publishing staff and patient surveys.
- The Modernisation Agency, which has a supporting role. The National Director of Clinical Governance and an NHS Clinical Governance Support Team are appointed to create, capture and spread best practice through health improvement programmes. At the time of writing, critical care improvement programmes are undergoing a 'weaning phase' where the representatives from the Modernisation Agency are slowly withdrawing the level of support. This assumes that staff/Trusts are now empowered and more independent.
- Local Trusts and Health Authorities, which have a professional obligation to implement guidelines.
- Integrated care pathways (ICP), which provide a framework for care and encourage the development and maintenance of a multidisciplinary team approach. Integrated care pathways are structured multidisciplinary care plans, which detail essential steps in the care of patients with a specific clinical problem. They are also a means of improving systematic collection of data for audit and promoting change in practice. If the care given should deviate from the pathway, a variance is recorded; this allows a record of what was done differently, why it was done differently, and what action was taken. Benefits to be gained from the use of integrated care pathways include improved communication, a reduction in documentation, improved clinical outcomes, a multidisciplinary review of practice, and less duplication of care, resulting in reduced cost and length of stay (Middleton and Roberts, 2000).

■ Strong leadership is an essential ingredient in the process of managing change (see Chapter 40). There are contradictions involved in operating a hierarchical power structure and attempting to develop an open and democratic framework of clinical governance. These can result in a 'blame and shame' culture, rather than a supportive environment in which healthcare professionals can critically appraise practice (Crinson, 1999).

Implications for practice

■ All practice areas have an obligation to provide high-quality care
■ Standards of care need to be agreed and in place
■ A Clinical Governance Committee should be present within each Trust.

Summary

In an attempt to improve quality of service to the patient, all Trusts are expected to adopt the principles of clinical governance. A lot of work has already gone into making it successful, but for many the hard work has only just begun.

Bibliography

Further reading

McSherry and Pearce (2002) is written in a way that is easily understood, and provides working examples for the implementation of clinical governance. It is a useful resource.

Useful sources

www.doh.gov/riskman.htm
www.chi.nhs.uk
http://hiru.mcmaster.ca/cochrane/cdsr.htm
www.doh.gov.uk
http://www.doh.gov.uk/essenceofcare

Chapter 37

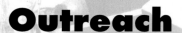

Outreach

Debbie Higgs

Contents

Learning outcomes

After reading this chapter you will be able to:

- Understand and appreciate the concept of outreach, its aims and objectives
- Identify the main early warning signs of critical illness
- Understand how the early warning score is applied to the acutely ill patient.

Introduction

The aim of this chapter is to explore the subject of critical care outreach services and the use of early warning scoring systems to detect developing critical illness. Outreach services are in part a result of recommendations made by the document produced by the Department of Health (2000a), *Comprehensive Critical Care*. Outreach is part of a new approach to critical care, which is based on a patient's need, rather than their location in the hospital. This is a relatively new concept, and is currently a topical issue that is influencing care and services in acute wards throughout the UK.

Background

During the past few years evidence has begun to emerge suggesting that some hospital patients exhibit premonitory signs of cardiac arrest, which may be observed by nursing and medical staff but are frequently not acted upon (Franklin and Mathew, 1994; Rich, 1999). Similar findings have been observed in relation to deterioration in the patients' condition prior to admission to ICU (Goldhill, 1997; McQuillan et al., 1998; Goldhill et al., 1999a; McGloin et al., 1999). These studies suggest that early recognition and treatment of these signs may prevent the necessity for some ICU admissions, thus reducing morbidity and mortality, and making better uses of costly intensive care resources. As patients admitted from hospital wards have a higher overall percentage mortality than patients admitted from other areas of the hospital (Goldhill and Sumner, 1998), an improvement in the management of seriously ill patients prior to ICU admission could potentially improve outcome.

A frequently cited study by McQuillan et al. (1998) examined the quality of care received by 100 patients prior to admission to intensive care. This two-centred study conducted structured interviews with the referring and intensive care clinical teams. The investigators completed a questionnaire that focused on the recognition, investigation, monitoring and management of each patient's airway, breathing and circulation. Two external assessors evaluated the questionnaires. The results demonstrated that 54 per cent of the cohort received sub-optimal care before admission to ICU. The assessors believed that this had a significant impact on individual morbidity and mortality. A similar study by McGloin et al. (1999) confirmed these findings: 37 per cent of their patients received sub-optimal care, with a significantly increased mortality. These papers provoked widespread discussion. Whilst many clinicians and senior nurses welcomed the study's findings, it must be recognised that some inconsistencies were evident in the methods used. McQuillan et al. (1998) did not define sub-optimal care, but relied on the subjective opinion of the assessors – who were aware of the eventual outcome, which may have biased their opinion. McGloin et al. did provide a definition for sub-optimal care but, as the data were collected contemporaneously, the assessors had to rely upon the quality of documentation to detect whether an abnormality had been recognised. The authors did identify this as a limitation of the study. It should be appreciated, however, that to provide a robust definition of sub-optimal care would be extremely difficult, as individual interpretation of practice varies between clinicians. Additionally, in the McGloin study only clear-cut cases of poor management were deemed sub-optimal:

Care was not deemed sub-optimal if medical and nursing ward management were considered satisfactory, even though abnormalities may have persisted for more that 12 hours.

(McGloin et al., 1999: 256)

Hence, potentially a patient's condition could have deteriorated to such an extent to warrant a higher level of care without being deemed sub-optimal.

Several strategies for reducing the occurrence of sub-optimal care and improving the early identification of sick patients have been proposed. These focus predominantly on the identification of patients at risk of critical illness and the provision of some form of critical care outreach service to provide expert advice in the management of these patients (Daffurn *et al.*, 1994; Lee *et al.*, 1995b; Goldhill, 1997; Morgan *et al.*, 1997; Audit Commission, 1999; Goldhill *et al.*, 1999b; Department of Health, 2000d).

Recognising that previous studies had identified pre-monitoring signs of cardio-pulmonary arrest, in an attempt to improve outcome and to prevent such arrests Lee *et al.* (1995b) introduced the concept of a Medical Emergency Team (MET) in Australia. This involved a team of multidisciplinary staff that responded to pre-defined physiological criteria. Goldhill *et al.* (1999a) support this concept. They found in their study that critically ill patients needed to be identified and managed expertly, recommending the use of a medical emergency team as developed by Lee *et al.* (1995b). Indeed, the Royal London team went on to establish a Patient at Risk Team (PART) to respond to patients admitted from wards in the hospital, to prevent further physical deterioration and to improve outcomes in intensive care (see Box 37.1)

Box 37.1   Patient at Risk Team (PART)

The Royal London Hospital established a Patient at Risk Team to respond to patients admitted from wards in the hospital, to prevent further physical deterioration and to improve outcomes in intensive care. The PART assessed patients who fulfilled certain criteria, as well as other patients who were causing concern to medical and nursing staff. The PART aimed to improve care for these patients by providing advice and support to those responsible for them on the wards, by facilitating early intensive care unit admission when appropriate, and by preventing unnecessary ICU admissions – thereby releasing valuable beds for use by patients in greater need of comprehensive critical care (Department of Health, 2000a)

Studies to evaluate the services provided by both teams have been carried out, and both centre on the success of the calling criteria designed to indicate to the teams those patients at risk of critical illness. Several other authors have attempted to devise early warning scoring systems for detecting patients at risk of developing critical illness (Morgan *et al.*, 1997; Stenhouse *et al.*, 2000; Welch, 2000), which rely on the observation of various physiological parameters. These will be discussed later in this chapter.

While much of the cited literature supports and highlights the view that seriously ill ward patients are often missed or inappropriately managed, it must be acknowledged why this phenomenon has arisen. In recent years, technological developments have led to an increase in the number of procedures carried out in day surgery. Those patients who are now cared for in acute general wards are therefore often older, undergoing major surgical procedures, or are acutely ill. Also, advances in anaesthetic and critical care techniques have enabled higher risk patients to undergo major surgical procedures that previously would have been inappropriate. The ability of critical care units to cope with this influx of sick patients continues to be a problem, with capacity far outstripped by demand. In addition, the demand for critical care beds not infrequently results in significantly reduced stays for certain patients because of the need to make the bed available for the next admission. This practice, as highlighted by Daly *et al.* (2001), can put patients at risk, with early discharges in certain groups of patients causing an increase in mortality. The net effect of these occurrences is an increase in the acuity and dependency of patients being cared for in acute general wards (Coad and Haines, 1999). Meanwhile, difficulties in the recruitment and retention of qualified staff have led to a dilution of the skill mix in many areas. Therefore, inexperienced junior staff may frequently be expected to care for more highly dependent patients.

Outreach teams

Whilst the literature on the critical care providers produced to date had a considerable impact, the main influences on the changes that followed in critical care were the Audit Commission Report (1999) and *Comprehensive Critical Care* (Department of Health, 2000a) The Audit Commission Report set out a number of recommendations for staff to consider when reviewing critical care provision. One such approach was to reduce cost through flexibility in using resources effectively. Improving ward care and recognising critical illness as it develops, it suggested, would potentially prevent admissions or make them much more timely, resulting in shorter stays. This view was echoed in *Comprehensive Critical Care* (Department of Health, 2000a). An expert group comprising experienced practitioners from relevant professional bodies was established by the Department of Health to meet and develop a framework for the future organisation and delivery of adult critical care services. The outcome was the publication of *Comprehensive Critical Care* in March 2000. It resulted in a number of proposals that described a service that would meet the needs of patients, delivered by professionals and specialities working in partnership. The document also re-classified patients' dependencies. This has since been expanded in agreement with the Department of Health and the Intensive Care Society (2002) in order to provide greater clarity of the levels. Their vision for future critical care services included the establishment of an outreach team to provide and support the care of level 1 patients on general wards, and critical care facilities to meet the needs of level 2 and 3 patients.

This reinforced the view that it is the patients who hold the dependency level, and not the beds. It also called for the flexible use of beds and provision of support services for long-term patients and those requiring follow-up. It stated that outreach services are an integral part of comprehensive critical care, and have three essential objectives:

1   To avert admissions by identifying patients who are deteriorating and either helping to prevent admission or ensuring that admission to a critical care bed happens in a timely manner to ensure best outcome

2   To enable discharges by supporting the continuing recovery of discharged patients on wards and post discharge from hospital, and also their relatives and friends

3   To share critical care skills with staff in wards and the community, ensuring enhancement of training opportunities and skills practice, and to use information gathered from the ward and community to improve critical care services for patients and relatives.

Comprehensive Critical Care (Department of Health, 2000a)

Outreach services should, it stated, be provided by a team trained not only in the clinical aspects of care but also in effective ways of sharing their skills so that ward staff feel supported and not disempowered (Department of Health, 2000a). A key contributor to the development of outreach teams is the Department of Health Modernisation Agency. Through the National Patient Access Team, the modernisation agency has supported conferences, study days, research and audit in promoting and developing the work of outreach teams. Created to help local staff across the service to make radical sustainable changes, the agency has been instrumental in facilitating the recommendations of *Comprehensive Critical Care*, its goal being 'to improve access, experience and outcomes for patients with potential or actual need for critical care'. The introduction of critical care networks, designed to bring together trusts in regional areas, has also helped in sharing best practice and providing parity of service provision.

Outreach teams have also been pivotal in sharing critical care skills. Evidence produced in the interim report by the National Outreach Forum (2003) indicates that 94 per cent of respondents reporting on critical care outreach services include educational activity as part of their services. Such provision ranges from bedside teaching to multidisciplinary courses such as Acute Life Threatening Events – Recognition and Treatment (ALERT, see Smith *et al.*, 2000). Many authors also report the setting up of ward-based courses for the management of critically ill patients within the ward environment (Haines and Coad, 2001; O'Riordan *et al.*, 2003). Such courses provide information and training on a wide range of clinical practices, such as tracheostomy care, central line management and non-invasive ventilation.

The publication of *Comprehensive Critical Care* saw an influx in the development of outreach teams across the country. However, due to the differing priorities, needs and resources of individual Trusts, the teams themselves vary considerably in the way they deliver services. Some are nurse-led, others are multidisciplinary, and some are simply individuals charged with the task of delivering all the demands of an outreach service. The National Outreach Forum (2002), with representation from all critical care networks, published the interim findings of a study looking at the distribution and configuration of outreach services across the country; the completed report (NHS Modernisation Agency, 2003) is available at www.modern.nhs.uk/criticalcare.

Early warning scoring systems

As mentioned previously, many authors have developed early warning scoring systems based on pre-defined physiological criteria. These systems are designed to help nursing and medical staff based in ward areas to identify quickly those patients at risk of developing critical illness. This view is based on the assumption that those sick patients demonstrate changes in their physiological status some-times hours before they require admission to ICU. Vital sign measurement is an important aspect of inpatient care. Observations provide a trend of the patient's progress, which allows for the prompt detection of deterioration or improvement in their condition. One of the first scoring systems to be introduced was the early warning scoring system (Morgan *et al.*, 1997), which focused on five physiologi-cal parameters: pulse rate, respiratory rate, systolic blood pressure, temperature and AVPU score (see Table 37.1). This has since been modified by Stenhouse *et al.* (2000) to include urine output, and relative deviation from patient's normal blood pressure. Scores are allocated to each abnormal parameter, resulting in a total score, which may or may not indicate a need to call for assistance. Valida-tion of the modified early warning system (MEWS) score by Subbe *et al.* (2001) gave the opinion that, whilst further multicentre study needed to be undertaken, as a simple bedside tool the MEWS could help identify some of those patients at risk of deterioration and in need of more active intervention (see Box 37.2).

Whilst such systems have yet to demonstrate sensitivity, specificity and useful-ness (Goldhill, 2000), it is important to highlight the use of such systems. For the

Table 37.1 The early warning scoring system – a score of 3 or more requires a referral

Score	3	2	1	0	1	2	3
HR (bpm)		<40	41–50	51–100	101–110	111–130	130
SBP (mmHg)	<70	71–80	81–100	101–199	>200		
RR (per min)		<8		9–14	15–20	21–29	>30
Temp (°C)		<35	35.1–36.5	36.6–37.4	>37.5		
CNS				A	V	P	U

Source: Morgan *et al.* (1997).

Key:
A, Alert; V, response to verbal stimulus; P, response to pain; U, unconscious.

Box 37.2   Modified early warning system (MEWS)

Queen's Hospital, Burton on Trent, has developed a modified early warning system (MEWS) to provide an early accurate predictor of clinical deterioration. 'At risk' patients are scored, and any member of the multidis-ciplinary team (doctors, nurses, physiotherapists) can trigger MEWS for any other patient.

Comprehensive Critical Care (Department of Health, 2000a)

outreach teams to be successful, they will rely in part on ward-based staff identifying to them those patients at risk of developing serious illness. These physiological criteria are in many cases a valuable tool for staff to use, if only to support their own thoughts and interpretations. Goldhill *et al.* (1999a: 534) comments:

> Our data suggest that respiratory rate, heart rate and the adequacy of oxygenation are the most important physiological indicators of a critically ill ward patient. The level of consciousness and presence of renal failure may also be important indicators.

This view is supported by as yet unpublished data from the Burton on Trent team, who found in their study that increases in respiratory rate were by far the most important trigger for identifying critical illness, closely followed by alterations in heart rate and blood pressure.

The ability to recognise critical illness must not be underestimated. All the systems of support mentioned rely on staff being able to identify sick patients. It should not be presumed that nurses or doctors do this well. Arguably, if early detection and intervention occurred, patients could be either prevented from moving to a critical care area, or could receive clinical management intervention early.

Implications for practice

- Outreach can support the care of critically ill patients throughout the hospital
- Outreach offers ward staff the opportunities to develop skills and knowledge further
- Some critically ill patients being cared for on wards will inevitably become more sick, necessitating admission to intensive care and other specialist areas; outreach teams can help to identify patients at risk, and hasten the transfer of patients to more appropriate areas
- Outreach services should be easily available and accessible to wards.

Summary

The concept of outreach has been embraced enthusiastically by many acute hospitals throughout the country. Instinct tells us that it must be a good idea. Early recognition of potential or actual critical illness and the consequent correction of abnormalities should improve the patient experience and outcome. The collaboration between the outreach team (whatever its model definition) and the multidisciplinary team actively contributes to the concept of 'seamless care' supported by *Comprehensive Critical Care* (Department of Health, 2000a), bridging the gap between critical care and the ward areas. Unfortunately, the rapid process of hospitals acquiring such teams has resulted in outreach services being set up with minimal development and preparation time. The lack of clear supporting evidence for outreach has provoked some criticism, with calls for caution. Cuthbertson (2003) suggests the need for research into the 'development of validated, sensitive and specific scoring systems', the definition of a standard of care and a framework for future outreach services.

However, as the interim National Outreach Forum Report indicates, outreach is more than just a service to help identify sick patients. Many teams provide significant support in terms of education and training for nursing and junior medical staff, and the allied professions. They may work in close co-operation with the resuscitation team, involving decisions about resuscitation status. Many teams support the respiratory teams in delivering ward-based non-invasive ventilation. Others are involved with providing follow-up services for patients discharged from the critical care units and the hospital. In addition, many outreach teams have been instrumental in providing guidelines and protocols for clinical practice within their own areas. Such activities support the continuum of care for patients, staff and relatives.

Research projects looking at the role of outreach and its impact on patient care are being undertaken. A large nationally funded project is about to start, which should provide useful information on outreach as a model of service delivery. Only time will provide the evidence needed to evaluate outreach services properly. They should not be seen as a substitute for a well-resourced critical care unit, but hopefully it will be demonstrated that they enhance, support and improve the quality of care acutely ill patients receive in hospital.

Bibliography

Further reading

Department of Health (2000a).
McQuillan *et al.* (1998).

Useful sources

www.doh.gov.uk/about/modagency.htm
www.sdo.lshtm.ac.uk

Chapter 38

Reflection

Tina Moore

Contents

Learning outcomes

After reading this chapter you will be able to:

- Develop self-awareness in the areas of personal and professional development
- Understand the benefits and problems associated with reflection
- Demonstrate knowledge of various models for reflection and determine the usefulness of each.

Introduction

Specialised knowledge is essential for professional practice and will manifest in professional competence. Schön (1995) suggests that self-consciousness (reflection) and continual self-critique (critical reflection) are crucial components of competence.

Using reflection as a means of enhancing professional practice originated from the work of Schön (1983). He described clinical practice as 'swampy lowlands' containing confusing, messy, complex problems that are often not clear-cut.

As illustrated in Box 38.1, nursing actions are not simply a matter of right or wrong. However, nurses need to make sense of their practices and clinical decision-making, and reflection is seen as a means of enabling them to achieve this. It is a way of encouraging experiential knowledge. Nurses may perform at different levels, with both formal theory and experience contributing to their decision-making.

Box 38.1   Clinical reflection

A patient who has had a large acute myocardial infarction with complicating left ventricular failure and cardiogenic shock continues to complain of severe chest pain despite active intervention to relieve it. What should the course of action be? Giving analgesia may reduce the pain, but may create additional life-threatening complications (large dosages of analgesia may compromise the patient's respiratory and cardiovascular status). If analgesia is withheld, the patient may deteriorate due to the effects of the pain. If, for humanitarian reasons, analgesia is given and the patient dies from the complicating effects, there is a possibility that feelings of guilt for the nurse administering the analgesia may become evident. These feelings should be explored and meaning(s) derived from the situation.

The Nursing and Midwifery Council (NMC) (2002b), as part of its framework for post-registration education and practice (PREP), expects all nurses to engage in some form of reflective activity and to provide written accounts within a Personal Professional Portfolio. The encouragement for a system of life-long learning for Nurses and Midwives has been echoed in a number of other documents (DOH, 1997; DOH, 1998c; Council of Deans and Heads, 1998). Life-long learning reinforces the necessity for nurses to reflect; hence, 'reflection' and 'reflective practice' are terms that have become familiar to many, and have in some instances become central to contemporary nursing practice.

This chapter will explore the concept of reflection and identify the benefits and problems associated with it. Suggestions on how to develop reflective practice are offered.

Time out 38.1

What do you understand by the terms 'reflection' and 'reflective p

Definitions

There is in existence a wealth of literature relating to reflection. Despite this the concept remains poorly defined, with a lack of clarity regarding its meaning (Scanlan and Chernomas, 1997; Pierson, 1998), thus making it difficult to put into operation (Atkins and Murphy, 1993).

Existing definitions suggest reflection is the process of learning to gain new understanding/knowledge from experience (Boyd and Fales, 1983; Boud et al., 1985; Wilkinson, 1999), and is stimulated by perceived discrepancies between an individual's beliefs/values, assumptions, and understanding or insight (Teekman, 2000). This can result in a reactionary process triggered by uncomfortable feelings/thoughts (Atkins and Murphy, 1993).

Three different levels of reflection have been described:

1   Reflection-*in*-action (thinking on one's feet simultaneously as practice occurs) involves devising and testing solutions when a problem is encountered (Schön, 1991). This is a form of tacit knowledge.
2   Reflection-*on*-action (retrospective thinking about an experience) (Schön, 1991) involves looking back at what has been done and learning lessons from what did, or did not, work.
3   Reflection-*before*-action as an important preparatory element of reflective learning (Greenwood, 1998).

Various models have been devised to guide the process of reflection, e.g. Johns (2000) which integrates Carper's 'four ways of knowing' (empirical, aesthetic, ethical and personal) (Carper, 1978). Kolb and Fry (1975) proposed an experiential learning cycle, which begins with a concrete experience followed by observation and reflection. Boud et al. (1985) considered retrospective reflection, which enables learning, with corresponding changes in attitudes and behaviour. The cyclical nature of this model suggests that these outcomes are then available to stimulate further reflections.

Process of reflection

Reflective models may help nurses to structure their reflection – particularly those who are junior and new to critical care nursing. Models will help nurses to complete the reflective cycle. Often the last stage (below) is omitted. However, a reflective model is not an essential tool (Rich and Parker, 1995); indeed, many nurses are experienced in the process of reflection and have developed their own model.

Most reflective models in existence generally follow the same process:

■   Stage 1 – a description of what happened: an event/situation creates an awareness of some kind of emotional response, e.g. puzzlement, surprise or discomfort
■   Stage 2 – applying existing theory and knowledge to the situation described: analysis of a situation, involving examination of current knowledge, perceptions and assumptions

■ Stage 3 – returning to the situation and improving: outcome of the analysis may include new understanding.

(Atkins and Murphy, 1993; Cranton, 1994; Kim, 1999)

Time out 38.2

1 Think of a situation that you have recently been involved in and which was meaningful to you. It could be a situation that created an unresolved issue or one that could have been dealt with better, or it may have been a positive experience.

2 Write a description in relation to each of the stages outlined above.

3 Consider the exercise you have just undertaken. What do you think are the aims of reflection?

Reflection: a justification

Possible reasons why nurses do not reflect include:

■ When competence has grown to a point of being over-confident in one's own knowledge and hence being unresponsive to suggestions to improve practice

■ Negative habitualisation resulting in routine and coping-dominated practice

■ Impulse, tradition and/or authority-guided practice

■ Acceptance of the realities of daily practice, concentrating upon discovering the most effective and efficient way of solving problems, often missing opportunities for reflection.

(Ferry and Ross-Gordon, 1998)

In a number of key areas reflection is claimed to be of benefit to the practitioner and the practice of nursing. However, these claims tend to be anecdotal and lack empirical evidence. Justifications for reflective practice are outlined below.

Generation of knowledge

A key function of reflective practice is to increase knowledge and understanding. Carper's (1978) seminal work describes four ways of 'knowing' in nursing, but her work has not been updated since publication and, to reflect contemporary changes, needs to include legal knowing (see Chapter 41).

The critical care experience for the patient and their family is a unique experience. Nurses need to learn from this in order to develop their clinical practice. Whilst there have been significant developments in the application of empirical knowing, learning form the 'lived experience' is sadly lacking.

Practice–theory gap

Reflection, in nursing, has been advocated as a way of overcoming the divergence between theory and practice and as a means of articulating and developing knowledge embedded within practice (Benner *et al.*, 1996).

Used effectively, reflection can answer questions about the nature of nursing and can be used to generate nursing theory (Boud *et al.*, 1985; Schön, 1991). The NHSE indicates that there is a lack of evidence demonstrating theory being generated from practising nurses (NHSE, 1998; see also Chapter 39).

Critical thinking

Reflection encourages critical thinking (Durgahee, 1998). This is seen as an essential component of professional practice, and is perhaps the most distinguishing attribute of an expert nurse. Lack of critical thinking relates to performing task-oriented care (Benner *et al.*, 1996).

Critical thinking involves:

- Cognitive skills (challenging assumptions)
- Self-regulated thinking
- Careful evaluation of data (Fowler, 1998)
- Motivation to look beyond what is known to the unknown
- Perseverance
- Fair-mindedness.

A sound knowledge base is the foundation of critical thinking, but experience in similar situations also influences patterns of thinking. Critical thinkers are flexible, open-minded, and willing to admit limitations and learn from errors in judgment. Unless critical analysis is achieved (which reviews and links experience to the past or future), reflection will not occur (Scanlan and Chernomas, 1997).

Enhancing clinical practice

The process of reflection should enable a greater insight into the meaning of practice and the creation of links between theory to practice, resulting in enhanced, patient-centred care (Bellman, 1996). However, there is little evidence to demonstrate that personal benefits are transmitted to patients, making it impossible to conclude that reflection improves patient care (Andrews *et al.*, 1998). It does, however, enable nurses to explore and come to understand the nature and boundaries of their own role and that of other health professionals (Johns, 2000).

Currently there is a shortage of empirical evidence supporting the claims made by reflective theory and its advocates, but empirical data may not be possible because of the nature of reflection – i.e. there are too many variables that could influence validity and reliability. Indeed, if nursing waits for 'credible evidence' to emerge, practice development may be stunted. Some scrutiny of professional practice, must, on the whole, be a positive undertaking.

Intuition and expert practice

Research from Benner (1984) and Benner and Tanner (1987) drew attention to the tacit nature of some aspects of nursing and explored how expert nurses use intuition in their practice. Saylor (1990) focused on intuitive nursing practice and recommended ways in which reflective practice can help nurses access tacit knowledge to complement technical rationality. She advised self-evaluation using a portfolio and some form of supervision; both are endorsed by the NMC (2002b).

Benner *et al.* (1996) describes intuition as judgment without a rationale. Intuition is also described in terms of vivid personal images, such as gut feelings, sixth sense, insight, instinct, common sense, inner feelings, hunches.

The role of intuition in Benner *et al.*'s (1996) description of the expert nurse (characterised by reasoning that is mature and practical in origin, accompanied by an intuitive grasp of the patient's situation) is the focus of much ongoing debate. English (1993) is critical of the concept of intuition in relation to the expert practitioner, claiming it is ambiguous. He suggests that in the absence of empirical evidence, intuition has limited applicability in nursing. English (1993), however, fails to support his claims through empirical evidence.

Problems associated with reflection

- Individuals have the right not to engage in reflection as self-protection against anxiety. Reflection may be seen as a form of surveillance (Gilbert, 2001). The process of reflection may lead practitioners to relive painful experiences that they may prefer to defend against. Indeed, the process of writing reflective experiences may be therapeutic (Johns, 2000), and should complement clinical supervision. Critics indicate that avoiding self-awareness is detrimental to good nursing practice (Barber, 1994).
- Dilemmas may arise as a result of role conflict, i.e. support or policing practice. This may result in practitioners hiding mistakes. Supervisors may be inexperienced and/or incompetent to provide adequate support when dealing with emotions. This could result from lack of adequate preparation for the role. Lack of time (Heath, 1998) would add to these problems.
- Uncertainties in the accuracy and recall of events, together with hindsight bias and the interfering effects of anxiety, can mean that sometimes people may not always do as they say they do (Andrews *et al.*, 1998). This indicates that reliance on memory is problematic (Wallace, 1996). When caring for critically ill patients there is so much to remember, so many variables to consider when making clinical decisions, that it is virtually impossible for nurses to remember every fine detail.
- The ethics of reading a document that contains potentially very sensitive and personal information has been questioned by Rich and Parker (1995), as constituting an invasion of privacy. Reflective accounts are personal, and the decision to make them public should be voluntary. Conflict may arise regarding confidentiality and professional implications. If an action/entry is in conflict with the NMC professional conduct guidelines, then appropriate action

needs to be taken. Ground rules should be agreed at the beginning (e.g. that the supervisor cannot guarantee confidentiality if matters arise of a professional nature).

■ The lack of clarity in the literature about confidentiality requires urgent attention and guidance from sources with ethical expertise. Whilst some ethical considerations arise from the literature, this is frequently a passing comment rather than a comprehensive analysis. Many authors provide guidance on reflective teaching and learning, but fail to mention/acknowledge that issues of a professional nature may arise (e.g. Kember *et al.*, 2001).

Developing reflective practice

Limited experience may restrict the use of reflection, but this should not be viewed as a barrier. Reflective skills have been identified by Atkins and Murphy (1993) as self-awareness, description, critical analysis, synthesis and evaluation.

Strategies to promote critical thinking, identified by Fowler (1998), include facilitation of:

■ Reflection
■ Comparisons of clinical situations
■ Forward thinking
■ Reasoned thinking
■ Learning from others
■ Peer/group learning.

Effective supervisory support networks need to be established. The use of mixed groups may possibly enhance the development of skills of reflection (Hawkins and Shohart, 1989).

Controversy surrounds the use of guidelines to structure reflection. For example Burns (1994) found that while students wanted guidance, staff were unwilling to provide it, fearing that, however unique the original experience, guides would produce uniformity. However, nurses who are faced with any new concept need guidance, and problems arise when inflexibility sets in.

Encouraging practitioners to reflect by writing about experiences (critical incidence, stories, drawing pictures) may help. The aim is to help nurses to clarify the knowledge underpinning their actions. Writing encourages self-involvement in the learning process, as the authors are involved in describing meaningful experiences and then deconstructing them to ascertain areas for learning. The scrutiny of practice has sometimes been experienced as too 'painful and disturbing', so lateral and critical thinking could not be promoted (Durgahee, 1998). A 'dumping of baggage' session may need to occur before the process of reflection begins. It may be seen as part of the reflective process.

Problem-based learning (PBL) has been identified as one way to facilitate the development of reflection and critical reflection (Alavi, 1995). This process engages learners in activities that reveal their thinking processes so that they can monitor the effectiveness of their ability to analyse, reason and acquire knowledge; facilitate the development of interpersonal collaborative skills – particularly listening, questioning and summarising; and enable them to assume increasing control for their own reflective learning.

Implications for practice

- Reflection depends on active strategies such as reflective writing
- Supervision by peers, one-to-one or in a group, appears to be the most effective form of clinical supervision to facilitate reflection
- Practice-generated theory accessed through reflection can challenge existing theory/practices
- All experience should be considered as a potential precursor to reflection, particularly habituated experiences
- Reflective practice should encompass critical analysis of personal self-awareness
- Caution should be expressed about the ethical challenges of becoming a reflective practitioner in relation to professional issues
- Practitioners reflecting should consider sharing their experiences with others.

Summary

Reflection involves the integration of practice experience and academic knowledge, and the reassessment of old perspectives, enabling the rejection of some views and ideas whilst others are retained. The culture within nursing is moving from the earlier acceptance of information to the questioning and critiquing of arguments and professional assumptions (particularly concerning their relevance and appropriateness for practice).

The value and development of nurturing practice knowledge is a key concern. In the absence of empirical evidence, reflection is still a useful way to identify strengths and deficiencies within practice, enabling practitioners to assess their professional needs and development accordingly. It also aids the supervision and guidance of nurses. However, reflection can only occur when the validity of prior learning is challenged (Mezirow, 1991).

Bibliography

Key reading

Kember *et al.* (2001) provides practical guidance to educationalist/mentors in facilitating reflection, but omits professional issues.

Suggested reading

Gilbert (2001) provides a critical view of clinical supervision and reflection.

Chapter 39

Practice development

Philip Woodrow

Contents

Learning outcomes

After reading this chapter you will be able to:

- Understand the historical contexts of practice
- Increase your understanding of possible aspects of practice development
- Identify strategies that enable the development of practice.

Introduction

Nightingale's school of nursing established an apprenticeship system of training. This system of learning 'on the job' from experienced practitioners remained essentially unchanged through the introduction of statutory professional regulation in 1911 and the birth of the National Health Service in 1948. Whatever merits apprenticeship has, it fosters an ethos of ritualised practice (Walsh and Ford, 1989; Ford and Walsh, 1994). Towards the end of the twentieth century,

society, governments and the healthcare professions themselves increasingly scru-
tinised the delivery of health care. This included demands to evaluate whether
health care was based on sound principles and evidence (DOH, 1999a). Nurses
are now individually professionally accountable for their actions (NMC, 2002a),
with a legal duty to base their practice on sound and current evidence (Tingle,
2002a).

Development of 'critical care without walls' has acknowledged that highly
dependent (level 2) and sometimes critically ill (level 3) patients are cared for in
various wards, so the knowledge and skills of staff need developing further. Con-
currently, promotion of evidence-based practice and concerns that much practice
is based on ritual rather than rationale have identified further needs for practice
development. The role of the practice development nurse is a way to meet the
needs of nurses, nursing and health care.

Developing practice

Public expectations may be high, but nursing has inherited an educational system
that has not always met the needs of nursing practice (Mulhall, 2002), while heavy
workloads leave nurses little time or energy for unpaid self-directed study in their
own leisure time. In an attempt to meet expectations, many specialist nursing roles
have been developed in recent decades. Some of these roles have been developed in
response to government or other 'top-down' initiatives; some have been driven by
local initiatives of individuals who were themselves either in a vaguely defined post
or keen to develop practice, using a 'bottom-up' approach to change (see Chapter
40). The continuing emergence of new roles indicates that initial hopes for previous roles have not always been fully met, and while some roles have evolved,
others have disappeared. Recently the UK government's Department of Health
promoted the role of Practice Development Nurse (Garbett and McCormack,
2002a), notably as an integral part of the NHS Plan (DOH, 2000e).

Nursing history suggests that practice does need development, but what practice development means and entails is open to interpretation and debate. Literature on practice development, and the role of practice development nurses, often
contains strong views but weaker evidence. This chapter presents personal views
on practice development from the author's perspective as a Practice Development
Nurse.

Governmental promotion of a role often brings funding, so many healthcare
Trusts applied for funding to appoint Practice Development Nurses. However,
the roles of post-holders often vary considerably, even within a single Trust. In
the UK, the term 'practice development' is used widely but inconsistently (Garbett
and McCormack, 2002b). Garbett and McCormack (2002b) found that most
literature expected practice development to:

- Improve patient care
- Transform the contexts and cultures in which nursing care takes place
- Apply systematic approaches to changing practice
- Facilitate change.

Chambers (2002: 101), echoing Kitson *et al.* (1996), suggests that practice development should integrate 'clinical practice, education and research for the advancement of evidence-based nursing, theory generation and scholarship within an environment of collaboration and shared ownership'. Joyce (1999) viewed the aim of practice development as examining and evaluating care delivery to improve quality and efficiency.

Such aims may be laudable, but whether they are achievable within one role or person is debatable. While Practice Development Nurses should facilitate practice development, all nurses remain individually accountable for their practice and so should participate in practice development. Practice development is not the sole responsibility of, and should not be confined to, Practice Development Nurses. Turner (2001) identifies two aspects to practice development: people, and their role.

The aims of the role will only be fulfilled if suitable people are appointed. Too often in recent nursing history, roles have failed because senior people have been shifted from one role to another to meet the needs of employers to offer comparable salaries and status, rather than because the individuals appointed meet the needs of healthcare provision. If strong leadership improves outcomes (Manley, 2000), impoverished leadership presumably brings impoverished outcomes.

Aims identified in literature tend to emphasise measurable behaviouristic objective markers (such as producing research) rather than the more subjective, but also possibly more humanistic, benefits (such as quality and morale). While evidence-based practice is desirable, nursing should value intuition as well, combining it with analysis (Goding and Edwards, 2002). There is a danger that 'evidence-based practice' may become one more mantra, leading to dismissal of practice that is not evidence-based without considering whether it might still have some validity. Rituals – the legacy of apprenticeship – may have survived because they work. Evidence passed on by role models/experts may have value (le May, 1999), so should be examined and analysed before being dismissed.

The theory–practice gap

A gap between the theory and practice of nursing persists (Cook, 1991; Upton, 1999; Mulhall, 2002). Currently, much theory generated by nursing academia questions existing practices; the almost inevitable clichéd conclusion of research is that 'more research is needed'. While questioning can be valuable, nurses in clinical practice need to provide care to their patients, and cannot withhold actions because 'more research is needed'. Nursing academia fails to meet the need of nurses in practice for unambiguous answers to immediate practical problems (Mulhall, 2002), and in so doing, too often fails to meet the needs of nursing practice.

Despite advocacy of evidence-based practice, there is often little or weak evidence for practice. Evidence is sometimes viewed as being unquestionable, and so is applied to practice uncritically (Ballinger and Wiles, 2001). All evidence is questionable, and some is faulty. Evidence-based practice requires nurses to be able to evaluate evidence, weighing the risks against the benefits of each option for each individual patient (DiCenso *et al.*, 1998). However, clinical nurses have little time (Palfreyman *et al.*, 2003) and may have limited skills to be able to sift and evaluate evidence. The large volume of evidence published and otherwise available necessitates some preliminary sifting. Nurses in clinical practice tend to rely on individuals whom they trust to provide reliable information, rather than searching through texts and electronic sources (Thomson *et al.*, 2002). Linking theory and practice can only be achieved if those promoting theory have clinical credibility (Murray and Thomas, 1998).

Some sifting is already available through meta-analyses – systematic reviews of research that critically synthesise comparable studies to accumulate evidence from an overall far larger number of patients and events. Meta-analyses are widely viewed as the most reliable form of evidence, and are widely available through journals and the Internet. Cochrane Reviews, the 'gold standard' for evidence-based practice, began as medical meta-analyses, but there are now Cochrane Reviews of nursing topics (Zwarenstein *et al.*, 1999). Cochrane Reviews are also available on the Internet. However, passive acceptance of any 'gold standard' creates a danger of establishing a new orthodoxy, and new rituals. Although generally reliable and of high quality, Cochrane Reviews may be fallible, as shown in the now discredited (Boldt, 2000; Wilkes and Navickis, 2001) review of albumin (Cochrane Injuries Group Albumin Reviewers, 1998).

While practice should be based on current and reliable evidence, nursing theory should also be generated from nursing practice. Successive Chief Nursing Officers in the UK have emphasised that practitioners should learn from practice (Garbett and McCormack, 2002a). Practice development is concerned directly with clinical practice (Manley and McCormack, 2003), so should enable nurses in practice to research and promote practice-based evidence.

There are many disincentives that hinder clinical staff from reading professional literature, including:

■ Heavy workloads
■ Often little support in study time or funding
■ Exhaustion
■ Geographical distance of some healthcare libraries from places of work
■ The sheer volume of literature currently being generated ('information overload').

Nurses seeking information find their colleagues are more accessible and useful than books or other resources (Thomson, 2002). After their immediate colleagues, nurses value people who are still linked with clinical practice, such as specialist and link nurses (Thomson, 2002). Practice development nurses should therefore have the skills to sift and critically analyse evidence, bringing relevant issues to the attention of clinical nurses and provoking discussion and critical thinking, so that nurses in clinical practice can make informed, evidence-based decisions.

So far this chapter has focused on the 'higher-level' skills of analysing evidence. However, nursing is a practice-based profession, and so in addition to cognitive skills, nurses need psychomotor skills to provide quality care. Many nurses in practice considered that the UK's Project 2000 system of pre-registration education failed adequately to develop the practical skills of qualifying nurses (Carlisle *et al.*, 1999; Howard, 2001). Therefore practice development should include developing nurses' skills.

A personal perspective

The author of this chapter is currently employed primarily to teach a short course for qualified ward nurses on the principles of caring for critically ill patients. This course develops practice through enabling ward staff to provide better, more efficient evidence-based care. It also helps develop those nurses as individual practitioners.

Practice development should include maintaining a current knowledge base (see Box 39.1). Through the employer's library service, the author regularly (each issue) follows over 150 journals. Evidence is integrated into course material, but is also taken back to practice or passed on to colleagues as appropriate. Wider dissemination is achieved through publication. In addition to writing books and articles, the author reviews for professional journals and publishers, and encourages colleagues to present their work for publication.

Box 39.1   Practice development

Some nurse authors and lecturers persist in emphasising the significance of Korotkoff sounds for blood pressure assessment. In most wards, sphygmomanometers have been replaced by automated blood pressure monitors. The Medical Devices Agency may soon warn against possession of mercury-containing equipment (Meekin and Allyn, 2001).

Rather than trying to develop skills in obsolete practices, practice development could include encouraging staff to monitor mean arterial pressure (see Chapter 32). Mean arterial pressure is the best indicator of perfusion pressure (Darovic, 2002a), so is more useful than either diastolic or systolic blood pressure for managing the hypotension that often occurs in critical illness. Historically this was not used in ward areas, presumably because it involved making a mathematical calculation. Most automated monitors calculate mean arterial pressure.

Credibility among clinical colleagues understandably partly relies on current clinical practice (Murray and Thomas, 1998). Unfortunately the practice of some theorists is obviously dated, and despite calls from such influential bodies as the NHS Executive, there has been little formal support for nurse educators to return to practice (Cutler, 2002).

To maintain clinical credibility, the author works clinically for one shift each week. This clinical work involves directly caring for patients; not teaching in the clinical area or attending meetings with clinical staff, which has sometimes been used to claim maintenance of current clinical practice (Clifford, 1993).

Strategies for developing practice

Increasing demands and constraints make proactive and dynamic development problematic, but not impossible. With high morale, staff are more likely to be motivated to develop themselves and their clinical area. Practice leaders, including managers, have an important role in motivating and maintaining morale, such as through:

- Auditing available resources in the clinical area, and raising awareness among staff of what is available
- Disseminating relevant information from literature, employers and other organisations, ensuring it remains readily available
- Developing guidelines, competencies and other mechanisms to guide the team
- Providing a teaching programme for staff as well as students
- Developing a 'learning zone', where some relevant journals and books are available
- Encouraging staff to make copies of coursework and other projects available in the 'learning zone'
- Encouraging individual staff members to develop a specialist interest in a topic, including displaying posters or other material in the 'learning zone'
- Identifying funding for a networked computer terminal, with access to Internet resources and databases
- Providing health information for patients and relatives; this could be through nationally produced booklets (such as those produced by the British Heart Foundation), or in-house posters and handouts
- Ensuring an effective individual performance review (IPR) mechanism exists to identify staff's continuing professional development needs, and ways these can be supported.

Implications for practice

- Practice development should be led by nurses who maintain clinical credibility by providing direct patient care
- Roles should remain flexible enough to meet local needs
- Practice Development Nurses have the potential to lead practice development, but should not be considered a substitute for development by others
- Practice development is the responsibility of all practising nurses.

Summary

This chapter has largely focused on the role of Practice Development Nurses, written from the personal perspectives and experiences of the author. Practice development may be viewed as one more of a long list of roles that, so far, have failed to fulfil initial expectations, or as a challenging alternative to the traditional tripartite divisions between clinical practice, management and education.

Evidence-based practice is desirable, but evidence for practice needs to be practice-based and should be critically evaluated. Practice development provides opportunities to promote a culture of analytical evidence-based practice. Practice Development Nurses can be a conduit for this to occur. Whatever labels are given to people who are empowered to be nursing leaders, practice will only progress if those leaders have the qualities necessary to fulfil expectations.

Exercise

1   List the ten aspects that you consider are most important to practice development in your area of work. Identify why you consider these to be priorities.
2   What would be needed for these aspects to be implemented (e.g. people, resources)? Which of these needs can be realistically achieved at present within your Trust? Consider whether there are any external organisations or resources that could be approached.
3   If you were to be appointed Practice Development Nurse in your ward, identify:

   - Your priorities for the next six months
   - How you will seek to implement them
   - What problems you expect
   - How you might resolve those problems.

Bibliography

Key reading

Garbett and McCormack's (2002a, 2002b) research provides comprehensive syntheses of views surrounding practice development.

Goding and Edwards (2002) examine issues surrounding the current high profile of 'evidence-based practice'.

Manley's work has largely created current concepts of practice development. Manley and McCormack (2003) summarises her work.

Further reading

The NHS Plan (DOH, 2000e) outlines government expectations of how UK health care will develop in the first decade of the twenty-first century, including 10 key roles identified for nurses. Although most readers will probably have seen or heard summaries of the plan, it is useful to look at the original document rather than rely on second-hand reports.

Hamer and Collinson (1999) provides a useful text about evidence-based practice.

Chapter 40

Managing change

Tina Moore

Contents

Learning outcomes

After reading this chapter you will be able to:

- Appreciate the need for change
- Understand the process of change management and indicate potential problems
- Develop a proactive strategy in the management of change.

Fundamental knowledge

Nature of HDU nursing (Chapter 1).

Introduction

Nurses have a professional and legal responsibility to provide and maintain a safe and acceptable standard of care. If nurses fail to do so, they will need to provide justification. Change is seen to be a natural process in the development and maintenance of standards.

Over the past decade there has been a number of developments within critical care (see Chapter 1). Many of these changes have been as a result of the government's vision of a new NHS, offering a fast and convenient but at the same time individual and useful service to a consistently high standard (DOH, 2000e).

Health care is a culture in which change is expected and/or inevitable, often occurring at a phenomenal rate and without apparent rationale. Change should reflect a proactive rather than a reactive philosophy. However, some changes may have been prompted by complaints, possibly through the Patient Advocacy and Liaison Service (DOH, 2001c) now appointed to every hospital. Change may also result from an independent regime of healthcare regulations, audit and inspection (DOH, 2001c).

Constant change, particularly without evaluation, and 'change made for change's sake' precipitate a 'turmoil' situation. There is a significant chance that the same difficulties will recur in spite of change. Change can be uncomfortable for many, and will gather casualties during its process. Therefore, change should only be implemented for a good reason. An example might be the implementation of an evidence-based approach to care that has been proven to make working practices more efficient and effective. Suctioning (Chapter 31) is one such example.

Most of the resistance to change is not a response to the innovation but to the way the change is managed. This chapter will therefore concentrate on the process of managing planned change.

Time out 40.1

1 Before reading further, think of changes that have occurred within your area of practice during the past year.
2 Write down how the changes were implemented (the process).
3 Do you think the change was implemented adequately? Give reasons for your answer.

Planned/unplanned change

Unplanned change contains less predictability and certainty than planned change. This causes a feeling of loss of control and increases anxiety. High resistance may occur, resulting in unsuccessful implementation. Human resource problems may arise, including loss of staff, recruitment problems, sickness and absenteeism. Careful planning and a collaborative approach are essential to help secure successful implementation of change.

As far as possible, planned change should occur at a pace to which staff are able to adjust comfortably. As the change is expected, there should be minimal surprises (but this can never be guaranteed). The involvement of staff in planning the change is essential. This process should identify early resistance, and enables the adoption of appropriate strategies to address the related issues. A proactive, non-restrictive leadership style facilitates acceptance and commitment, resulting in higher risk-taking and creativity.

A model for change

Change is a complex process that can be difficult and demanding but also exciting, and therefore needs to be managed effectively. A model of change may help in this process. There are various models for managing change available, such as Lewin's model based on Field Force Analysis Theory, and Action Research.

A model proposed by Ketefian (1978) indicates that there are five components to the planned change process (Figure 40.1). It is simple to follow, and considers most factors involved in the change process. Ketefian does not explicitly include evaluation (a crucial part of the change process); therefore this should be built into the model.

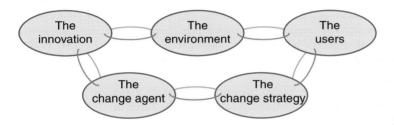

Figure 40.1 **Planned change process**

Together, these components make an interlinked chain. In order for the change to be successful, all these components need to be addressed – ensuring no gaps.

Time out 40.2

1 Reflect on the poorly implemented situation you may have identified in Time out 40.1. How do you think that particular process could have been improved?
2 Was the innovation considered useful in aiding the care of patients?

Innovation

As previously discussed, change needs to be adopted for a good reason, such as enhancing the quality of care. Initial assessment of a situation will help to identify the areas of practice to be developed. An evaluation of the compatibility/relevancy of the proposed innovation can help to identify problem areas (e.g. assessment of patient, fluid management). Together, staff should examine their former position (past), where they are now (present), and where they want to be (future).

The innovation needs to show a benefit and not be a case of 'change for change's sake'. Hence, change needs to be observable in practice (e.g. improvements in care) – for example, a move away from routinised approaches such as hourly observations performed on all level 2 patients and adopting an individualised approach where frequency of monitoring will be done on an individual basis.

Whatever the innovation, it needs to be compatible with the existing values and beliefs of the people involved in the change (directly or indirectly). Exceptions to this are outdated or dangerous practices where there are professional implications. For example, in one critical care unit it was still routine to wash all the patients in the early hours of the morning. Many staff resisted proposed changes to this practice, even though it was potentially detrimental to the patients.

Consultation and collaboration is an essential element of the change process. Significant time must be spent on strengthening relationships, communicating with the staff about the idea for change, and providing a rationale for making the change (human beings usually seek relevancy). In order to promote a sense of control, worth, belonging and consequently ownership, a non-judgmental, democratic approach to leadership/management is crucial in the first instance. However, if the rate of implementation is too slow, or is stifled, then an autocratic approach may be justified.

Minor changes are easier to implement than major ones. If the innovation is complex, implementation may need to be broken down into manageable stages.

Time out 40.3

1   Following from Time out 40.2, write down the staff's reaction to the change.

Environment

To aid successful implementation a culture of blame should be minimised, ideally eroded altogether and replaced by a culture of openness. Questioning, challenging and critical reflection should be nurtured. The change agent should have the courage and confidence not to take any negativity personally (resistance is usually directed at process rather than people). Trusting relationships between staff are essential. If trust is lacking, change will not succeed. Changing the environment may prove to be the most challenging part of the change process, so time may need to be spent addressing these issues.

Users

Several characteristics and personalities emerging within the change process have been identified by Rogers and Shoemaker (1971); see Figure 40.2.

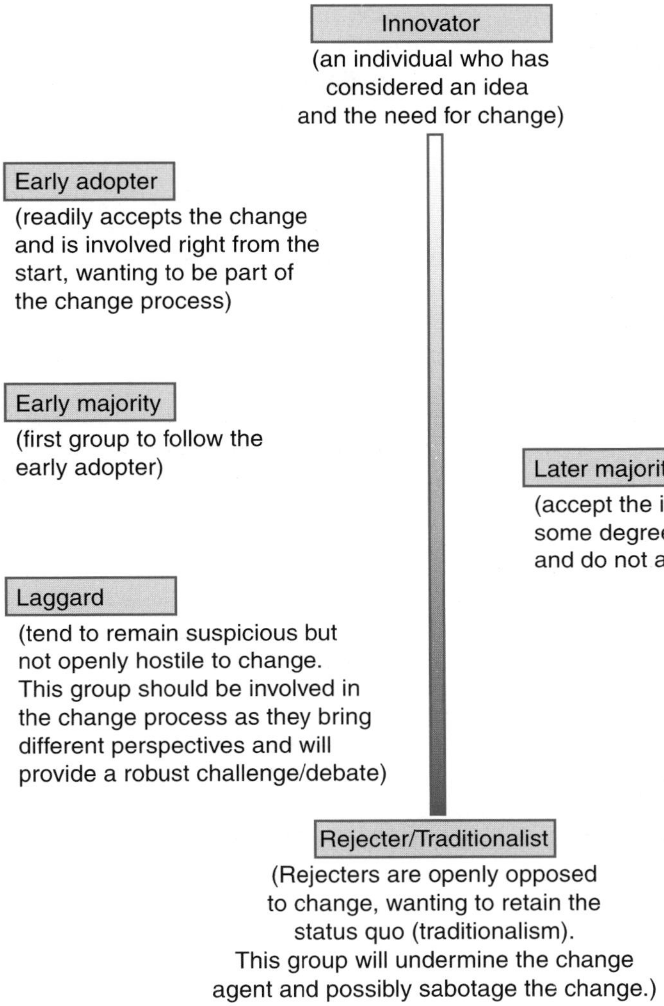

Innovator

(an individual who has
considered an idea
and the need for change)

Early adopter

(readily accepts the change
and is involved right from the
start, wanting to be part of
the change process)

Early majority

(first group to follow the
early adopter)

Later majority

(accept the innovation with
some degree of scepticism
and do not actively resist)

Laggard

(tend to remain suspicious but
not openly hostile to change.
This group should be involved in
the change process as they bring
different perspectives and will
provide a robust challenge/debate)

Rejecter/Traditionalist

(Rejecters are openly opposed
to change, wanting to retain the
status quo (traditionalism).
This group will undermine the change
agent and possibly sabotage the change.)

Figure 40.2 **Users of change**

Change agent

A change agent is considered to be someone who can initiate, lead and implement a change. There are some individuals who are 'visionary' but lack strategic capabilities, and will involve co-opted members to implement the change. Ideally the change agent should lead in all stages, enabling continuity, consistency and commitment to the idea.

Effective leadership, management, communication and interpersonal skills are integral parts of being a change agent. Supporting and directing staff requires taking on a facilitative role; the ability to team-build and network successfully.

Successful change cannot occur without the involvement and commitment of others. Change agents need personal commitment, enthusiasm, and the ability to stimulate and excite others. Change agents also need to be creative thinkers, prepared to undertake risks, to have a clear vision of the goal they want to achieve, and to be able to nurture a culture of change.

The innovation, users and environment all influence the type of change agent required. External agents usually bring objectivity to a situation, but also a tendency towards authoritarian behaviour (possibly due to lack of time to build up relationships). 'In-house' change agents tend to be accepted by the group (as they have already established relationships and are possibly part of the team), but may lack objectivity. As a result, authority may not be used appropriately.

Time out 40.4

1   Identify some of the reasons why you think people resist change.
2   How would you minimise the barriers of change?

Resistance to change

Change can be destabilising, and often generates stress. The avalanche of changes affecting nursing is one reason for this (Ootim, 1997). Here, resistance could be a normal reaction and may be an inevitable part of change.

Reasons for resistance to change include:

- Feeling threatened, fear of personal loss (Daft, 2002)
- Uncertainty (King and Anderson, 1995)
- Lack of understanding about what the change involves (Daft, 2002)
- Individual practice being under scrutiny and being criticised
- Reluctance to take risks, feeling secure with the status quo (Muchinsky, 2000)
- Complacency
- Not understanding the need to change.

Much of the resistance to change relates to how the change affects the individual, or how the change is being/has been managed.

Positive attitudes towards change may take some time to develop. Anxieties encourage avoidance behaviour, particularly when individuals are required to adopt a totally new approach.

Achieving ownership for everyone is essential, but may not be achieved. Where possible, changes should be designed to develop existing systems, procedures, cultures and traditions, enabling staff gradually to alter/adapt as they get used to the change. The aim is to create as little disruption as possible.

Resistance to change may result in a breach of the *Code of Conduct* (NMC, 2002a). Disciplinary action may be required, particularly if poor practice exists. Before this happens, managers need to demonstrate that they have tried to address the issues through means such as performance appraisals and reviews; altering roles and responsibilities; increasing clinical supervision; and education and training. Evidence needs to be provided to justify disciplinary action, as it can give the impression of victimisation.

The current Labour Government has indicated that best practice can no longer be optional for NHS staff, and stipulates that managers and clinicians must make change happen (DOH, 2000e). The *Code of Conduct for NHS Managers* (DOH, 2002b) is a contractual agreement that includes involvement in the change process.

Change strategies

A number have already been discussed, but there are four main strategies:

1   Rational empirical (i.e. via research) – the belief is that people will listen to and be guided by rational/reasoning and empirical evidence.
2   Power – coercive (top-down) represents the traditional model of healthcare management; changes are imposed, often with little or no rationale. Change is not permanent; once the change agent has gone, previous practices return (i.e. 'when the cat's away the mice will play').
3   Normative – re-educative (bottom-up) relies on the group's perception of the need for change and so change may not occur.
4   Combined (combination of all mentioned).

(Lancaster, 1999)

There is no ultimately right or wrong strategy. The strategy should be selected in accordance with the innovation, the type of environment in which the change is to occur and the users of the change. Longer-lasting change requires a bottom-up, non-directive approach with an open and facilitative style of leadership.

A people-centred approach is usually adopted, through early involvement of staff, enabling joint diagnosis and getting them to critique the status quo. Staff should be involved in the decision-making processes as appropriate (DOH, 2002b); this should occur early rather than when decisions have been made and cannot be influenced. Effective communication channels and regular meetings are required so that all those involved can be informed. A sense of control allows for a willingness to accept change. This process can also help anticipated resistance as early as possible. Time needs to be built in for this to happen – a realistic timetable for events need to be planned. If this approach fails, a top-down approach may be justified.

Change can only begin when one thing ends and something new starts. For this to happen, there is a need to let go of the old even though the future is unpredictable (Clarke, 1994). Change can initiate the process of letting go. Several factors that appear to help people move through the transition process include:

■   Recognising that something has ended and allowing the grieving process to occur, preserving the positive aspects

■ Being given time to think about or 'hypothesise' a change, imagining what the new situation will be like before it happens (being proactive)

■ Consciously managing an 'in between' phase of transition, recognising that sometimes there will be uncertainty.

(Clarke, 1994)

Whatever strategy is adopted, evaluation is an essential feature that needs to be built in, enabling the identification of issues that need attention. It is also a way of allowing staff to recognise the strengths and identify areas for development.

SWOT analysis

The SWOT analysis (identifying Strengths, Weaknesses, Opportunities and Threats) technique is used analyse an organisation/individual in terms of quality (usually associated with business). It is a simple and effective technique. This approach can create a proactive management style that is linked to clinical excellence and high quality (see Box 40.1).

Box 40.1   SWOT analysis

S (internal) – Identifies advantages, practices that are conducted well. It usually relates to staff/experience/skills/product quality

W (internal) – Identifies which areas need special attention (thus turning them into strengths). Considering what could be improved; what is done badly; what should be avoided. Usually relates to lack of skills/no experience/lack of finance

O (external) – Need to be proactive and adopt strategies to enable changes in practice. Relates to gaps in the market/ new market. Risk assessment is designed to achieve this

T (external) – Identifies obstacles being faced. Need to be monitored carefully and action taken, if necessary, relates to competition

---

Leadership

The concepts of management and leadership are often confused. There is a difference:

Leadership is out of the spirit, compounded of personality and vision; its practice is an art; management is of the mind, a matter of accurate calculation . . . its practice is a science. Managers are necessary; leaders are essential.

(Field Marshal Slim, cited in McSherry and Pearce, 2002)

A good team leader is the most essential ingredient when effecting a successful change, where groups of people can be co-ordinated to work in harmony toward a mutual goal (Ford and Walsh, 1994).

Leadership is concerned with heading and facilitating development and innovation in practice, enhancing professional standards, being a pacemaker and developer, influencing practice and policy. Management is about organising self and others towards a goal. Change agents need to be effective managers as well as leaders.

The type of leadership style adopted will influence the rate of adoption of an innovation by staff, and thus its success (see Box 40.2).

Box 40.2 Leadership styles	
Leadership style	*Characteristics in relation to change*
Autocratic	Provides structure and directs in the decision-making process; not willing to delegate responsibility. This approach is restrictive and controlling, and generally impedes change
Democratic	Involves others early and provides a structure that is not constrained; enables the development of a collaborative, empowered and trusting environment. Leader needs to be comfortable with delegation and be able to delegate appropriately. Considered the best approach to facilitate change
Laissez-faire	Concerned with allowing group members to express themselves; does not impose but allows suggestions. Potentially there is little control and limited direction. Success is dependent upon the strength and competence of the group

Implications for practice

- All nurses have a professional obligation to be involved in the change process – this should be built into the appraisal system
- Staff should not be excluded from the change process
- Nurses must keep themselves abreast of the changes occurring at a national and local level
- Existing beliefs and values need to be synonymous with the philosophy of change
- Change should occur for a good reason, and the change process should be planned
- Evaluation is crucial and should be a natural part of the change process.

Summary

Health care has been, still is, and will always be a recipient of change. In order to moderate the difficulties associated with this process, an appropriate implementation plan needs to be developed and followed. Consideration needs to be given to professional implications, time, users' ability/motivation, perceived and actual standards of practice and, of course, leadership style.

Exercise

1   Conduct a SWOT analysis within your clinical environment in relation to caring for the critically ill patient.
2   Work out strategies to try and turn the identified weaknesses into strengths.
3   What strategies will you plan in order to manage this change.

Bibliography

Key reading

Rehtmeyer (2000).

Further reading

Curtis and White (2002) provides a useful insight into the common reasons why people resist change. Detailed strategies to overcome this are offered.

Chapter 41

Professional issues

Tina Moore

Contents

Learning outcomes

After reading this chapter you will be able to:

- Consider the criteria for nursing as a profession
- Understand the implications of professional accountability and role expansion
- Understand the doctrine of informed consent, and how it relates to the critically ill.

Fundamental knowledge

Read Chapters 1, 10 and 12.

Introduction

Since the beginning of the nineteenth century, nursing has experienced a widening of role boundaries. Today nurses are involved in more complex decision-making processes and care delivery (including invasive procedures), and as a result must understand the professional and legal implications of their role.

This chapter will discuss the issues and implications of professional accountability, particularly in relation to the scope of professional practice and the issue of informed consent. Advocacy, although a professional role, will not be discussed, as this was addressed in Chapter 1.

Nursing as a profession

> **Time out 41.1**
>
> 1 What do you consider to be the characteristics of a profession? Write them down.
> 2 Now compare your answers to Pyne's (1998) definition.

The criteria for defining a profession have been put forward by Pyne (1998) (Box 41.1), who states that an occupational group must fulfil not some but *all* of those listed.

Box 41.1   Criteria for a profession

1 Practice is based on a recognised body of learning
2 The profession establishes an independent body for the perusal of aims and objectives
3 Admission to corporate membership is based on strict standards of competence attested by examinations and assessed experience
4 It recognises that its practice must be for the benefit of the public as well for the benefit of its practitioners
5 It recognises a responsibility to advance and extend the body of knowledge on which it is based
6 It recognises its responsibility in the provision of education and training
7 It recognises the need for its members to conform to high standards of ethics and a Professional Code of Conduct

---

Whilst the set of criteria in Box 41.1 have been achieved by nursing, it is incomplete. Nursing is a caring profession, and therefore requires the integration of vocational values of caring as identified by Roache (1987) – i.e. compassion, commitment, conscience, confidence and commitment. This integration will help achieve the compassion and the rigour of professionalism.

Role expansion

Expanded roles are now seen as a natural progression of the nurse's existing role; this is coupled with increased accountability under the guidance of the *Code of Professional Conduct* (NMC, 2002a).

A number of DOH and NHS executive reports suggest greater co-operation between nursing and medical staff, particularly in areas where roles are overlapping. Subsequent documents have been produced outlining the role and legal responsibilities of the nurse. This has been a growth area in nursing. The NHS plan envisages that appropriately qualified nurses will undertake a wider range of clinical tasks (DOH, 2000e), including ordering investigations and diagnostic tests in addition to roles in prescribing and discharge.

On consenting to role expansion, nurses should consider issues relating to professional accountability. There is no defence in criminal or civil law that allows nurses to say that someone ordered them to do a potentially harmful or unlawful act. Nurses should challenge practices and decisions that they believe are improper, for their own as well as the patients' benefit.

Therefore, role expansion should be accepted with caution and only if it is in the best interest of the patient. There is concern that vital aspects of nursing will be lost if nurses begin to undertake functions that were once considered to be the domain of doctors. For example, 'basic' nursing care (e.g. undertaking observations, catheter care, prevention of pressure sores etc.) may be neglected while nurses are instead giving all the patients on the ward their intravenous medication.

Post-registration education and practice

Role expansion requires appropriate education and clinical support. There should be opportunities for continuous professional development (CPD).

The PREP (post-registration education and practice) standard is a professional requirement set by the Nursing and Midwifery Council (NMC, 2002b). It includes statutory (legal) requirements that nurses must achieve in order for registration to be renewed.

- The PREP (practice) standard states that nurses must have worked in some capacity during the previous 5 years for a minimum of 100 days (750 hours), or have successfully completed a return to practice course
- The PREP (CPD) standard states that nurses should undertake and record professional development (at least 5 days over the past 3 years). An audit will be conducted by the NMC before renewal of registration.

PREP is in place to help nurses provide the highest possible standard of care. A variety of approaches could be undertaken to meet the requirements – e.g. a visit to another clinical setting (considered to be a centre of excellence), perhaps a respiratory care unit. The purpose of the visit would be to increase knowledge on certain aspects of care, e.g. NIV therapy.

Individual study days could be undertaken (e.g. tracheostomy care/wound care), where nurses should learn about evidence-based approaches, and updated guidelines/policies and practices. This information could then be discussed with colleagues. Following this, the nurse might wish to produce an information poster or leaflet or conduct a teaching session on the topic.

Taking on role expansion is seen to make care more personal, effective and holistic. This can be facilitated through mechanisms such as clinical supervision and reflection.

Time out 41.2

1 Write down your understanding of the terms 'responsibility' and 'accountability' (separate lists).
2 Now compare what you have written. Do you think that they mean the same, or can you identify any differences in meaning?

Professional accountability

Accountability is an integral part of professional practice, requiring the nurse to give explanations and justification for actions and omissions in relation to care. Definitions of accountability reflect the expectation that justification should be evidence-based.

Accountability implies that a situation has been assessed, a plan has been made and carried out, and the results evaluated. Accountability assumes the nurse has the necessary knowledge, skill, experience, and therefore subsequent authority, to carry out the plan.

Arenas of accountability include:

■ *Patient:* nurses are primarily accountable to the patients within their care; they have a legal and professional duty to act in the best interest of the patient (civil liability)
■ *Professional body:* NMC – Professional Conduct Committee (professional liability)
■ *Employers:* nurses in breach of employment contract may face an industrial tribunal
■ *Public:* nurses can be tried in the criminal law courts (criminal liability) if a crime is suspected of being committed (Dimond, 2002)
■ *Themselves* (Walsh, 1997).

Informed consent

Time out 41.3

1 List the different types of consent available. Which mode do you mainly use?
2 What type of patients do you gain consent from? What set of criteria do you use?

Critically ill patients may present a challenge for nurses in terms of balancing the respect for patient autonomy and the duty of care. Conflict arises when on the one hand nurses may wish to make a decision and respect the patient's autonomy, and on the other there is the possibility of being open to the charge of negligence or failure of duty to care (Tingle and Cribb, 1995). For instance, a competent patient may develop severe pain post-operatively following an invasive procedure and refuse analgesia. The patient's coping mechanisms fail and he demonstrates signs of neurogenic shock. As a result, he is harmed by the effects of pain (resulting from refusal to receive analgesia).

There is the risk of *assuming* that the majority of critically ill patients are unlikely to understand the implications of treatment; therefore healthcare professionals adopt the advocacy role, often providing care in a manner they feel would be most beneficial to the patient. This approach, where consent is not actively obtained, implies paternalism.

Consent means a voluntary, uncoerced decision, made by a sufficiently competent or autonomous person on the basis of adequate information and deliberation, to accept rather than reject some proposed course of action that will affect them.

For consent to be valid it must comply with the following:

1   *Be voluntary without any form of coercion or influence from others.* This may at times be difficult to achieve. Being critically ill creates a stressful situation for patients, and consequently they have poor concentration and often are unable to recall information received. This could be due to the degree of illness, anxiety, medication, or sleep/sensory deprivation. Some patients will exercise their autonomy not to be autonomous, and select an advocate.

    Patients will vary in the amount and type of information they want. Nurses should be present when the patient is being given information, in order to be in a position to clarify and expand upon that information.

2   *The person must be competent in order to make an autonomous decision.* When patients are competent to give their informed consent they have all the qualities and abilities necessary to make autonomous decisions about their care management. Whether any patient can achieve this is debatable. There is an inconsistent approach to gaining consent, and a lack of accepted standards on the principle of competence (Welie and Welie, 2001).

3   *Be specific to the treatment proposed.* Generally, simple treatments require the absorption and analysis of simple concepts, whereas more complex treatments will require greater comprehension. There may be a number of factors influencing patients' ability to perceive and retain information, e.g. environmental stress, medication, anxiety about their illness.

4   *Assessment of patients' decision-making competence must also be specific to this situation.* For consent to be valid, patients must be mentally competent. If the competency of a patient is in doubt, three tests should be applied:

    ■   Could the patient comprehend and retain the necessary information?
    ■   Was he able to believe it?

■ Was he able to weigh the information, balancing risks and needs so as to arrive at a choice? (Dimond, 2002).

Establishing a patient's competency (determined through understanding) is a subjective process and is open to assessor variability. Generalised labelling of a patient as incompetent must be avoided. Consent should be viewed as a continuous process rather than an outcome to be achieved. Constant reassessment of the level of competence is required, as this can change intermittently

5 *Patients should be provided with information of sufficient quality, scope and choice to enable them to make an informed autonomous decision.* This must include all risks and hazards associated with the procedure in addition to disclosure of alternatives

Nurses have a professional obligation to provide information and the opportunity for consent. A patient who is legally competent can understand and retain treatment information, and can use it to make an informed choice (NMC, 2002a). The principle of informed consent is in place to respect the patient's right to be autonomous and the recognition that healthcare professionals have a duty to provide the patient with sufficient information. This is also echoed in a number of government guidelines, e.g. DOH (2001b).

Common law in tort clearly states that the professional has a right to withhold some or all information, if it is in the patient's best interest to do so (Buka and Fletcher, 2001). This is known as therapeutic privilege.

Critically ill patients require the use of simple, easy-to-understand language. This should help to prevent confusion and aid actual understanding. A patient can withdraw consent at any time. It is considered good practice to explore the reasons with the patient (if possible) before terminating treatment (DOH, 2001d).

Failure to obtain patient consent or to inform a patient fully of the reasons for a procedure can result in a legal case of assault, trespass and battery. Exceptions include emergency situations where a patient is treated against his or her will.

Defences to not gaining informed consent could include:

■ Consent (i.e. consenting not to be informed)
■ Necessity
■ Making a lawful arrest
■ Acting under a statutory power, e.g. Mental Health Act (1983)
■ Parental powers.

Failure to provide information according to the Bolam Test (1957) could, if harm were to occur, leave the individual/Trust open to litigation (see p. 407).

Time out 41.4

Consider Mrs Brown, who has been admitted following bowel surgery. Pre-operatively she was in a debilitated state. Post-operatively she has developed hypovolaemic shock. The nurse assigned to care for Mrs Brown was busy helping another nurse with her patient; she was also in charge of the unit. During the course of the shift, Mrs Brown's condition deteriorates. Subsequently she suffers a cardiac arrest. During the resuscitation procedure the wall suction is found not to be working, and the portable machine is in use. Finally, the patient dies.

1 Do you consider negligence to have occurred?
2 Give reasons for your answer.
3 Write down your understanding of negligence.

Negligence

There are occasions when patients sue healthcare professionals for damages owing to harm that they have suffered. The law of negligence is the most commonly used legal concept in maintaining standards. It is based on the law of tort, and refers to a civil wrong. Patients have a range of rights that will be protected by the civil courts.

When an individual considers suing for damages for harm suffered, the burden of proof, according to law, lies with that individual. This burden of proof depends on a balance of probabilities.

The law of negligence can be used in two different ways:

1   To sue another person for compensation for harm or damage
2   To indicate that behaviour has fallen below required standards.

To succeed in an action, the plaintiff must show:

■   That the existence of a duty to care was owed to the plaintiff by the defendant
■   Breach of that duty by the defendant
■   That as a result the plaintiff suffered damage (and the harm suffered must have been reasonably foreseeable).

Duty of care

A 'duty of care' to someone is to be obliged to take his or her interest into account. The person who has the duty must take reasonable care to avoid acts or omissions that can reasonably be foreseen which will cause injury/harm.

A duty of care is owed when:

- Any person is voluntarily attended by a nurse in an emergency situation, whether on or off duty (Kent v Griffiths and others, 2002)
- Any patient presents themselves to a hospital and nurses have knowledge of that patient.

(In the case of Mrs Brown, because of the contractual agreement between patient and nurse a legal duty of care is owed.)

Breach of duty of care

The standard of care owed to the patient needs to be identified and examined. Patients depend upon nurses and their standards of professional conduct. The standard of care for any professional person must be of a high level. The courts require a reasonable standard to be followed, a standard that would be supported by competent professional opinion and practice (Dimond, 2002). Thus the nurse is expected to exhibit the expertise normally demonstrated by competent nurses – i.e. to comply with the Bolam Test (see Box 41.2).

Courts rely on expert evidence to give an opinion of what is deemed to be a reasonable action and the accepted practice in such a situation. It is assumed that experts' opinions will be based on current evidence in order to provide a logical basis for their expert opinion. Documentation for consultation in regarding an acceptable standard of performance would be NMC documentation, policies, procedures and national guidelines.

In the case of role expansion, a medical standard of care may be looked for (Tingle, 2002a, 2002b). The law would not find it acceptable to say that in doing a medical activity a nurse would be legally expected to perform at a lower standard of care. Some situations require deviation from the normal accepted procedures. Nurses can deviate from accepted standards, but need to document why clearly (Dimond, 2002).

Box 41.2 The Bolam Test

- Ordinary skilled person exercising and professing to have that skill
- A reasonably competent practitioner
- Acting in accordance with practice accepted at that time as proper by a reasonable body of professional opinion.

Source: Bolam v Friern Barnet, 1957

(In the case of Mrs Brown it needs to be established if the nurse involved was suitably qualified and experienced (competent) and whether current guidance was followed.)

Did the nurse in charge put Mrs Brown at risk?

Causation

This seeks to examine the causal link between the failure of the defendant to follow the approved practice and the harm suffered by the patient that must be reasonably foreseeable (Dimond, 2002). There is a need to establish a causal link between the breach of duty of care by the nurse, and the harm suffered by the patient.

(It could be argued that there was no causal link between the actions of the nurse and the suction machine not working. Mrs Brown's condition was so critical that even if the suction was in order she may have died anyway. Therefore, whilst there may be evidence of poor practice, the criteria for negligence are not fulfilled.)

Implications for practice

- Nurses should undertake role expansion with caution and be assessed as competent
- Nurses will be judged in accordance with their actions (which must be of a reasonable professional standard)
- Professional practice should be within the designated boundaries of the discipline
- Patients should know the nature, purpose, risks and benefit of the proposed procedure.

Summary

If nurses are going to continue to expand their professional role they will need to accept the increases in accountability and professional implications. Continuous Professional Development needs to be undertaken in order to maintain and enhance standards of care. By doing so, nurses will be in a strong position to defend practices.

Bibliography

Key reading

Buka and Fletcher (1999) describes a legal framework for application to clinical practice.

Dimond (2002), Tingle (2002a, 2002b) and Tingle and Cribb (1995) are the authoritative books which are more professionally directed.

The British Journal of Nursing Professional series is very useful and also provide examples of professional conduct cases.

Recommended sources

Nursing Midwifery Council Professional Advice Service, 020-73336538 or email advice@nmc-uk.org

Conclusion

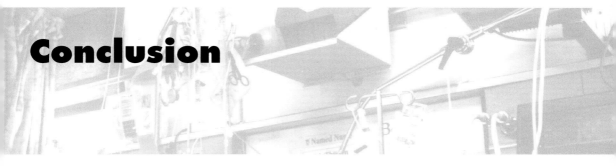

Approaches to caring for highly dependent patients have undergone radical change (DOH, 2000a). These changes not only affect nurses working in critical care units, but also those who are working in areas such as general/specialist wards/units, accident and emergency departments and community care. Due to the diversity of caring required for patients with level 2 needs, ward nurses in particular are now in a situation where they have experienced increases in the complexity of care required by their patients.

These changes result in expanding roles for nursing, often within more technological roles (Goldman, 1999). Whilst technology should be made available to benefit patients, the importance of the humanistic approach also needs to be highlighted (Ashworth, 1990). A careful balancing of knowledge, skills and responsibilities should be undertaken together with the wider context of high dependency care. *High Dependency Nursing Care* has adopted a holistic style to help the reader identify components of competent, safe and sensitive practice, not only for the patients but also for their families.

Limitations to this holistic approach have been highlighted by many people, indicating the need for more evidence, such as with cultural issues. This holistic theme is also reflected in the different perspectives discussed within the book, whether within practice, management, education or policy, and these areas are all underpinned by evidence.

Patient outcomes can be improved by early recognition and prompt appropriate intervention (Goldhill and Sumner, 1998). Nurses have a moral, professional and legal obligation to provide competent, safe and sensitive care. *High Dependency Nursing Care* has provided information to enable nurses to identify/ recognise clinical features relating to common disorders and provide appropriate intervention based on evidence offered.

As clinical developments grow, particularly in the areas of research, technology and practice, education and training has to be a lifelong experience. It is anticipated that through a rigorous educational process (theory and practice), nurses will be capable of retaining, developing and maintaining their clinical competence when looking after critically ill patients. This book offers some input on the various strategies that can be undertaken to facilitate nurses developing their practice, thus enabling them to accept the challenges ahead.

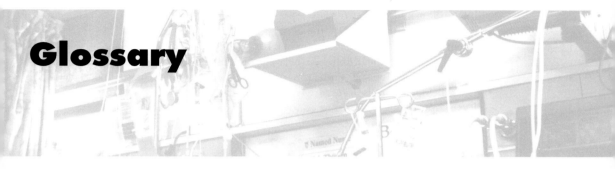

Glossary

ARDS   Acute Respiratory Distress Syndrome

atelectasis   collapse of alveoli

cardioversion   defibrillation as an elective procedure to alter pathological rhythms (e.g. atrial fibrillation)

collateral circulation   blood vessels that develop to bypass complete or incomplete obstruction to blood flow. Collateral blood vessels are weak, tortuous and friable, so liable to rupture

CPAP   Continuous Positive Airway Pressure

cytokine   'cell killer' – intracellular chemicals which regulate cell life; excessive cell damage releases large numbers into the plasma, causing pathological damage

D-dimers   a fibrin degradation product (FDP), released when clot breakdown (lysis) occurs. Normal D-dimer levels are <250 ng/ml or μg/l. Normal levels are sometimes reported as 'negative'

dead space   space between where air or gas enters the airway and the alveoli where gas exchange occurs (average physiological adult dead space = 150 ml)

dyne   unit of force needed to drive 1 g of mass at a speed of 1 cm/second

dysphoria   opposite to euphoria – anxiety, restlessness

ethical dilemma   occurs when two (or more) morally acceptable courses of action are present and to choose one action prevents the selection of another. Here the individual experiences tension because the moral obligations resulting from the dilemma create differing and opposing demands (Beauchamp and Childress, 2001)

gluconeogenesis   increased hepatic glucose synthesis from amino acids

glycogenolysis   conversion of glycogen into glucose

haemoptysis   blood in sputum

hypercapnia   high (arterial) blood carbon dioxide (>6.0 kPa)

joule   the work involved by one newton moving one metre

Ketogensis   production of ketones

kilocalorie (kcal) the energy needed to warm 1 kg of water by 1°C. 1 kcal = 4.184 kJ

melaena black, tar-like stools, containing blood

myocyte cardiac muscle cell

NIV non-invasive ventilation

parenchyma functional tissue of an organ

polymers tiny molecules strung in a long repeating chain

pulse pressure the difference between arterial systolic and diastolic pressure. High pulse pressure indicates poor vessel compliance (e.g. atherosclerosis), while narrow pulse pressure (e.g. 20) indicates hypovolaemia

PVC premature ventricular contraction

respiratory failure type 1 failure of oxygen exchange (PaO_2 <8.0, $PaCO_2$ <6.0 kPa)

respiratory failure type 2 failure of oxygen exchange (PaO_2 <8.0, $PaCO_2$ >6.0 kPa)

stroke volume amount of blood ejected with each contraction of the left ventricle

suppurate form pus

SVR resistance to blood flow by all of the systemic vasculature

tachypnoea fast breathing

tacit knowledge knowledge which is difficult to articulate

utility usefulness – what is right is what is most useful

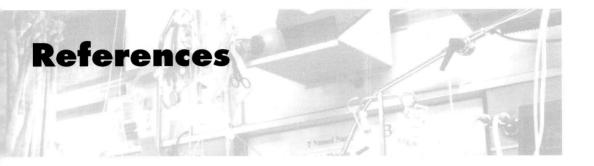

References

3M Health Care (2003) at www.3m.com/uk/littmann (accessed on 21 February 2003)

Abelow, B. (1998) *Understanding Acid Base*. Baltimore: Williams & Wilkins.

Acheson, D. (Chair) (1998) *Independent Inquiry into Inequalities in Health*. London: The Stationery Office.

Adam, S. (2002) The role of nurse consultant in expanded critical care. *Nursing Times* 98(1): 34–36.

Adam, S.K., Osborne, C. (1997) *Critical Care Nursing: Science and Practice*. Oxford: Oxford Medical Publications.

Adam, S., Whitlock, M., Baskett, P., Bloomfield, P., Higgs, R. (1994) Should relatives be allowed to watch resuscitation? *British Medical Journal* 308(6945): 1687–1689.

Agnelli, G., Becattini, C., Kirschstein, T. (2002) Thrombolysis vs heparin in the treatment of pulmonary embolism: a clinical outcome-based meta-analysis. *Archives of Internal Medicine* 162(22): 2505–2688.

Akgul, S., Akyolcu, N. (2002) Effects of normal saline on endotracheal suctioning. *Journal of Clinical Nursing*, 11(6): 826–830.

Aksoy, S. (2000) Can the 'quality of life' be used as a criterion in health care services? *Bulletin of Medical Ethics* 162: 19–22.

Alavi, C. (1995) *Problem Based Learning in a Health Sciences Curriculum*. London: Routledge.

Albarran, J.W., Kapeluch, H. (2000) Role of the nurse in thrombolytic therapy – expanding the clinical horizons. In J.P. Cruickshank, M.A. Bradbury (eds) *Aspects of Cardiovascular Nursing*. London: Mark Allen, pp. 104–117.

Albarran, J.W., Salmon, D. (2000) Lesbian, gay and bisexual experiences within critical nursing 1988–1998: a survey of the literature. *International Journal of Nursing Studies* 37(5): 445–455.

ALG (2000) *Sick of being Excluded: Improving the Health of London's Black and Minority Ethnic Communities. The Report of the Race, Health and Social Exclusion Commission*. London: Association of London Government.

Allen, C.H., Ward, J.D. (1998) An evidence-based approach to management of increased intracranial pressure. *Critical Care Clinics* 14(3): 485–495.

Alleyne, J., Thomas, V. (1994) The management of sickle cell crisis pain as experienced by patients and their carers. *Journal of Advanced Nursing* 19(4): 725–732.

Allmark, P., Klarzynski, R. (1992) The case against nurse advocacy. *British Journal of Nursing* 1(12): 33–36.

Alspach, J.G. (1998) *Core curriculum for Critical Care Nursing*, 5th edn. Philadelphia: W.B. Saunders Co.

American College of Chest Physicians and The Society for Critical Care Medicine (1992) Consensus conference: definitions for sepsis and organ failure and guidelines for the use of innovative therapies. *Critical Care Medicine* 20(6): 864–874.

American Psychiatric Association (1994) *Diagnostic and Statistical Manual of Mental Disorders (DSM-1V)*, 4th edn. Washington, DC: American Psychiatric Association.

Andrew, C.M. (1998) Optimising the human experience: nursing the families of people who die in intensive care. *Intensive and Critical Care Nursing* 14(2): 59–65.

Andrews, M., Gidman, J., Humphries, A. (1998) Reflection: does it enhance professional nursing practice. *British Journal of Nursing* 7(7): 413–417.

Andrews, T., Waterman, H., Hillier, V. (1999) Blood gas analysis: a study of blood loss in intensive care. *Journal of Advanced Nursing* 30(4): 851–857.

Appleyard, N., Langan, S. (1997) Human resources and education. In D.R. Goldhill and P.S. Withington (eds) *Textbook of Intensive Care*. London: Chapman and Hall, pp. 761–766.

Appleyard, M.E., Gavaghan, S.R., Gonzalez, C., Ananian, L., Tyrell, R., Carroll, D. (2000) Nurse-coached intervention for the families of patients in critical care units. *Critical Care Nurse* 20(3): 40–48.

Ardley, C. (2002) Should relatives be denied access to the resuscitation room? *Intensive and Critical Care Nursing* 19(1): 1–10.

Armstrong, P.J., Sinclair, S.J., Campanella, C. (1993) The transtracheal Doppler probe. *British Journal of Intensive Care* 3(5): 175–182.

Armstrong, S.C., Cozza, KL., Watanabe, K.S. (1997) The misdiagnosis of delirium. *Psychosomatics* 38(5): 433–439.

Ashdown, M. (1985) Sudden death. *Nursing Mirror* 161(18): 22–24.

Ashworth, P. (1980) *Care to Communicate*. London: Royal College of Nursing.

Ashworth, P. (1990) High technology and humanity for intensive care. *Intensive Care Nursing* 6(3): 150–160.

Association of Surgeons of Great Britain and Ireland, Association of Upper Gastro-Intestinal Surgeons of Great Britain and Ireland, British Society of Gastroenterology, and the Pancreatic Society of Great Britain and Ireland (1998) UK Guidelines for the management of acute pancreatitis. *Gut* 42(suppl. 2): S1–S13.

Atkins, S., Murphy, K. (1993) Reflection: a review of the literature. *Journal of Advanced Nursing* 18(8) 1188–1192.

Attard, A.R., Corlett, M.J., Kidner, N.J., Leslie, A.P., Fraser, C.A. (1992) Safety of early pain relief for acute abdominal pain. *British Medical Journal* 305(6853): 554–556.

Attia, J., Ray, J.G., Cook, D.J., Douketis, T., Ginsberg, J.S., Geerts, W.H. (2001) Deep vein thrombosis and its prevention in critically ill adults. *Archives of Internal Medicine* 161(10): 1268–1279.

Audit Commission (1999) *Critical to Success, The place of efficient and effective critical care services within the acute hospital.* London: Audit Commission.

Australian NHMRC (1999) *Acute Pain Management: Scientific Evidence Report.* National Health and Medical Research Council (Australia). Also at www.health. gov.au/nhmrc/publications.

B v. *Secretary for Health* (2002) ALL ER 449.

Bach, P.B., Brown, C., Gelfand, S.E., McCrory, D.D. (2001) Management of acute exacerbations of chronic obstructive pulmonary disease: a summary and appraisal of published evidence. *Annals of Internal Medicine* 134(7): 600–620.

Baigent, C., Collins, R., Appleby, P., Parish, S., Sleight, P., Peto, R. ISIS-2 Collaborative Group (1998) 10-year survival among patients with suspected acute myocardial infarction in randomised comparison of intravenous streptokinase, oral aspirin, both or neither. *British Medical Journal* 316(7141): 1337–1343

Baird, M.S. (2001) Hematological. In P. Swearingen, J. Keen (eds) *Manual of Critical Care Nursing,* 4th edn. St. Louis: Mosby.

Baldasseroni, S., Opasich, C., Gorini, M. *et al.* (2002) Left bundle branch block is associated with increased 1-year sudden and total mortality rate in 5517 outpatients with congestive heart failure: a report from the Italian Network on Congestive Heart Failure. *American Heart Journal* 143(3): 398–405.

Baldwin, M. (2003) Patient advocacy: a concept analysis. *Nursing Standard* 17(21): 33–39.

Ball, C. (2002) The devil is in the detail. *Intensive and Critical Care Nursing* 18(2): 71–72.

Ball, P. (2001) Critical care of spinal cord injury. *Spine* 26(24S): S27–S30.

Ballantyne, J.C., McKenna, J.M., Ryder, E. (2003) Epidural analgesia – experience of 5628 patients in a large teaching hospital derived through audit. *Acute Pain* 4(3–4): 89–97.

Ballinger, C., Wiles, R. (2001) A critical look at evidence-based practice. *British Journal of Occupational Therapy* 64(5): 253–255.

Banks, P.A. (1998) Acute and chronic pancreatitis. In M. Felman, B.F. Scharschmidt, M.H. Sleisenger (eds) *Sleisenger and Fordtran's Gastrointestinal and Liver Disease.* Philadelphia: W.B. Saunders Co., pp. 809–862.

Barber, P. (1994) *Who Cares for the Carers? Distance Learning Centre.* London: South Bank University.

Barczak, N.L. (1998) Anatomy and physiology of the renal system. In C.M. Hudak, B.M Gallo, P.G. Morton (eds) *Critical Care Nursing. A Holistic Approach.* Philadelphia: Lippincott

Bar-El, Y., Ross, A., Kablawi, A., Egenburg, S. (2001) Potentially dangerous negative intrapleural pressure generated by ordinary pleural drainage systems. *Chest* 119(2): 511–514.

Barnard, A., Sandelowski, M. (2001) Technology and humane nursing care: (ir) reconcilable or invented difference? *Journal of Advanced Nursing* 34(3): 367–375.

Baron, T.H. (1999) Acute necrotizing pancreatitis. *New England Journal of Medicine* 340(18): 1412–1417.

Barrett, J.R. (2001) *Assessment Made Incredibly Easy,* 2nd edn. Springhouse: Springhouse.

Barry, B. (1998) Acute renal failure. In P. Murphy (ed.) *Handbook of Critical Care*. London: Science Press.

Baskett, P.J. (1994) Doctors need to be trained to work in public. *British Medical Journal* 308(6945): 1687–1689.

Bateman, N.T., Leach, R.M. (1998) Acute oxygen therapy. *British Medical Journal* 317(7161): 798–801.

Baudouin, S.V. (2002) The pulmonary physician in critical care. 3: Critical care management of community acquired pneumonia. *Thorax* 57(3): 267–271.

Baxendale, B.R., Yeoman, P.M. (1997) Spinal injury. In D.R. Goldhill, P.S. Withington (eds) *Textbook of Intensive Care*. London: Chapman and Hall Medical, pp. 639–651.

Beauchamp, T., Childress, F. (2001) *Principles of Biomedical Ethics*, 5th edn. New York: Oxford University Press.

Beckingham, I.J., Bornman, P.C. (2001) Acute pancreatitis. *British Medical Journal* 322(7286): 595–598.

Beckingham, I.J., Ryder, S.D. (2001) Investigation of liver and biliary disease. *British Medical Journal* 322(7227): 33–36.

Beers, M.H., Berkow, R. (eds) (1999) *The Merck Manual of Diagnosis and Therapy*. 17th edn. New Jersey: Merck Research Laboratories.

Beevers, G., Lip, G.Y.H., O'Brien, E. (2001a) Blood pressure measurement. *British Medical Journal* 322(7292): 981–985.

Beevers, G., Lip, G.Y.H., O'Brien, E. (2001b) *ABC of Hypertension*. London: BMJ Books.

Behrendt, C.E. (2000) Acute respiratory failure in the United States. *Chest* 118(4): 1100–1105.

Belanger, M.A., Reed, S. (1997) A rural community hospital's experience with family-witnessed resuscitation. *Journal of Emergency Nursing* 23(3): 238–239.

Bell, J.M., Wright, L.M. (1990) Flaws in family nursing education. *The Canadian Nurse* 86(6): 28–30.

Bell, R.L., Ovadia, P., Abdullah, F., Spector, S., Rabinovici, R. (2001) Chest tube removal; end-inspiration or end-expiration? *Journal of Trauma* 50(4): 674–677.

Bellman, L.M. (1996) Changing nursing practice through reflection on the Roper, Logan and Tierney model: the enhancement approach to action research. *Journal of Advanced Nursing* 24(1): 129–138.

Bellomo, R. (2003) Acute renal failure. In A.D. Bersten, N. Soni (eds) *Intensive Care Manual*, 5th edn. Edinburgh: Butterworth-Heinemann, pp. 453–458.

Benner, P. (1984) *From Novice to Expert: Excellence and Power in Clinical Nursing Practice*. Menlo Park, California: Addison-Wesley.

Benner, P., Tanner, C. (1987) How expert nurses use intuition. *American Journal of Nursing* 87(1): 23–31.

Benner, P., Tanner, C.A., Chelsa, C.A. (1996) *Expertise in Nursing Practice: Caring, Clinical Judgement and Ethics*. New York: Springer.

Bennett, O. (2001) Cardiovascular problems in the diabetic patient. *Professional Nurse* 16(9): 1339–1343.

Benson, A., Latter, S. (1998) Implementing health promoting nursing: the integration of interpersonal skills and health promotion. *Journal of Advanced Nursing* 27(1): 100–107.

Bettany, G.E., Powell-Tuck, J. (1997) Nutritional support in surgery. *Surgery* 15(10): 233–237.

Bickley, L. and Hoekelman, R. (1999) *Bates Guide to Physical Examination*, 7th edn. Philadelphia: Lippincott.

Blackmore, E. (1996) Developments in practice. The needs of relatives during the patients stay in intensive care following routine cardiac surgery. *Nursing in Critical Care* 1(5): 230–236

Blackwood, B. (1999) Normal saline instillation with end tracheal suctioning: primum non nocere (first do no harm). *Journal of Advanced Nursing* 29(4): 928–934.

Blazys, D. (1999) Oxygen saturation readings. *Journal of Emergency Nursing* 25(5): 386–387.

Bloe, C. (2001) Nurse initiated coronary thrombolysis. *Nursing Times* 97(15): 40–42.

BMA (2001) *Withholding and Withdrawing Life-prolonging Medical Treatment*, 2nd edn. London: British Medical Journal Books.

BMA/RCN (1993) *Cardiopulmonary Resuscitation: a Statement from the BMA and RCN*. London: BMA and RCN.

BNF (2002) *British National Formulary 44*. London: British Medical Association/ Royal Pharmaceutical Society of Great Britain.

Bochud, P., Calandra, T. (2003) Science, medicine, and the future: pathogenesis of sepsis: new concepts and implications for future treatment. *British Medical Journal* 362(7383): 262–266.

Bodernham, A.R., Barry, B.N. (2001) The role of tracheostomy in ICU. *Anaesthesia and Intensive Care Medicine* 2(9): 336–339.

Bolam v. *Friern Barnet HMC* (1957) ALL ER 118.

Boldt, J. (2000) The good, the bad, and the ugly: should we completely banish human albumin from our intensive care units? *Anaesthesia and Analgesia* 91(4): 887–895.

Bone, R.C., Grodzin, C.J., Balk, R.A. (1997) Sepsis: a new hypothesis for pathogenesis of the disease process. *Chest* 112(1): 235–243.

Borgbom-Engberg, I. (1991) Giving up and withdrawal by ventilator treated patients: nurses' experiences. *Intensive Care Nursing* 7: 2000–2005.

Bothma, P.A., Joynt, G.M., Lipman, J. *et al.* (1996) Accuracy of pulse oximetry in pigmented patients. *South African Medical Journal* 86(5): 594–596.

Boud, D., Keogh, R., Walker, D. (1985) *Reflection: Turning Experience into Learning*. New York: Kogan Page.

Bove, L.A. (1994) How fluids and electrolytes shift after surgery. *Nursing* 24(8): 34–39.

Bove, L.A. (1996) Restoring electrolyte balance: calcuim and phosphorous. *Registered Nurse* 59(3): 47–52.

Boyd, E.M., Fales, A.W. (1983) Reflective learning: key to learning from experience. *Journal of Humanistic Psychology* 23(2): 99–117.

Bradley, C. (2001) Stress ulcer prevention – the controversy continues. *Intensive and Critical Care Nursing* 17(1): 58–60.

Brans, Y.W. (1991) Biomedical technology: To use or not to use? *Clinics in Perinatology* 18(3): 389–401.

Bray, J., Cragg, P., Macknight, A. *et al.* (1999) *Lecture Notes of Human Physiology*, 4th edn. Oxford: Blackwell Science.

Brearley, S. (1990) *Patient Participation*. London: Scutari Press.

Breshers, V.L., Davey, S.S. (1998) Structure and function of the respiratory system. In K.L. McCance, S.E. Huether (eds) *Pathophysiology: The Biologic Basis for Disease in Adults and Children*, 3rd edn. St. Louis: Mosby.

Brewin, A. (1997) Comparing asthma and chronic obstructive pulmonary disease (COPD). *Nursing Standard* 12(4): 49–55.

Bridges, M.J., Middleton, R. (1997) Direct arterial vs oscillometric monitoring of blood pressure: stop comparing and pick one. *Critical Care Nurse* 17(3): 58–72.

Briggs, M. (1995) Principles of acute pain assessment. *Nursing Standard* 9(19): 23–27.

Briggs, D. (1996) Nasogastric feeding in intensive care units: a study. *Nursing Standard* 49(10): 45–54.

British Society of Gastroenterology Endoscopy Committee (2000) Non-variceal upper gastrointestinal haemorrhage guidelines. *Gut* 51 (suppl. IV): iv1–iv6.

British Thoracic Society (1997a) BTS guidelines for the management of chronic obstructive pulmonary disease. *Thorax* 52(suppl. 5).

British Thoracic Society (1997b) The British guidelines on asthma management (1995): review and position statement. *Thorax* 52(suppl. 1): S1–S20.

British Thoracic Society (1997c) Suspected acute pulmonary embolism: a practical approach. *Thorax* 52(suppl. 4).

British Thoracic Society (2002) Non-invasive ventilation in acute respiratory failure. *Thorax* 57(3): 192–211.

Brooks, N. (2000) Quality of life and the high dependency unit. *Intensive and Critical Care Nursing* 16(1): 18–32.

Broomhead, R. (2002) Percutaneous tracheostomy. *Anaesthesia and Critical Care* 3(6): 210–212.

Brown, S.B. (1999) Managing sleep disorders. *Clinical Review* 9: 51–69.

BTS/SIGN (British Thoracic Society/Scottish Intercollegiate Guidelines Network) (2003) British Guideline on the Management of Asthma. *Thorax* 58: Supplement 1.

Buckman, R. (1988) *I Don't Know What to Say*. London: Pan.

Budd, K., Langford, R. (1999) Tramadol revisited. *British Journal of Anaesthesia* 82(4): 493–495.

Buka, P., Fletcher, L. (1999) *A Legal Framework for Caring*. Basingstoke: Macmillan Press Ltd.

Burchiel, K.J., Hsu, F.P. (2001) Pain and spasticity after spinal cord injury: mechanisms and treatment. *Spine* 26(24S): S146–S160.

Burke, C., Seeley, M.G. (1994) An oncology unit's initiation of bereavement support programme. Oncology Forum. *Nursing* 21(10): 1657–1680.

Burns, S. (1994) Assessing reflective learning. In A. Palmer, S. Burns, C. Buhman (eds) *Reflective Practice in Nursing. The Growth of the Professional Practitioner*. Oxford: Blackwell Science.

Burr, G. (1998) Contextualizing critical care family needs through triangulation: An Australian study. *Intensive and Critical Care Nursing* 14(4): 161–169.

Bushnell, D. (2003) *Ventilation and Perfusion Lung Imaging for Diagnosis of Pulmonary Embolism*, at http://www.vh.org/adult/provider/radiology/icmrad/nuclear/O2PulmonaryEmbolism.ht1. . . Accessed: 11/07/2003.

Buus-Frank, M. (1999) Nurses versus machine: slaves or masters of technology? *Journal of Obstetric, Gynaecologic and Neonatal Nursing* 28(4): 401–433.

Calzia, E., Radermacher, P. (1997) Airway pressure release ventilation and biphasic positive airway pressure. *Clinical Intensive Care* 8(6): 296–301.

Campbell, B. (1997) Arterial waveforms: monitoring changes in configuration. *Heart and Lung* 26(3): 204–214.

Campbell, P. (1990) Psychiatry and personal autonomy. *Clinical Public Health* 4: 11–15.

Capovilla, J., VanCouwenberghe, C., Miller, W.A. (2000) Noninvasive blood gas monitoring. *Critical Care Nursing Quarterly* 23(2): 79–86.

Caraceni, P., Van Thiel, D.H. (1995) Acute liver failure. *Lancet* 345(8943): 163–169.

Carlisle, C., Luker, K.A, Davies, C., Stilwell, J., Wilson, R. (1999) Skills competency in nurse education: nurse managers' perceptions of diploma level preparation. *Journal of Advanced Nursing* 29(5): 1256–1264.

Carmack, B.J. (1997) Balancing engagement and detachment in caregiving. *Image – the Journal of Nursing Scholarship* 29(2): 139–143.

Carnevale, F. (1991) High technology and humanity in intensive care: finding a balance. *Intensive Care Nursing* 7(1): 23–27.

Carper, B.A. (1978) Fundamental patterns of knowing in nursing. *Advances in Nursing Science* 1(1): 13–23.

Carr, E. (1997) Factors influencing the experience of pain. *Nursing Times* 93(39): 53–54.

Carr, E.C.J. (2000) Exploring the effect of postoperative pain on patient outcomes following surgery. *Acute Pain* 3(4): 183–191.

Carr, K. (2002) Ward visits after intensive care discharge: why? In R.D. Griffiths, C. Jones (eds) *Intensive Care Aftercare*. Oxford: Butterworth-Heinemann, pp. 69–82.

Carroll, P. (1997) Pulse oximetry at your fingertips. *Registered Nurse* 60(2): 22–27.

Carroll, P. (2000) Exploring chest drain options. *Registered Nurse* 63(10): 50–54.

Carroll, P. (2002) A guide to mobile chest drains. *Registered Nurse* 65(5): 56–60.

Casey, G. (2001) Oxygen transport and the use of pulse oximetry. *Nursing Standard* 15(47): 46–55.

Cates, C. (2001) Chronic asthma. *British Medical Journal* 323(7319): 976–979.

Cathcart, F. (1988) Seeing the body after death. *British Medical Journal* 297(6655): 997–998.

Cavanagh, J.D., Colvin, B.T. (1997) Bleeding and clotting disorders. In D.R. Goldhill, P.S. Withington (eds) *Textbook of Intensive Care*. London: Chapman & Hall, pp. 545–554.

Chadda, K., Louis, B., Benaïssa, L. *et al.* (2002) Physiological effects of decannulation in tracheostomized patients. *Intensive Care Medicine* 28(12): 1761–1767.

Chadwick, R., Tadd, W. (1992) *Ethics and Nursing Practice*. Basingstoke: Macmillan.

Challinor, P. (1998) Renal physiology and acute renal failure. In P. Challinor and J. Sedgewick (eds) *Principles and Practice of Renal Nursing*. London: Stanley Thornes.

Chambers, M. (2002) Nursing informatics and practice development. *NTresearch* 7(2): 101–115.

Chan, F.K.L., Leung, W.K. (2002) Peptic-ulcer disease. *British Medical Journal* 360(9337): 933–941.

Chandler, G. (1991) Creating an environment to empower nurses. *Nursing Management* 22(8): 20–23.

Channer, K., Morris, F. (2002) Myocardial ischaemia. *British Medical Journal* 324(7344): 1023–1026.

Charalambous, C., Schofield, I., Malik, R. (1999) Acute diabetic emergencies and their management. *Care of the Critically Ill* 15(4): 132–135.

Charnock, Y., Evans, D. (2001) Nursing management of chest drains. *Australian Critical Care* 14(4): 156–160.

Chen, Y.C. (1990) Psychological and social support systems in intensive and critical care. *Intensive Care Nursing* 6(1): 59–66.

Chevallier, A. (1996) *The Encyclopaedia of Medicinal Plants*. London: Dorling Kindersley.

Clark, S. (1993) Psychological needs of the critically ill patients. In J.M. Clochesy, S. Cardin, E.B. Rudy, A.A. Whittaker (eds) *Critical Care Nursing*. Philadelphia: W.B Saunders.

Clarke, A. (1991) Nurses as role models and health educators. *Journal of Advanced Nursing* 16(10): 1178–1184.

Clarke, G.M. (1997) Severe sepsis. In T.E. Oh (ed.) *Intensive Care Manual*, 4th edn. Oxford: Butterworth-Heinemann, pp. 525–539.

Clarke, L. (1994) *The Essence of Change*. London: Prentice Hall.

Clifford, C. (1985) Helplessness: A concept applied to nursing practice. *Intensive Care Nursing* 1(1): 19–24.

Clifford, C. (1993) The clinical role of the nurse teacher in the UK. *Journal of Advanced Nursing* 18(2): 281–289.

Clinical Standards Advisory Group (1999) *Services for Patients with Pain*. London: HMSO.

Coad, S. (1996) Cardiovascular needs. In C. Viney (ed.) *Nursing the Critically Ill*. London: Baillière Tindall, pp. 77–119.

Coad, S., Haines, S. (1999) Supporting staff caring for critically ill patients in acute care areas. *Nursing in Critical Care* 4(5): 245–248.

Coakley, J.H. (1997) Polyneuropathy. In D.R. Goldhill, P.S. Withington (eds) *Textbook of Intensive Care*. London: Chapman and Hall Medical, pp. 503–506.

Coates, S., Tivey, M., Stenhouse, C., Allsop, P. (2000) Introduction of a modified early warning score to surgical wards to improve detection of patients developing critical illness. *Journal of Integrated Care* 4: 41–42.

Cochrane Injuries Group Albumin Reviewers (1998) Human albumin in critically ill patients: systemic review of randomised control trials. *British Medical Journal* 317(7153): 235–240.

Cole, L. (2002) Unravelling the mystery of acute pancreatitis. *Dimensions of Critical Care Nursing* 21(3): 86–89.

Collin, C., Daly, G. (1998) Brain injury. In Stokes M (ed.) *Neurological Physiology*. St. Louis: Mosby.

Collins, P.M., Benedict, J.L. (1996) Pleural effusion. *American Journal of Nursing* 96(7) 38–39.

Collins, T. (2000) Understanding shock. *Nursing Standard* 14(49): 35–39.

Compton, P. (1991) Critical illness and intensive care: what it means to the client. *Critical Care Nurse* 11(1): 50–56.

Connolly, M.J. (1996) Obstructive airways disease: a hidden disability in the aged. *Age and Ageing* 25(4): 265–267.

Connors, A.F., Speroff, T., Dawson, N.V. *et al.* (1996) The effectiveness of right heart catheterisation in the initial care of critically ill patients. *JAMA* 276(11): 889–897.

Contrino, J., Hair, G., Kreutzer, D.L, Rickles, F.R. (1996) In situ detection of tissue factor in vascular endothelial cells: correlation with the malignant phenotype of human breast disease. *Nature Medicine* 2(2): 209–215.

Cook, D., Guyatt, G., Marshall, J. *et al.* (1998) A comparison of sucralfate and ranitidine for the prevention of upper gastrointestinal bleeding in patients requiring mechanical ventilation. *New England Journal of Medicine* 338(12): 791–797.

Cook, D.J., Guyatt, G.H., Jaeschke, R. *et al.* (1995) Determinants in Canadian health care workers of the decision to withdraw life support from the critically ill. *JAMA* 273(9): 703–708.

Cook, N. (2003) Respiratory care in spinal cord injury with associated traumatic brain injury: bridging the gap in critical care nursing interventions. *Intensive and Critical Care Nursing* 19(3): 143–153.

Cook, S. (1991) Mind the theory/practice gap in nursing. *Journal of Advanced Nursing* 16(12): 1462–1469.

Coolican, M.B. (1994) Families facing the sudden death of a loved one. *Critical Care Clinics of North America* 6(3): 607–612.

Coombs, M. (2001) Making sense of arterial blood gases. *Nursing Times* 97(27): 36–38.

Cooper, M.C. (1993) The intersection of technology and care in the ICU. *Advances in Nursing Science* 15(3): 23–32.

Cooper, N. (2002) Oxygen therapy – myths and misconceptions. *Care of the Critically Ill* 18(3): 74–77.

Copnell, B., Furgusson, D. (1995) Endotracheal suctioning: time-worn ritual or timely intervention? *American Journal of Critical Care* 4(2): 100–105.

Council of Deans and Heads (1998) *Breaking the Boundaries: A Position Paper*, University London. Faculties for Nursing, Midwifery and Health Visiting.

Courtney, R. (1995) Community partnership primary care: a new paradigm for primary care. *Public Health Nursing* 12(6): 366–373.

Covinsky, K.E., Wu, A.W., Landefeld, C.S. *et al.* (1999) Health status versus quality of life in older patients: does the distinction matter? *American Journal of Medicine* 106(4): 435–440.

Cox, C.L., McGrath, A. (1999) Respiratory assessment in critical care units. *Intensive and Critical Care Nursing* 15(4): 226–234.

Cranton, P. (1994) *Understanding and Promoting Transformative Learning*. San Francisco: Jossey-Bass.

Crimlisk, J.T., Horn, M.H., Wilson, D.J., Merino, B. (1996) Artificial airways: a survey of cuff management practices. *Heart and Lung* 25(3): 225–235.

Crinson, I. (1999) Clinical governance: the new NHS, new responsibilities? *British Journal of Nursing* 8(7): 449–453.

Crockett, A. (2002) The burden of COPD: counting the cost. *Geriatric Medicine* 32(10): 19–23.

Crosby, L., Parsons, C. (1992) Cerebrovascular response of closed head-injured patients to a standardized endotracheal tube suctioning and manual hyperventilation procedure. *Journal of Neuroscience Nursing* 24: 40–49.

Curtis, E., White, P. (2002) Resistance to change: causes and solutions. *Nursing Management* 8(10): 15–20.

Curtis, T. (1999) Climbing the walls. *Nursing in Critical Care* 4(2): 18–22.

Cuthbertson, B.H. (2003) Outreach critical care – cash for no questions? *British Journal of Anaesthesia* 90(1): 5–6.

Cutler, L.R. (2002) From ward-based critical care to educational curriculum 2: a focused ethnographic case study. *Intensive and Critical Care Nursing* 18(5): 280–291.

Cutler, L., Garner, M. (1995) Reducing relocation stress after discharge from the Intensive Therapy Unit. *Intensive and Critical Care Nursing* 11(6): 333–335.

Czarnik, R.E., Stone, K.S., Everhart, C.G., Preusser, B.A. (1991) Differential effects of continuous verses intermittent suction on tracheal tissue. *Heart and Lung* 20(2): 144–157.

Daffurn, K., Lee, A., Hillman, K.M., Bishop, G.F., Bauman, A. (1994) Do nurses know when to summon emergency assistance? *Intensive and Critical Care Nursing* 10(2): 115–120.

Daft, R.L. (2002) *The Leadership Experience*. London: Dryden Press.

Daly, K., Beale, R., Chang, R.W.S. (2001) Reduction in mortality after inappropriate early discharge from intensive care unit: logistic regression triage model. *British Medical Journal* 322(7297): 1274–1276.

Danis, M. (1998) Improving end-of-life care in the intensive care unit: what's to be learned from outcomes research? *New Horizons* 6(1): 110–118.

Dar, K., Williams, T., Aitken, R., Woods, K.L., Fletcher, S. (1995) Arterial versus capillary sampling for analysing blood gas pressure. *British Medical Journal* 310(6971): 24–25.

Darovic, G.O. (2002a) Physical assessment of the pulmonary system. In Darovic, G.O. (ed.) *Hemodynamic Monitoring: Invasive and Noninvasive Clinical Application*, 2nd edn. Philadelphia: W.B. Saunders Company, pp. 59–76.

Darovic, G.O. (2002b) Cardiovascular anatomy and physiology. In Darovic, G.O. (ed.) *Hemodynamic Monitoring: Invasive and Noninvasive Clinical Application*, 2nd edn. Philadelphia: W.B. Saunders Company, pp. 77–118.

Davidson, B. (1999) *What's All This About Stress?* Wirral: Tudor Business Publishing Limited.

Dawson, D. (2000) Neurological care. In M. Sheppard, M. Wright (eds) *High Dependency Nursing*. London: Baillière Tindall, pp. 145–182.

Day, C.P. (2002) Alcohol and the liver. *Medicine* 30(11): 18–20.

Day, T., Wainwright, S., Wilson-Barnett, J. (2001) An evaluation of a teaching intervention to improve the practice of end tracheal suctioning in intensive care units. *Journal of Clinical Nursing* 10(5): 682–696.

Day, T., Farnell, S., Wilson-Barnett, J. (2002) Suctioning: a review of current research recommendations. *Intensive and Critical Care Nursing* 18(2): 79–89.

Dean, B. (1997) Evidence based suction management in Accident and Emergency: vital component of airway care. *Accident and Emergency Nursing* 5(2): 92–98.

De Beaux, I., Chapman, M., Fraser, R. *et al.* (2001) Enteral nutrition in the critically ill: a prospective survey in an Australian Intensive Care Unit. *Anaesthesia and Intensive Care* 29(6): 619–622.

Department of Health (1992) *The Patient's Charter; Raising the Standards.* London: The Stationery Office.

Department of Health (1993) *The Citizen's Charter.* London: The Stationery Office.

Department of Health (1995) *Study of the Provision of Intensive Care in England.* London: The Stationery Office.

Department of Health (1997) *The New NHS: Modern, Dependable.* London: The Stationery Office.

Department of Health (1998a) *Quality in the New NHS.* London: The Stationery Office.

Department of Health (1998b) *Reducing junior doctors' continuing action to meet New Deal standards: rest periods and working arrangements, improving catering and accommodation for junior doctors and other action points.* London: DOH.

Department of Health (1998c) *A First Class Service.* London: DOH Stationery Office.

Department of Health (1999a) *Making a Difference: Strengthening the Nursing, Midwifery and Health Visiting Contribution to Health and Healthcare.* London: DOH.

Department of Health (1999b) *Saving Lives: Our Healthier Nation.* London: DOH.

Department of Health (2000a) *Comprehensive Critical Care: A Review of Adult Critical Care Services.* London: The Stationery Office.

Department of Health (2000b) *Heart Attacks and Other Acute Coronary Syndromes: Modern Standards and Service Models.* London: DOH.

Department of Health (2000c) *An Organisation with a Memory; Report of an Expert Group on Learning from Adverse Incidents in the NHS, chaired by the Chief Medical Officer.* London: DOH.

Department of Health (2000d) *Modernising Critical Care Services.* Health Service Circular 2000/017. London: NHS Executive.

Department of Health (2000e) *The NHS Plan: A Plan for Investment. A Plan for Reform.* London: DOH.

Department of Health (2001a) *The Nursing Contribution to the Provision of Comprehensive Critical Care for Adults; A Strategic Plan of Action.* London: The Stationery Office.

Department of Health (2001b) *Essence of Care.* London: Department of Health.

Department of Health (2001c) *Departmental Report 2002–3.* London: DOH.

Department of Health (2001d) *Good Practice in Consent Implementation Guide: Consent to Examination and Treatment.* London: DOH.

Department of Health (2002a) *Realising the Potential of Critical Care Nurses.* London: DOH.

Department of Health (2002b) *Code of Conduct for NHS Managers.* London: DOH.

DiCenso, A., Cullum, N., Ciliska, D. (1998) Implementing evidence-based nursing: some misconceptions. *Evidence-Based Nursing* 1(2): 38–40.

Dickson, A. (2002) Caring for a patient with a respiratory disorder. In M. Walsh (ed.) *Watson's Clinical Nursing and Related Sciences,* 6th edn. London: Baillière Tindall.

Dickson, S.L. (1995) Understanding the oxygen dissociation curve. *Critical Care Nurse* 15(5): 54–58.

Dillon, A., Lyon, J., Coombs, M.A. (1997) *Haemodynamic Profiles and the Critically Ill Patient: A Practical Guide.* Oxford: Bios Scientific Publishers.

Dimond, B. (2002) *Legal Aspects in Nursing.* 3rd edn. London: Prentice Hall.

Dinges, D.F., Douglas, S.D., Zaugg, L. *et al.* (1994) Leukocytosis and natural killer cell function parallel neurobehavioral fatigue induced by 64 hours of sleep deprivation. *Journal of Clinical Investigation* 93(5): 1930–1939.

Distenfield, A., Woermann, U. (2002) Sickle cell anaemia, available at www.emedicine.com/med/topic216.htm.

Docherty, B., Bench, S. (2002) Tracheostomy management for patients in general ward settings. *Professional Nurse* 18(2): 100–104.

Doering, L.V. (1999) Pathophysiology of acute coronary syndromes leading to acute myocardial infarction. *Journal of Cardiovascular Nursing* 13(3): 1–20.

Dolan, S. (2000a) Respiratory therapy. In J. Mallett, L. Dougherty (eds) *Manual of Clinical Nursing Procedures*. Oxford: Blackwell Science, pp. 517–526.

Dolan, S. (2000b) Vascular access devices. In J. Mallett, L. Dougherty (eds) *Manual of Clinical Nursing Procedures*, 5th edn. Oxford, London, Edinburgh: Blackwell Science.

Dolan, S. (2003) Severe sepsis – a major challenge for critical care (editorial). *Intensive Care Medicine* 19(2): 63–67.

Donnison, P., Criswell, J. (2002) Renal protection during abdominal aortic aneurysm surgery. *Care of the Critically Ill* 18(6): 175–180.

Downie, R.S., Tannahill, C., Tannahill, A. (1996) *Health Promotion: Models and Values*, 2nd edn. Oxford: Oxford Medical Publications.

Doyal, L., Dowling, S., Cameron, A. (1998) *Challenging Practice. An Evaluation for Innovatory Nursing Posts in the South West*. Bristol: Policy Press.

Dracup, K.A., Cannon, M.P. (1999) Combination treatment strategies for management of acute myocardial infarction: New directions with current therapies. *Critical Care Nurse* (Suppl.): 3–15.

Drew, K., Brayton M., Ambrose, A., Bernard, G. (1998) End-tidal carbon dioxide monitoring for weaning patients: a pilot study. *Dimensions of Critical Care Nursing* 17(3): 127–134.

Durgahee, T. (1998) Facilitating reflection: from a sage on stage to a guide on the side. *Nurse Education Today* 18(2): 158–164.

Dusheiko, G. (1999) Hepatitis C. *Surgery* 27(1): 37–39.

Dyer, I. (1991) Meeting the needs of visitors – a practical approach. *Intensive Care Nursing* 7(3): 135–147

Dyer, I. (1995) Preventing the ITU syndrome, or how not to torture an ITU patient! Part 1. *Intensive and Critical Care Nursing* 11(3): 130–139.

Dyer, I. (1997) Research into visitor needs using Molter's tool: time to move on. *Nursing in Critical Care* 2(6): 285–290.

Eastland, J. (2001) A framework for nursing the dying patient in ICU. *Nursing Times* 97(3): 36–39.

Eddleston, J., Macdonald, I., Littler, C. (1997) Withdrawal of sedation in critically ill patients. *British Journal of Intensive Care* 7(6): 216–222.

Edwards, S. (1996) *Nursing Ethics: A Principle-Based Approach*. Basingstoke: Macmillan.

Edwards, S. (2001) Regulation of water, sodium and potassium: implications for practice. *Nursing Standard* 15(22): 36–45.

Eichhorn, D.J., Meyers, T.A., Mitchell, T.G., Gazzetti, C. (1996) Opening the doors:

family presence during resuscitation. *Journal of Cardiovascular Nursing* 10(4): 59–70.

Ellin, R.J. (1994) Magnesium: the 5th but forgotten electrolyte. *Clinical Chemistry* 102: 616–622.

Elliott, M.W. (2002) Acute non-invasive ventilation: where are the current indications? *Scottish Medical Journal* 32(4): 266–274.

Ellis, A., Cavanagh, S. (1992) Aspects of neurological assessment using the Glasgow coma score. *Intensive and Critical Care Nursing* 8(2): 94–99.

Ellison, G. (1992) A private disaster. *Nursing Times* 88(52): 52–53.

Emmanuel, E.J., Fairclough, D.L., Emanuel, L.L. (2000) Attitudes and desires related to euthanasia and physician-assisted suicide among terminally ill patients and their caregivers. *JAMA* 284(19): 2460–2468.

English, I. (1993) Intuition as a function of the expert nurse: a critique of Benner's novice to expert model. *Journal of Advanced Nursing* 18(3): 387–393.

Epstein, O., Perkin, D., de Bono, D., Cookson, J. (2003) *Clinical Examination*, 3rd edn. London: Mosby.

European Resuscitation Council (2001) Guidelines 2000 for adult and paediatric basic life support and advanced life support. *Resuscitation* 48: 199–239.

Ewins, D., Bryant, J. (1992) Relative comfort. *Nursing Times* 88(52): 61–63.

Eynon, C.A., Menon, K.D. (2002) Critical care management of head injury. *Anaesthesia & Critical Care* 3(4): 135–139.

Fallah, M.A, Prakah, C., Edmundowica, S. (2000) Acute gastrointestinal bleeding. *Medical Clinics of North America* 4(5): 1183–1208.

Farquhar, M. (1995) Definitions of quality of life: a taxonomy. *Journal of Advanced Nursing* 22(3): 502–508.

Farrell, M. (1989) Dying and bereavement. The role of the critical care nurse. *Intensive Care Nursing* 5(1): 39–45.

Farrell, M. (1999) The challenge of breaking bad news. *Intensive and Critical Care Nursing* 15(2): 101–110.

Fehrenbach, C. (2002) Chronic obstructive pulmonary disease. *Nursing Standard* 17(10): 45–51.

Feied, C., Handler, J.A. (2002) Pulmonary embolism, at http: //www.emedicine.com/ EMERG/topic490.htm. (accessed 2 April 2003).

Fennerty, T. (1997) Pulmonary embolism. *British Medical Journal* 314(7078): 425–429.

Fernandez del Castillo, C. (1993) Acute pancreatitis. *Lancet* 342: 475–478.

Ferrin, M. (1996) Restoring electrolyte balance: magnesium. *Registered Nurse* 59(5): 31–35.

Ferry, N., Ross-Gordon, J. (1998) An inquiry into Schon's epistemology or practice: exploring the links between experience and reflective practice. *Adult Education Quarterly* 48: 98–112.

Field, D. (1997a) Cardiovascular assessment – part 2. *Nursing Times* 93(39): 55–57.

Field, D. (1997b) Cardiovascular assessment. *Nursing Times* 93(35): 45–47.

Field, D. (2000) Respiratory care. In M. Sheppard, M. Wright (eds) *Principles and Practice of High Dependency Nursing*. London: Baillière Tindall, pp. 69–109.

Field, L. (1996) Are nurses still underestimating patient's pain post-operatively? *British Journal of Nursing* 5(13): 778–784.

Finlay, I., Dallimore, D. (1991) Your child is dead. *British Medical Journal* 302(6791): 1524–1525.

Fiorentini, A. (1992) Potential hazards of tracheobronchial suctioning. *Intensive Critical Care Nursing* 8(4): 217–226.

Fitzgerald, G., Patrono, C. (2001) The coxibs, selective inhibitors of cyclooxygenase-2. *New England Journal of Medicine* 345(6): 433–442.

Fitzgerald, M. (2001) Acute asthma. *British Medical Journal* 323(7317): 841–845.

Flanning, H. (2000) Fluid and electrolyte balance. In K. Manley, L. Bellman (eds) *Surgical Nursing: Advancing Practice*. Edinburgh: Churchill Livingstone, pp. 538–555.

Fleckman, A.M. (1993) Diabetic ketoacidosis. *Endocrinology and Metabolism Clinics of North America* 22(2): 181–207.

Flint, G. (1999) Head injuries. *British Journal of Theatre Nursing* 9(1): 15–21.

Flynn, J.B., Bruce, N.P. (1993) *Introduction to Critical Care Skills*. St. Louis: Mosby.

Ford, P., Walsh, M. (1994) *New Rituals for Old*. Oxford: Butterworth-Heinemann.

Forrester, D.A., Murphy, P.A., Price, D.M. (1990) Critical care family needs: nurse–family members confederate pairs. *Heart and Lung* 19(6): 655–661.

Fowler, L. (1998) Improving critical thinking in nursing practice. *Journal for Nurses in Staff Development* 14(4): 183–187.

Fox, M. (1999) The importance of sleep. *Nursing Standard* 13(24): 44–47.

Fox, V., Gould, D., Davies, N., Owen, S. (1999) Patients' experiences of having an underwater seal chest drain: a replication study. *Journal of Clinical Nursing* 8(6): 684–692.

Franklin, C., Mathew, J. (1994) Developing strategies to prevent in hospital cardiac arrest: analysing responses of physicians and nurses in the hours before the event. *Critical Care Medicine* 22(2): 244–247.

Frausing, E., Jorgen, H., Phanareth, K., Kok-Jensen, A., Dirksen, A. (2001) Peak flow as predictor of overall mortality in asthma and chronic obstructive pulmonary disease. *American Journal of Respiratory and Critical Care Medicine* 163(3 part 1): 690–693.

Freebairn, R.C., Oh, T.E. (1997) Pulmonary embolism. In T.E. Oh (ed.) *Intensive Care Manual*, 4th edn. Oxford: Butterworth-Heinemann, pp. 280–290.

Friedemann, M.L. (1989) The concept of family nursing. *Journal of Advanced Nursing* 14(3): 211–216.

Fukatsu, K., Zarzaur, B.L., Johnson, C.D., Lundberg, A.H., Wilcox, H.G., Kudsk, K.A. (2001) Enteral nutrition prevents remote organ injury and death after a gut ischaemia insult. *Annals of Surgery* 233(5): 660–668.

Fulbrook, P., Allan, D., Carroll, S., Dawson, D. *et al.* (1999) On the receiving end: experiences of being a relative in critical care (part 1). *Nursing in Critical Care* 4(3): 138–145.

Fulbrook, S. (1998) Legal implications of relatives witnessing resuscitation. *British Journal of Theatre Nursing* 7(10): 33–35.

Gallant, M.H., Beaulieu, M.C., Carnevale, F.A. (2002) Partnership: an analysis of the concept within the nurse–client relationship. *Journal of Advanced Nursing* 40(2): 149–157.

Gallon, A. (1998) Pneumothorax. *Nursing Standard* 13(10): 35–39.

Ganong, W.F. (2003) *Review of Medical Physiology*, 21st edn. Connecticut: Appleton and Lange.

Garbett, R., McCormack, B. (2002a) The qualities and skills of practice developers. *Nursing Standard* 16(50): 33–36.

Garbett, R., McCormack, B. (2002b) A concept analysis of practice development. *NTresearch* 7(2): 87–100.

Garfield, M.J., Jeffrey, R., Ridley, S.A. (2000) An assessment of staffing level required for a high dependency unit. *Anaesthesia* 55: 137–143.

Geisser, M., Roth, R., Bachman, J., Eckert, T. (1996) The relationship between symptoms of post-traumatic stress disorder and pain, affective disturbance and disability among patients with accident and non-accident related pain. *Pain* 66(2–3): 207–214.

Gelling, L. (1999) Causes of ICU psychosis: the environmental factors. *Nursing in Critical Care* 4(1): 22–26.

Ghost, S., Watts, D., Kinnear, M. (2002) Management of gastrointestinal haemorrhage. *Postgraduate Medical Journal* 78(915): 4–14.

Giacchino, S., Houdek, D. (1998) Ruptured varices: act fast. *Registered Nurse* 61(5): 33–36.

Gilbert, T. (2001) Reflective practice and clinical supervision: meticulous rituals of the confessional? *Journal of Advanced Nursing* 36(2): 199–205.

Gillies, P. (1998) Effectiveness of alliances and partnerships for health promotion. *Health Promotion International* 13(2): 99–120.

Gillon, R. (1985) *Philosophical Medicine Ethics*. Chichester: Wiley.

Gimson, A.E.S., Ramage, J.K., Panos, M.L. *et al.* (1993) Randomised trial of variceal banding ligation vesus injection sclerotherapy of bleeding oesophageal varices. *Lancet* 342(8868): 391–394.

Glasby, M.A., Myles, L.M. (2000) Applied physiology of the CNS. *Surgery* 18(9): iii–vi.

Glass, C., Grap, M. (1995) Ten tips for safe suctioning. *American Journal of Nursing* 5(5): 51–53.

Godden, J., Hiley, C. (1998) Managing the patient with a chest drain: a review. *Nursing Standard* 12(32): 35–39.

Goding, L., Edwards, K. (2002) Evidence-based practice. *Nurse Researcher* 9(4); 45–57.

Goh, J., Gupta, A.K. (2002) The management of head injury and intracranial pressure. *Current Anaesthesia and Critical Care* 13(3): 129–137.

Goldfrad, C., Rowan, K. (2000) Consequences of discharges from intensive care at night. *Lancet* 355(9210): 1138–1142

Goldhill, D.R. (1997) Introducing the postoperative care team: Additional support, expertise and equipment for general postoperative patients. *British Medical Journal* 314(7078): 389.

Goldhill, D.R. (2000) Medical emergency teams. *Care of the Critically Ill* 16(6): 209–212.

Goldhill, D.R., Sumner, A. (1998) Outcome of intensive care patients in a group of British intensive care units. *Critical Care Medicine* 26(8): 1337–1345.

Goldhill, D.R., White, S.A., Sumner, A. (1999a) Physiological values and procedures in the 24 hours before ICU admission from the ward. *Anaesthesia* 54(9): 529–534.

Goldhill, D.R., Worthington, L., Mulcahy, A., Tarling, M., Sumner, A. (1999b) The patient-at-risk team: identifying and managing seriously ill ward patients. *Anaesthesia* 54(9): 853–860.

Goldhill, D.R., McNarry, A. (2002) Intensive care outreach services *Current Anaesthesia and Critical Care* 13: 356–361.

Goldman, H.G. (1999) Role expansion in intensive care: survey of nurses' view. *Intensive and Critical Care Nursing* 15(6): 313–323.

Golembiewski, J.A., O'Brien, D. (2002) A systematic approach to the management of postoperative nausea and vomiting. *Journal of Perianesthesia Nursing* 17(6): 364–376.

Gonce Morton, P. (1998) Anatomy and physiology of the respiratory system. In C.M. Hudak, B.M. Gallo, P. Gonce Morton (eds) *Critical Care Nursing: A Holistic Approach*, 7th edn. Philadelphia: Lippincott.

Gorman, K. (1999) Sickle cell disease: do you doubt your patient's pain? *American Journal of Nursing* 99(3): 38–43.

Gosling, P. (1995) Albumin and the critically ill. *Care of the Critically Ill* 11(2): 57–61.

Gosling, P. (1999) Fluid balance in the critically ill: the sodium and water audit. *Care of the Critically Ill* 15(1): 11–16.

Graham, A. (1996) Chest drain insertion. *Care of the Critically Ill* 12(5): centre insert.

Gramlich, T. (1992) Pulse oximetry. *Emergency* 24(8): 25–27.

Granberg, A., Engberg, I.B., Lundberg, D. (1996) Intensive care syndrome: a literature review. *Intensive and Critical Care Nursing* 12(3): 173–182.

Granberg-Axèll, A., Bergbom, I., Lunberg, D. (2001) Clinical signs of ICU syndrome/delirium: an observational study. *Intensive and Critical Care Nursing* 17(2): 72–93.

Gray, E. (2001) Pain management for patients with chest drains. *Nursing Standard* 14(23): 40–44.

Green, A. (1996) An exploratory study of patients' memory recall of their stay in an adult intensive therapy unit. *Intensive and Critical Care Nursing* 12(3): 131–137.

Green, L., Raeburn, J. (1990) Contemporary developments in health promotion; definitions and challenges. In N. Bracht (ed.) *Health Promotion at the Community Level*. London: Sage.

Greenwood, J. (1998) The role of reflection in single and double loop learning. *Journal of Advanced Nursing* 27(5): 1048–1053.

Griggs, A. (1998) Tracheostomy: Suctioning and humidification. *Nursing Standard* 13(2): 49–53, 55–56.

Guenter, P.A., Settle, R.G., Perlmutter, S. *et al.* (1991) Tube feeding-related diarrhoea in acutely ill patients. *Journal of Parenteral and Enteral Nutrition* 15(3): 277–280.

Gunning, K., Rowan, K. (1999) Outcome data and scoring systems. *British Medical Journal* 319(7204): 241–244.

Gupta, N. (2001) Pneumothorax: is chest tube clamp necessary before removal? *Chest* 119(4): 1292–1293.

Gustafsson, U., Ek, A. (1992) The relevance of sleep, circadian rhythm and lifestyle, related to a holistic theory of health. *Scandinavian Journal of Caring Sciences* 6(1): 29–35.

Guyton, A.C., Hall, J.E. (2000) *Textbook of Medical Physiology*, 10th edn. Philadelphia: W.B. Saunders.

Guzman, J.A., Kruse, J.A. (2001) Targeting the gut in shock and organ failure. *Clinical Intensive Care* 12(5,6): 203–209.

Hadley, M.N. (2002) Management of acute spinal cord injuries in an intensive care unit or other monitored setting. *Neurosurgery Online* 50(3): S51–S57.

Hafsteindóttir, T.B. (1996) Patients' experience of communication during the respiratory treatment period. *Intensive and Critical Care Nursing* 12(5): 261–271.

Haider, A.W., Larson, M.G., Franklin, S.S., Levy, D. (2003) Systolic blood pressure, diastolic blood pressure, and pulse pressure as predictors of risk for congestive heart failure in the Framingham study. *Annals of Internal Medicine* 138(1): 10–16.

Haines, S., Coad, S. (2001) Supporting ward staff in acute care areas: expanding the service. *Intensive and Critical Care Nursing* 17(2): 105–109.

Hale, A.S., Moseley, M.J., Warner, S.C. (2000) Treating pancreatitis in the acute care setting. *Dimensions of Critical Care Nursing* 19(4): 15–21.

Hall, B., Hall, D.A. (1994) Learning from the experience of loss: people bereaved during intensive care. *Intensive and Critical Care Nursing* 10(4): 265–270.

Hall, M., Jones, A. (1997) Reducing morbidity from insertion of chest drains: clamping may be appropriate to prevent discomfort and reduce risk of oedema. *British Medical Journal* 315(7103): 313.

Haller, M., Zollner, C., Briegel, J., Forst, H. (1995) Evaluation of a new continuous thermodilution cardiac output monitor in critically ill patients: a prospective criterion standard study. *Critical Care Medicine* 23(5): 860–866.

Halloran, T.H. (1995) Spinal cord trauma. In N.A. Urban, K.K. Greenlee, J.M. Krumberger, C. Winkelman (eds) *Guidelines for Critical Care*. St. Louis: Mosby, pp. 92–99.

Halm, M.A. (1990) Effects of support groups on family members during critical illness. *Heart and Lung* 19(1): 62–71.

Hamer, S., Collinson, G. (eds) (1999) *Achieving Evidence-Based Practice*. London: Baillière Tindall.

Hampton, J.R. (2003a) *The ECG in Practice*, 4th edn. Edinburgh: Churchill Livingstone.

Hampton, J.R. (2003b) *The ECG Made Easy*, 6th edn. Edinburgh: Churchill Livingstone.

Hampton, J.R. (2003c) *150 ECG Problems*, 2nd edn. Edinburgh: Churchill Livingstone.

Hand, H. (2000) The development of diabetic ketoacidosis. *Nursing Standard* 15(8): 47–52, 54–55.

Hanley, D. (1997) Intracranial hypertension. In T.E. Oh (ed) *Intensive Care Manual*, 4th edn. Oxford: Butterworth-Heinemann, pp. 395–402.

Hanson, C., Strawser, D. (1992) Family presence during cardiopulmonary resuscitation: Foote Hospital emergency department's nine-year perspective. *Journal of Emergency Nursing* 18(2): 104–106.

Harding, S., Balarajan, R. (1996) Patterns of mortality in second generation Irish people living in England and Wales: Longitudinal Study. *British Medical Journal* 312(7043): 1389–1392.

Harkin, D.W., Barros, A.A.B., McCallion, K., Hoper, M., Halliday, M.I., Campbell, C.F. (2001) Bacterial permeability-increasing protein attenuates systemic inflammation and acute lung injury in porcine lower limb ischaemia reperfusion injury. *Annals of Surgery* 234(2): 233–244.

Harris, A., Misiewicz, J.J. (2001) Management of *Helicobacter pylori* infection. *British Medical Journal* 323(7320): 1047–1050.

Harvey, M.G. (1992) Humanizing the intensive care unit experience. *Clinical Issues in Perinatal & Women's Health Nursing* 3(3): 369–376.

Hatchett, R. (1994) Should relatives watch resuscitation? A successful American programme. *British Medical Journal* 309(6951): 407.

Hatchett, R. (2002) Clinical observation and monitoring devices. In R. Hatchett, D. Thompson (eds) *Cardiac Nursing: a Comprehensive Guide*. Edinburgh: Churchill Livingstone, pp. 69–96.

Hawker, F. (2003) Hepatic failure. In A.D. Bersten, N. Soni (eds) *Intensive Care Manual*, 5th edn. Edinburgh: Butterworth-Heinemann, pp. 431–441.

Hawkins, P., Shohart, R. (1989) *Supervision in the Helping Profession*. Buckingham: Open University Press.

Hawthorne, J., Redmond, K. (1998) *Pain: Causes and Management*. Oxford: Blackwell.

Hawton, K., Townsend, E., Deeks, J. *et al.* (2001) Effects of legislation restricting pack size of paracetamol and salicylate on self poisoning in the United Kingdom: before and after study. *British Medical Journal* 322(7296): 1203–1207.

Heath, H. (1998) Reflection and patterns of knowing in nursing. *Journal of Advanced Nursing* 27(5): 1054–1059.

Hegarty, A., Portenoy, R.K. (1994) Pharmacotherapy of neuropathic pain. *Seminars in Neurology* 14(3): 213–224.

HELP Booklet (2002) adapted from ALERT™ course manual. ISBN 1 86137 196 9. University of Portsmouth.

Henderson, N. (1997) Central venous lines. *Nursing Standard* 11(42): 49–54.

Hess, D., Kacmarek, R.M. (1993) Techniques and devices for monitoring oxygenation. *Respiratory Care* 38(6): 646–671.

Hewitt, J. (2002) A critical series of the arguments debating the role of the nurse advocate. *Journal of Advanced Nursing* 37(5): 439–445.

Hickey, J.V. (1997a) Intracranial pressure: theory and management of intracranial pressure. In J.V. Hickey (ed.) *The Clinical Practice of Neurological and Neurosurgical Nursing*, 4th edn. Philadelphia: Lippincott, pp. 295–328.

Hickey, J.V. (1997b) Craniocerebral injuries. In J.V. Hickey (ed) *The Clinical Practice of Neurological and Neurosurgical Nursing*, 4th edn. Philadelphia: Lippincott, pp. 385–417.

Higgins, D.J., Singer, M. (1993) Transoesophageal Doppler for continuous haemodynamic monitoring. *British Journal of Intensive Care* 3(10): 376–378.

Higgs, R. (1994) Relatives' wishes should be accommodated. *British Medical Journal* 308(6945): 1688.

Hillberg, R.E., Johnson, D.C. (1997) Noninvasive ventilation. *New England Journal of Medicine* 337(24): 1746–1752.

Hilling, L., Bakow, E., Fink, J., Kelly, C., Sobush, D., Southorn, P. (1992) Nasotracheal suctioning. *Respiratory Care* 37: 898–901.

Hinds, C.J., Watson, D. (1996) *Intensive Care*, 2nd edn. London: W.B. Saunders.

Hinds, C.J., Watson, D. (1999) ABC of intensive care – circulatory support. *British Medical Journal* 318(7200): 1749.

Hirschl, M.M., Binder, M., Gwechenberger, M. *et al.* (1997) Non-invasive assessment of cardiac output in critically ill patients by analysis of the finger blood-pressure waveform. *Critical Care Medicine* 25(11): 1909–1914.

Hoffbrand, A.V., Lewis, S.M., Tuddenham, G.D. (1999) *Post Graduate Haematology*, 4th edn. Oxford: Butterworth-Heinemann.

Hoffbrand, A.V., Pettit, J.E., Moss, P.A. (2001) *Essential Haematology*. Oxford: Blackwell Science.

Hofhuis, J., Bakker, J. (1998) Experiences of critically ill patients in the ICU: What do they think of us? *International Journal of Intensive Care* 98(5): 114–117.

Hogg, J.C., Senior, R.M. (2002) Chronic obstructive pulmonary disease C2: pathology and biochemistry of emphysema. *Thorax* 57(9): 830–834.

Holgate, S.T., Frew, A. (2002) Respiratory disease. In P. Kumar, M. Clarke (eds) *Clinical Medicine*, 5th edn. Edinburgh: W.B. Saunders.

Holland, K., Hogg, C. (2001) *Cultural Awareness in Nursing and Health Care*. London: Arnold.

Hoogenberg, K., Girbes, A.R. (1998) The use of dopamine and noradrenaline in ICU patients with special reference to renal function. *International Journal of Intensive Care* 5(3): 82–89.

Horne, J. (1998) *Why We Sleep*. Oxford: Oxford University Press.

Horne, M.M. (2001) Endocrinological dysfunctions. In P. Swearingen, J. Keen (eds) *Manual of Critical Care Nursing*, 4th edn. St. Louis: Mosby.

Horwood, A. (1990) Malnourishment in intensive care units, as high as 50%: are nurses doing enough to change this? *Intensive Care Nursing* 6(4): 205–208.

Hough, A. (2001) *Physiotherapy in Respiratory Care*, 3rd edn. Cheltenham: Nelson Thornes.

Houghton, A.R., Gray, D. (1997) *Making Sense of the ECG*. London: Edward Arnold.

Howard, D. (2001) Student nurses' experiences of Project 2000. *Nursing Standard* 15(48): 33–38.

Hubbard, J., Mechan, D. (1997) *The Physiology of Health and Illness*. Cheltenham: Stanley Thornes Ltd.

Hudak, C.M., Gallo, B.M., Morton, P.G. (eds) (1998) *Critical Care Nursing: a Holistic Approach*, 7th edn. Philadelphia: Lippincott.

Huddleston, S.S., Ferguson, S.G. (1997) *Critical Care and Emergency Nursing*, 3rd edn. Springhouse, Pennsylvania: Springhouse Corporation.

Hudsmith, J.G., Menon, K.D. (2002) Neuromuscular disorders: relevance to anaesthesia and intensive care. *Anaesthesia and Critical Care* 3(5): 169–173.

Huether, S.E. (1998a) The renal and urologic systems. In K.L. McCance, S.E. Huether (eds) *Pathophysiology: The Biologic Basis for Disease in Adults and Children*. St. Louis: Mosby.

Huether, S.E (1998b) The cellular environment: fluids and electrolytes, acids and bases. In K.L. McCance, S.E. Huether (eds) *Pathophysiology: The Biologic Basis for Disease in Adults and Children*. St. Louis: Mosby.

Huff, J. (1997) *ECG Workout*, 3rd edn. Philadelphia: Lippincott.

Humphreys, M. (2002) Hyperkalaemia: a dangerous electrolyte disturbance. *Connect* 2(1): 28–30.

Hund, E.F., Borel, C.O., Cornblath, D.R., Hanley, D.F., McKhann, G.M. (1993) Intensive management and treatment of severe Guillain–Barré Syndrome. *Critical Care Medicine* 21(3): 433–446.

Hyde, J., Sykes, T., Graham, T. (1997) Reducing morbidity from chest drains: knowledge of basic principles and use of appropriate equipment would help. *British Medical Journal* 314(7085): 914–915.

Hyers, T.M. (2003) Management of venous thromboembolism. *Archives of Internal Medicine* 163(7): 759–768.

Illich, I. (1976) *Limits to Medicine. Medical Nemesis.* London: Marion Boyars.

Intensive Care National Audit and Research Centre (1999) *The INCARC System of Patient-related Activities (SOPRA).* London: Intensive Care National Audit and Research Centre.

Intensive Care Society (1997) *Standards for Intensive Care.* London: Intensive Care Society.

Intensive Care Society (2002) *Levels of Critical Care for Adult Patients.* London: Intensive Care Society.

Intensive Care Society Standards (2002) *Introduction of Outreach Services.* London: Intensive Care Society.

International Association of the Study of Pain (1979) Pain terms: a list of definitions and usage. *Pain* 6: 249–252.

Inwald, D., Roland, M., Kuitert, L., McKenzie, S., Petros, A. (2001) Oxygen treatment for severe acute asthma. *British Medical Journal* 323(7304): 98–100.

Isbister, J.P. (2003) Haemostatic failure. In A.D. Bersten, N. Soni (eds) *Intensive Care Manual*, 5th edn. Edinburgh: Butterworth-Heinemann, pp. 941–953.

Isea, J.O., Poyant, D., O'Donnell, C., Faling, L.J. (1993) Controlled trial of a continuous irrigation suction catheter vs conventional intermittent suction catheter in clearing bronchial secretions from ventilated patients. *Chest* 103(4): 1227–1230.

Jablonski, R.S. (1994) The experience of being mechanically ventilated. *Qualitative Health Research* 4(2): 186–207.

Jackson, C. (1996) Humidification in the upper respiratory tract: a physiological overview. *Intensive and Critical Care Nursing* 12(1): 27–32.

Jackson, I. (1996) Critical care nurses' perception of a bereavement follow-up service. *Intensive and Critical Care Nursing* 12(1): 2–11.

Jackson, I. (1998) A study of bereavement in an intensive care unit. *Nursing in Critical Care* 3(3): 141–150.

Jackson, N., Wendon, J. (2000) The management of acute liver failure. *Clinical Intensive Care* 11(3): 127–135.

Jarvis, C. (1996) *Physical Examination and Health Assessment*, 2nd edn. Philadelphia: W.B. Saunders.

Jennett, B., Teasdale, G. (1974) Assessment of coma and impaired consciousness. *Lancet* ii(7872): 81–83.

Jensen, J.A., Onyskiw, J.E., Prasad, N.G.N. (1998) Meta-analysis of arterial oxygen saturation monitoring by pulse oximetry in adults. *Heart and Lung* 27(6): 387–408.

Johns, C. (2000) *Becoming a Reflective Practitioner: a Reflective and Holistic Approach to Clinical Nursing, Practice Development and Clinical Supervision.* Oxford: Blackwell Science.

Johnson, C.D. (1998) Severe acute pancreatitis: a continuing challenge for the intensive care team. *British Journal of Intensive Care* 8(4): 130–137.

Johnson, L. (1999) Factors known to raise intracranial pressure and the associated implications for nursing management. *Nursing in Critical Care* 4(3): 117–127.

Jolley, S. (2001) Managing post-operative nausea and vomiting. *Nursing Standard* 15(40): 47–52.

Jolliet, P., Abajo, B., Pasquina, P., Chevrolet, J.-C. (2001) Non-invasive pressure support ventilation in severe community-acquired pneumonia. *Intensive Care Medicine* 27(5): 812–821.

Jones, C., O'Donnell, K. (1994) After intensive care – what then? *Intensive and Critical Care Nursing* 10(10): 89–92.

Jones, D.W., Appel, L.J., Sheps, S.G. Roccella, E.J., Lenfant, C. (2003) Measuring blood pressure accurately. *JAMA* 289(8): 1027–1030.

Jones, I. (2003) Acute coronary syndromes: identification and patient care. *Professional Nurse* 18(5): 289–292.

Jonker, G. (1997) The many facets of Islam. In C.M. Parkes, P. Laungani, B. Young (eds) *Death and Bereavement Across Cultures.* London: Routledge, pp. 147–165.

Joyce, L. (1999) Development of practice. In S. Hamer, G. Collinson (eds) *Achieving Evidence-Based Practice.* London: Baillière Tindall, pp. 109–127.

Kacmarek, R.M. (1999) Newer ventilatory strategies. *Current Opinion in Anaesthesiology* 12(2): 113–141.

Kam, A.C., O'Brien, M., Kam, P.C.A. (1993) Pleural drainage systems. *Anaesthesia* 48(2): 154–161.

Kannan, S. (1999) Practical issues in non-invasive positive pressure ventilation. *Care of the Critically Ill* 15(3): 76–79.

Kaufman, D.A. (2001) Pulmonary ventilation/perfusion scan. http: /www.nlm.nih.gov/medlineplus/ency/article/003828.htm accessed: 11/07/2003.

Keays, R. (2003) Diabetic emergencies. In A.P. Bersten, N. Soni (eds) *Intensive Care Manual,* 5th edn. Edinburgh: Butterworth-Heinemann, pp. 551–558.

Keely, B.R. (1998) Preventing complications. Recognition and treatment of autonomic dysreflexia. *Dimensions in Critical Care Nursing* 17(4): 170–176.

Keen, J.H. (2001) Septic shock. In: P. Swearingen, J. Keen (eds) *Manual of Critical Care Nursing,* 4th edn. St. Louis: Mosby.

Kelly, D., Skidmore, S. (2002) Hepatitis C-Z: recent advances. *Archives of Disease in Childhood* 86(5): 339–343.

Kember, D., Jones, A., Loke, A.Y. (2001) *Reflective Teaching and Learning in the Health Professions.* Oxford: Blackwell Science.

Kennedy, J.F. (1997) Enteral feeding for the critically ill patient. *Nursing Standard* 11(33): 39–43.

Kent v. *Griffiths and others* (2002) 2 ALL ER 474.

Kerr, M.E., Rudy, E.B., Weber, B.B. *et al.* (1997) Effect of short-duration hyperventilation during endotracheal suctioning on intracranial pressure in severe head injured adults. *Nursing Research* 46(4): 195–201.

Kessenich, C. (2000) Teaching health assessment in advanced practice nursing programs. *Nurse Educator* 25(4): 170–172.

Kestevan, P., Saunders, P. (1993) Disseminated intravascular coagulation. *Care of the Critically Ill* 9(1): 22–27.

Ketefian, S. (1978) Strategies of curriculum change. *International Nursing Review* 25(1): 14–24.

Kiely, J.L., Deegan, P., Buckley, A., Shiels, P., Maurer, B., McNicholas, W.T. (1998) Efficacy of nasal continuous positive airway pressure therapy in chronic heart failure: importance of underlying cardiac rhythm. *Thorax* 53(11): 957–962.

Kiger, A.M. (1995) *Teaching for Health*, 2nd edn. Edinburgh: Churchill Livingstone.

Kim, H. (1999) Critical reflective inquiry for knowledge development in nursing. *Journal of Advanced Nursing* 29(5): 1205–1212.

Kincey, J., Pratt, D., Slater, R., Dixon, M. (2003) A survey of patterns and sources of stress among medical and nursing staff in an intensive care unit setting. *Care of the Critically Ill* 19(3): 83–87.

King, N., Anderson, N.R. (1995) *Innovation and Change in Organisations*. London: Routledge.

Kinloch, D. (1999) Instillation of normal saline during end tracheal suctioning: effects on mixed venous oxygen saturation. *American Journal of Critical Care* 8(4): 231–240.

Kinn, S., Scott, J. (2001) Nutritional awareness of critically ill surgical high-dependency patients. *British Journal of Nursing* 10(11): 704–709.

Kishen, R. (2002) Managing acute renal failure in the critically ill: Where are we today? *Care of the Critically Ill* 18(6): 170–172.

Kitson, A.L., Ahmed, L.D., Harvey, G., Seers, K., Thomson, D.R. (1996) From research to practice: open organisational model for promoting research based practice. *Journal of Advanced Nursing* 23(3): 430–440.

Kodiath, M., Kodiath, A. (1992) A comparative study of patients with chronic pain. *Clinical Nursing Research* 1(3): 278–291.

Kolb, D.A., Fry, R. (1975) Towards an applied theory of experiential learning. In C.L. Cooper (ed.) *Theories of Group Processes*. Chichester: John Wiley, pp. 33–57.

Krachman, S.L., D'Alonzo, G.E., Criner, G.J. (1995) Sleep in the intensive care unit. *Chest* 107(6): 1713–1720.

Kramer, N., Meyer, T.J., Meharg, J., Cece, R.D., Hill, N.S. (1995) Randomized, prospective trial on noninvasive positive pressure ventilation in acute respiratory failure. *American Journal of Respiratory and Critical Care Medicine* 151(6): 1799–1806.

Krumberger, J. (2002) When the liver fails. *Registered Nurse* 65(2): 26–29.

Kubitz, T. (1999) Increase the muscular mass and to lose corporeo fat during sleep (translated version). http://www.olypian.it/on/55.

Kubler-Ross, E. (1970) *On Death and Dying*. London: Routledge.

Kubler-Ross, E. (1991) *On Life after Death*. California: Celestial Arts.

Kudst, K.A. (2003) Effect of route and type of nutrition on intestine-derived inflammatory responses. *American Journal of Surgery* 185(1): 16–21.

Kuwabara, S., Ogawara, K., Sing, J.-Y. *et al.* (2002) Differences in membrane properties of axonal and demyelinating Guillain–Barré Syndromes. *Annals of Neurology* 52(2): 180–187.

LaBonte, R. (1994) Health promotion and empowerment: reflections on professional practice. *Health Education Quarterly* 21(2): 253–268.

Laitinen, H. (1996) Patients' experience of confusion in the intensive care unit following cardiac surgery. *Intensive and Critical Care Nursing* 12(2): 79–83.

Lancaster, J. (1999) (ed.) *Nursing Issues in Leading and Managing Change*. St Louis: Mosby.

Lancet (1998) Editorial. First lessons from the 'Bristol case'. *Lancet* 351(117): 1669.

Lanfear, J. (2002) The individual with epilepsy. *Nursing Standard* 16(4): 43–53.

Larvin, M. (1999) Acute pancreatitis. *Surgery* 17(11): 261–265.

Lee, A., Bishop, G., Hillman, K.M., Daffurn, K. (1995b) The medical emergency team. *Anaesthesia and Intensive Care* 23(2): 183–186.

Lee, B., Chang, R.W.S., Jacobs, S. (1990) Intermittent nasogastric feeding: a simple and effective method to reduce pneumonia among ventilated ICU patients. *Clinical Intensive Care* 1(3): 100–102.

Lee, B.Y., Karmaker, M.G., Herz, B.L., Sturgill, R.A. (1995a) Autonomic dysreflexia revisited. *Journal of Spinal Cord Medicine* 18(2): 75–87.

Leith, B.A. (1998) Transfer anxiety in critical care patients and their family members. *Critical Care Nurse* 18(4): 24–32.

le May, A. (1999) *Evidence-Based Practice*. London: Nursing Times Clinical Monographs (no. 1).

Leske, J.S. (1992) Needs of adult family members after critical illness. Prescriptions for interventions. *Critical Care Nursing Clinics of North America* 4(4): 587–595.

Levi, M., Cate, H. (1999) Disseminated intravascular coagulation: current concepts. *New England Journal of Medicine* 58(150): 592.

Levi, M., Evert, D., Tom, V. *et al.* (2000) Novel approaches to the management of disseminated intravascular coagulation. *Critical Care Medicine* 28(9): 20–24.

Lewin, K. (1951) *Field Theory in Social Science*. New York: Harper and Row.

Lewis, R. (2000) Diabetic emergencies. Part 2: hyperglycaemia. *Accident and Emergency Nursing* 8(4): 24–30.

Lewis, S.J., Egger, M., Sylvester, P.A., Thomas, S. (2001) Early enteral feeding versus 'nil by mouth' after gastro-intestinal surgery: systematic review and meta-analysis of controlled trials. *British Medical Journal* 323(7316): 773–776.

Lightowler, J.V., Wedzicha, J.A., Elliott, M.W., Ram, F.S. (2003) Non-invasive positive pressure ventilation to treat respiratory failure resulting from exacerbations of chronic obstructive pulmonary disease: Cochrane systematic review and meta-analysis. *British Medical Journal* 326(7382): 185–187.

Lindahl, B., Sandman, P. (1998) The role of advocacy in critical care nursing: a caring response to another. *Intensive and Critical Care Nursing* 14(4): 179–186.

Lindermann, E. (1994) Symptomatology and management of acute grief. *American Journal of Psychiatry* 151(6): 155–160.

Lindsay, G., Templeton, F. (2002) Investigating coronary heart disease in patients with angina. *Professional Nurse* 17(5): 300–303.

Lip, G.Y.H. (2003) *Clinical Hypertension*. London: The Royal Society of Medicine Press Limited.

Lip, G.Y.H., Beevers, D.G. (1995) History, epidemiology and importance of atrial fibrillation. *British Medical Journal* 311(7016): 1361–1363.

Liptzin, B., Levkoff, S.E. (1992) An empirical study of delirium subtypes. *British Journal of Psychiatry* 161: 843–845.

Lookinland, S. (1995) Stress management of staff, family and patients. In W.C. Shoemaker, A.M. Ayres, A. Grenvik, P.R. Holbrook (eds) *Textbook of Critical Care*, 3rd edn. Philadelphia: W.B. Saunders Company.

Lumb, A. (2000) *Nunn's Applied Respiratory Physiology*, 5th edn. Oxford: Butterworth-Heinemann.

Lumley J. (2002) *Surface Anatomy: The Anatomical Basis of Clinical Examination*, 3rd edn. Edinburgh: Churchill Livingstone.

Lynch, M. (2001) Pain as the fifth vital sign. *Journal of Intravenous Nursing* 24(2): 285–294.

Macintyre, P., Ready, L. (1996) *Acute Pain Management: A Practical Guide*. London: Saunders.

MacLachlan, M. (1997) *Culture and Health*. Chichester: Wiley.

Macleod Clark, J. (1993) From sick nursing to health nursing: evolution or revolution. In J. Wilson Barnett, J. Macleod Clark (eds) *Research in Health Promotion and Nursing*. Macmillan: Basingstoke.

MacPherson, G. (1994) *Blacks Medical Dictionary*, 37th edn. London: A and C Black.

Macrae, W. (2001) Chronic pain after surgery. *British Journal of Anaesthesia* 87(1): 88–98.

McArdle, J. (1999) Understanding oesophageal varices. *Nursing Standard* 14(9): 46–42.

McArdle, J. (2000) The biological and nursing implications of pancreatitis. *Nursing Standard* 14(48): 46–51.

McCaffery, M. (1965) *Nursing Practice Theories Related to Cognition, Bodily Pain and Man – Environment Interactions*. Los Angeles: University of California.

McCaffery, M., Ferrel, B. (1999) Opioids and pain management. What do nurses know? *Nursing* 29(3): 48–52.

McCaffery, M., Pasero, C. (1999) *Pain Clinical Manual*, 2nd edn. St. Louis: Mosby.

McCartney, J.R. (1994) Anxiety and delirium in the Intensive Care Unit. *Critical Care Clinics of North America* 10(4): 673–680.

McClave, S.A., Sexton, L.K., Spain, D.A. *et al.* (1999) Enteral tube feeding in the intensive care unit: factors impeding adequate delivery. *Critical Care Medicine* 27(7): 1252–1256.

McConnell, E.A. (1996) The future of technology in critical care. *Critical Care Nurse* 3(suppl.): 3–16.

McGloin, H., Adam, S., Singer, M. (1999) Unexpected deaths and referrals to intensive care of patients on general wards. Are some cases potentially avoidable? *Journal of the Royal College of Physicians of London* 33(3): 255–259.

McGrath, A., Cox, C.L. (1998) Cardiac and circulatory assessment in intensive care units. *Intensive and Critical Care Nursing* 14(6): 283–287.

McKinney, A., Deeny, P. (2002) Leaving the intensive care unit: a phenomenological study of the patients' experience. *Intensive and Critical Care Nursing* 18(6): 320–331.

McLeod, G.A., Davies, H.T.O., Munnoch, N., Bannister, J., Macrae, W. (2001) Postoperative pain relief using thoracic epidural analgesia: outstanding success and disappointing failures. *Anaesthesia* 56(1): 75–81.

McMahon-Parkes, K. (1997) Management of pleural drains. *Nursing Times* 93(52): 48–52.

McNeill, H.E. (2000) Biting back at poor oral hygiene. *Intensive and Critical Care Nursing* 16(6): 367–372.

McQuay, H., Moore, A. (1998) *An Evidence-based Resource for Pain Relief*. Oxford: Oxford Medical.

McQuillan, P., Pilkington, S., Allan, A. *et al.* (1998) Confidential inquiry into quality of care before admission to intensive care. *British Medical Journal* 316(7148): 1853–1858.

McSherry, R., Haddock, J. (1999) Evidence-based health care: its place within clinical governance. *British Journal of Nursing* 8(2): 113–117.

McSherry, R., Pearce, P. (2002) *Clinical Governance*. Oxford: Blackwell Science.

McWhirter, J.P., Pennington, C.R. (1994) Incidence and recognition of malnutrition in hospital. *British Medical Journal* 308(6934): 945–948.

Malacrida, R., Bettelini, C., Degrate, A. *et al.* (1998) Reasons for dissatisfaction: a survey of relatives of intensive care patients who died. *Critical Care Medicine* 26(7): 1187–1193.

Mallett, J., Dougherty, L. (eds) (2000) *The Royal Marsden Hospital Manual of Clinical Nursing Procedures*, 5th edn. Oxford: Blackwell Science.

Mallik, M. (1997) Advocacy in nursing: a review of the literature. *Journal of Advanced Nursing* 25(1): 130–138.

Malloch, K., Porter-O'Grady, T. (1999) Partnership economics: nursing's challenge in a quantum age. *Nursing Economics* 17(6): 299–307.

Mamberg, K., Ryden, I., Efendic, S. (1995) Randomised trial of insulin-glucose infusion followed by subcutaneous insulin treatment in diabetic patients with acute myocardial infarction (Digami Study): effects on mortality at one year. *Journal of the American College of Cardiology* 26(1): 57–65.

Manias, E., Botti, M., Bucknall, T. (2002) Observation of pain assessment and management – the complexities of clinical practice. *Journal of Clinical Nursing* 11(6): 724–233.

Manley, K. (1986) The dying patient in the intensive care unit – the problems. *Care of the Critically Ill* 2(4): 152–154.

Manley, K. (1997) A conceptual framework for advanced practice: an action research project operationalizing an advanced practitioner/consultant nurse role. *Journal of Clinical Nursing* 6(3): 179–190

Manley, K. (2000) Organisational culture and consultant nurse outcomes: part 2. *Nursing Standard* 14(37): 34–39.

Manley, K., McCormack, B. (2003) Practice development: purpose, methodology, facilitation and evaluation. *Nursing in Critical Care* 8(1): 22–29.

Mann, D.V., Hershman, M.J., Hittinger, R., Glazer, G. (1994) Multicentre audit of death from acute pancreatitis. *British Journal of Surgery* 81(6): 890–893.

March, K., Mitchell, P., Grady, S., Winn, R. (1990) Effect of backrest position on intracranial and cerebral perfusion pressures. *Journal of Neuroscience Nursing* 22(6): 375–381.

Marieb, E.N. (2004) *Human Anatomy and Physiology*, 5th edn. San Fransisco: Benjamin/Cummings Publishing Company Inc.

Marinac, J.S., Mesa, L. (2000) Using a severity of illness scoring system to assess intensive care unit admissions for diabetic ketoacidosis. *Critical Care Medicine* 28(7): 2238–2241.

Martinson, B.C., O'Connor, P.J., Pronk, N.P. (2001) Physical inactivity and short-term all-cause mortality in adults with chronic disease. *Archives of Internal Medicine* 161(9): 1175–1180.

Masip, J., Betbesé, A.J., Páez, J. *et al.* (2000) Non-invasive pressure support ventilation versus conventional oxygen therapy in acute cardiogenic pulmonary oedema: a randomised trial. *Lancet* 356(9248): 2126–2132.

Matamis, D., Papanikolaou, G. (1998) Blood gas exchange. *International Journal of Intensive Care*. Winter: 125–132.

Mattice, C. (1998) The best place to stick a pulse ox sensor. *Registered Nurse* 61(5): 63–65.

Mattison, L.E., Coppage, L., Alderman, D.F., Herlong, J.A., Sahn, S.A. (1997) Pleural effusions in the medical ICU. *Chest* 111(4): 1018–1023.

Maynard, S.J., Scott, G.O., Riddell, J.W., Adgey, A.A.J. (2000) Management of acute coronary syndromes. *British Medical Journal* 321: 220–223.

Medical Device Agency (MDA) (2001) *Equipped to Care: The Safe Use of Medical Devices in the 21st Century*. London: Medical Device Agency.

Meekin, J., Allyn, W. (2001) Over exposure. *Infection Control* (Supplement): 17–19.

Mehta, S., Jay, G.D., Woolard, R.H. *et al.* (1997) Randomized, prospective trial of bilevel versus continuous positive airway pressure in acute pulmonary edema. *Critical Care Medicine* 25(4): 620–628.

Mehta, S.H., Cox, A., Hoover, D.R. *et al.* (2002) Protection against persistence of hepatitis C. *Lancet* 359(9315): 1478–1483.

Melzack, R., Wall, P. (1988) *The Challenge of Pain*, 2nd edn. London: Penguin.

Mengelkoch, L.J., Martin, D., Lawler, J. (1994) A review of the principles of pulse oximetry and accuracy of pulse oximetry estimates during exercises. *Physical Therapy* 74(1): 40–49.

Menon, D.K. (1999) Cerebral protection in severe brain injury: physiological determinants of outcome and their optimisation. *British Medical Bulletin* 55(1): 226–258.

Mergener, K., Baillic, J. (1998) Acute pancreatitis. *British Medical Journal* 316(7124): 44–48.

Merlani, P., Garnerin, P., Diby, M., Ferring, M., Ricou, B. (2001) Linking guideline to regular feedback to increase appropriate requests for clinical tests: blood gas analysis in intensive care. *British Medical Journal* 323(7313): 620–624.

Merritt, S. (2000) Putting sleep disorders to rest. *Registered Nurse* 63(7): 26–31.

Messori, A., Trippoli, S., Vaiani, M., Gorini, M., Corrado, A. (2000) Bleeding and pneumonia in intensive care patients given ranitidine and sucralfate for prevention of stress ulcer: meta-analysis of randomised controlled trials. *British Medical Journal* 321(7269): 1103–1106.

Metheny, N. (1993) Minimising respiratory complications of nasogastric tube feedings. State of the science. *Heart and Lung* 22(3): 213–222.

Meyer, T.J., Eveloff, S.E., Bauer, M.S., Schwartz, W.A., Hill, N.S., Millman, R.P. (1994) Adverse environmental conditions in the respiratory and medical ICU settings. *Chest* 105(4): 1211–1216.

Meyers, T.A., Eichhorn, D.J., Guzzetta, C.E. *et al.* (2000) Family presence during invasive procedures and resuscitation. *American Journal of Nursing* 100(2): 32–41.

Mezirow, J. (1991) *Transformational Dimensions of Adult Learning*. San Francisco: Jossey Bass.

Middleton, S., Roberts, A. (2000) *Integrated Care Pathways: A Practical Approach to Implementation*. Oxford: Butterworth-Heinemann.

Miles, M.S., Funk, S.G., Carlson, J. (1993) Parental stressor scale: neonatal intensive care unit. *Nursing Research* 42(3): 148–152.

Miller, A. (1999) Pleural therapeutic procedures. *Medicine* 27(11): 174–176.

Miller, A.C., Harvey, E. (1993) Guidelines for the management of spontaneous pneumothorax. *British Medical Journal* 307(6896): 114–116.

Mirski, M.A., Muffleman, B., Ulatowski, J.A., Hanley, D.F. (1995) Sedation for the critically ill neurologic patient. *Critical Care Medicine* 23(12): 2038–2053.

Mitcham, C. (1994) *Thinking through Technology: The Path between Engineering and Philosophy*. Chicago: University of Chicago Press.

Molter, N.C. (1979) Needs of relatives of critically ill patients: a descriptive study. *Heart and Lung* 8(2): 332–339.

Moore, A., Edwards, J., Barden, J., McQuay, H. (2003) *Bandoliers Little Book of Pain*. Oxford: Oxford University Press.

Moore, F.A., Feliciano, D.V., Andrassy, R.J. *et al.* (1992) Early enteral feeding, compared with parenteral, reduces postoperative septic complications. *Annals of Surgery* 216(2): 172–183.

Moore, T. (1998) *Patient Participation in Intensive Care*. Unpublished dissertation.

Morgan, R.J.M., Williams, F., Wright, M.M. (1997) An early warning scoring system for detecting developing critical illness. *Clinical Intensive Care* 8: 100.

Morrison, P. (1994) *Understanding Patients*. London: Baillière Tindall.

Muchinsky, P.M. (2000) *Psychology Applied to Work*. London: Wadsworth.

Mulhall, A. (2002) Nursing research and nursing practice: an exploration of two different cultures. *Intensive and Critical Care Nursing* 18(1): 48–55.

Mulvey, D.A., Mallett, S.V., Browne, D.R.G. (1993) Endotracheal intubation. *Intensive Care World* 10(3): 122–128.

Munro, M.F., Gallant, M., MacKinnon, M. *et al.* (2000) The Prince Edward Island conceptual model for nursing: a nursing perspective of primary health care. *Canadian Journal of Nursing Research* 32(1): 39–55.

Murphy, P. (1998) Respiratory system. In P. Murphy (ed.) *Handbook of Critical Care*. London: Science Press.

Murray, C., Thomas, M. (1998) How can the clinical credibility of nurse lecturers be improved? *British Journal of Nursing* 7(8): 490–492.

NAC (2001a) *Press release: National Asthma Campaign Asthma Audit reveals rise in estimated asthma prevalence – from 3.4 to 5.1 million*. London: NAC, 11 September 2001.

NAC (2001b) *Asthma Audit 2001 Summary*. London: NAC (factsheet 18).

Naftchi, N.E., Richardson, J.S. (1997) Autonomic dysreflexia: pharmacological management of hypertensive crises in spinal cord injured patients. *Journal of Spinal Cord Medicine* 20(3): 355–360.

Naidoo, J., Wills, J. (1998) *Practising Health Promotion: Dilemmas and Challenges.* London: Baillière Tindall.

Nair, K.S., Patel, R.L. (2002) Radial artery pseudoaneurysm following arterial cannulation. *Care of the Critically Ill* 18(2): 57–58.

National Health Service Executive (1996) *The Development of Nursing. Health Visiting Roles in Clinical Practice: A Contribution to the Debate.* London: North Thames NHSE.

National Health Service Executive (1998) *Integrating Theory and Practice in Nursing.* A report commissioned by the Chief Nursing Officer/Director of Nursing, July. London: Department of Health.

National Health Service Modernisation Agency (2003) *Progress in Developing Services: Critical Care Outreach.* Department of Health.

National Service Framework for coronary heart disease, at www.doh.gov.uk/nsf/chd.

National Service Framework for diabetes, at www.doh.gov.uk/nsf/diabetes.

National Outreach Forum (2002) *Interim Results.* Department of Health.

Navran, D. (1996) *The big PLUS in ethical decision making,* at http: //www.cs.bgsu.edu/maner/heuristics/1998EthicsResourceCenter1.htm (accessed 5 August 2003).

Nazroo, J. (1997) *The Health of Britain's Ethnic Minorities.* London: Policy Studies Institute.

Neil, M (1992) Community participation in Quebec's Health System: a strategy to curtail community empowerment? *International Journal of Health Services* 22(2): 287–301.

Nelson, R.A., Yu, H., Ziegler, M.G., Mills, P.J., Clausen, J.L., Dinsdale, J.E. (2001) Continuous positive airway pressure normalizes cardiac autonomic and hemodynamic responses to a laboratory stressor in apneic patients. *Chest* 119(4): 1092–1101.

Ng, A., Hall, F., Atkinson, A., Kong, K.L., Hahn, A. (2000) Bridging the analgesic gap. *Acute Pain* 3(4): 194–199.

Nicholson, J.P., Wolmarans, M.R., Park, G.R. (2000) The role of albumin in critical illness. *British Journal of Anaesthesia* 85(4): 599–610.

Nieman, W., Smith, M.J. (1999) Arrhythmias post MI. *American Journal of Nursing* (suppl.): 44–47.

Niven, N. (2000) *Health Psychology for Health Care Professionals.* Edinburgh: Churchill Livingstone.

NMC (2002a) *Code of Professional Conduct for the Nurse, Midwife and Health Visitor,* 4th edn. London: Nursing and Midwifery Council.

NMC (2002b) *PREP Handbook.* London: NMC.

Nock, S.L. (1992) *Sociology of the Family.* New Jersey: Prentice Hall.

Nolan, J., Greenwood, J., Mackintosh, A. (1998) *Cardiac Emergencies: a Pocket Guide.* London: Butterworth-Heinemann.

Norman, J., Cook, A. (2000) Medical emergencies. In M. Sheppard, M. Wright (eds) *High Dependency Nursing.* London: Baillière Tindall, pp. 213–236.

Noronha, L., Matuschak, G. (2002) Magnesium in critical illness: metabolism, assessment and treatment. *Intensive Care Medicine* 28(6): 667–669.

North, B., Reilly, P. (1994) Management and manipulation of ICP. *Current Anaesthesia and Critical Care* 5(1): 23–28.

North, N. (1995) Economics and health care. In G. Moon, R. Gillespie (eds) *Society and Health*. London: Routledge, pp. 213–225.

O'Brien, E. (2001) Blood pressure measurement is changing! *Heart* 85(1): 3–5.

Odell, M. (1996) Intracranial pressure monitoring, nursing in a district general hospital. *Nursing in Critical Care* 1(5): 245–247.

Odell, M. (2000) The patients' thoughts and feelings about their transfer from intensive care to the general ward. *Journal of Advanced Nursing* 31(2): 322–329

O'Grady, J. (1999) Acute liver failure. *Medicine* 27(1): 80–82.

Oh, T.E (2003) Oxygen therapy. In A.D. Bersten, N. Soni (eds) *Intensive Care Manual*, 5th edn. Edinburgh: Butterworth-Heinemann, pp. 275–282.

O'Hanlon-Nichols, T. (1996) Commonly asked questions about chest drains. *American Journal of Nursing* 96(5): 60–64.

O'Hanlon-Nichols, T. (1997) Basic Assessment Series: The Adult Cardiovascular System. *American Journal of Nursing* 97: 12, 34–40.

O'Hanlon-Nichols, T. (1998a) Basic Assessment Series: The Adult Pulmonary System. *American Journal of Nursing* 98: 2, 39–45.

O'Hanlon-Nichols, T. (1998b) Basic Assessment Series: Gastrointestinal System. *American Journal of Nursing* 98: 4, 48–53.

O'Malley, P., Favalovo, R., Anderson, B., Anderson, M.L., Sicove, S. Benson-Landau, M. *et al.* (1991) Critical care nurse perceptions of family needs. *Heart and Lung* 20(2): 189–201.

O'Neill, D. (2003) Using a stethoscope in clinical practice in the acute sector. *Professional Nurse* 18(7): 391–394.

O'Neill, L.J., Carter, D.E. (1998) The implications of head injury for family relationships. *British Journal of Nursing* 7(14): 842–846.

Ootim, B. (1997) Effective change. *Nursing Management* 4(2): 10.

O'Riordan, B., Gray, K., McArthur Rouse, F. (2003) Implementing a critical care course for ward nurses. *Nursing Standard* 17(20): 41–44.

Owen, S., Gould, D. (1997) Underwater seal chest drains: the patient's experience. *Journal of Clinical Nursing* 6(3): 215–225.

Oxford Pain Research Trust (2003) *Acute Pain – Conclusions.* www.jr2.ox.ac.uk/bandolier/painrest/acpnconc/acpnconc.hlml.

Page, S.R., Hall, G.M. (1999) *Diabetes: Emergency and Hospital Management.* London: BMJ Books.

Paley, J. (2000) Asthma and dualism. *Journal of Advanced Nursing* 31(6): 1293–1299.

Palfreyman, S., Tod, A., Doyle, J. (2003) Comparing evidence-based practice of nurses and physiotherapists. *British Journal of Nursing* 12(4): 246–253.

Palmer, K.R., Penman, I.D., Paterson-Brown, S. (2002) Alimentary tract and pancreatic disease. In C. Haslett, E.R. Chilvers, N.A. Boon, N.R. Colledge (eds) *Davidson's Principles and Practice of Medicine*, 19th edn. Edinburgh: Churchill Livingstone, pp. 747–830.

Pang, D., Keeenan, S.P., Cook, D.J. (1998) The effect of positive pressure airway support on mortality and the need for intubation in cardiogenic pulmonary edema. A systematic review. *Chest* 114(4): 1185–1192.

Papadopoulos, I., Tilki, M., Taylor, G. (1998) *Transcultural Care: Issues for Health Professionals*. Trowbridge: Quay Books.

Parkes, C. (1996) *Bereavement: Studies of Grief in Adult Life*. London: Penguin.

Parsons, C.L., Sole, M.L., Byers, J.F. (2000) Noninvasive positive-pressure ventilation: averting intubation of the heart failure patient. *Dimensions of Critical Care Nursing* 19(6): 18–24.

Pasero, C. (1996) Pain during sickle-cell crises. *American Journal of Nursing* 96(1): 59–60.

Payne-James, J.J., Silk, D.B.A. (1992) Can artificial nutrition support for the critically ill be improved? In M. Rennie (ed.) *Intensive Care Britain*. London: Greycoat Publishing, pp. 88–93.

Pearce, C.B., Duncan, H.D. (2002) Enteral feeding: nasogastric, nasojejunal, percutaneous endoscopic gastrostomy, or jejunostomy: it's indications and limitations. *Postgraduate Medical Journal* 78(918): 198–204.

Perez, A. (1995) Restoring electrolyte balance: hypokalaemia. *Registered Nurse* 58(12): 33–36.

Perkins, J.M.T., Galland, B.B. (1999) Venous thrombosis and pulmonary embolism. Part 1: Prevention. *Care of the Critically Ill* 15(4): 140–143.

Perkins, L.A., Shortall, S.P. (2000) Ventilation without intubation. *Registered Nurse* 63(1): 34–38.

Pierson, W. (1998) Reflection and nursing education. *Journal of Advanced Nursing* 27(1): 165–170.

Pilcher, T., Odell, M. (2000) Position statement on nurse–patient ratios in critical care. *Nursing Standard* 15(12): 38–41.

Pinger, R.R., Payne, W.A., Hahn, D.B., Hashn, E.J. (1995) *Issues for Today: Drugs*, 2nd edn. St. Louis: Mosby.

Plant, P.K., Owen, J.L., Elliott, M.W. (2001) Non-invasive ventilation in acute exacerbation of chronic obstructive pulmonary disease: long term survival and predictors of in-hospital outcome. *Thorax* 56(9): 708–712.

Platt, O.S., Brambilla, D.J., Rosse, W.F. *et al.* (1994) Mortality in sickle cell disease: life expectancy and risk factors for early death. *New England Journal of Medicine* 330(23): 1639.

Playle, J. (1995) Humanism and positivism in nursing: contradictions and conflicts. *Journal of Advanced Nursing* 22(5): 979–984.

Polderman, K.H., Girbes, A.R.J. (2002a) Central venous catheter use. Part 1: Mechanical complications. *Intensive Care Medicine* 28(1): 1–17.

Polderman, K.H., Girbes, A.R.J. (2002b) Central venous catheter use. Part 2: Infection complications. *Intensive Care Medicine* 28(1): 18–28.

Poponcik, J.M., Renston, J.P., Bennett, R.P., Emerman, C.L. (1999) Use of a ventilatory support system (BiPAP) for acute respiratory failure in the emergency department. *Chest* 116(1): 166–171.

Porter, J., Jick, H. (1980) Addiction rare in patients treated with narcotics. *New England Journal of Medicine* 302: (2) 123.

Poulter, A. (1998) The patient with Guillain–Barré syndrome: implications for critical care nursing practice. *Nursing in Critical Care* 3(4): 182–189.

Pratt, R. (2003) Prevention and control of viral hepatitis. *Nursing Standard* 17(33): 43–52.

Preston, R. (2001) Introducing non-invasive positive pressure ventilation. *Nursing Standard* 15(26): 42–45.

Priestley, J. (1999) How critical care nurses identify and meet the needs of visitors to intensive care units. *Nursing in Critical Care* 4(1): 27–29.

Pritchard, A.J.M. (1994) Tracheostomy care. *Care of the Critically Ill* 10(2): 66–69.

Provan, D., Hemson, A. (1999) *ABC of Clinical Haematology*. London: BMJ.

Puntillo, K., Weiss, S.J. (1994) Pain: its mediators and associated morbidity in critically ill cardiovascular surgical patients. *Nursing Research* 43(1): 31–36.

Pyne, R. (1998) *Professional Discipline in Nursing, Midwifery and Health Visiting*. Oxford: Blackwell Science.

Qui, C., Winblad, B., Viitanen, M., Futiglioni, L. (2003) Pulse pressure and risk of Alzheimer Disease in persons aged 75 years and older. *Stroke* 34(3): 594–599.

Quinn, S., Redman, K., Begley, C. (1996) The needs of relatives visiting adult critical care units as perceived by relatives and nurses: Part 2. *Intensive and Critical Care Nursing* 12(4): 239–245.

Rafferty, K., Smith-Coggins, R., Chen, A. (1995) Gender-associated differences in emergency department pain management. *Annals of Emergency Medicine* 26(4): 414–421.

Raper, S., Maynard, N. (1992) Feeding the critically ill patient. *British Journal of Nursing* 1(6): 273–280.

Ravenscroft, A.J., Bell, M.D.D. (2000) 'End-of-life' decision making within intensive care – objective, consistent, defensible? *Journal of Medical Ethics* 26(6): 435–440.

RCN (2000) *Clinical Governance: How Nurses can get Involved*. London: RCN.

RCN (2003) *Guidance for Nursing Skills in Critical Care*. London: RCN.

RCN Critical Care Forum (1997) *The Nature of Intensive Care Nursing Work in Intensive Care*. London: RCN.

Redeker, N.S (2000) Sleep in acute care settings: An integrated review. *Journal of Nursing Scholarship* 32(1): 31–38.

Redeker, N.S., Wykpisz, E. (1999) Effects of age on activity-rest after coronary artery bypass surgery. *Heart and Lung* 28(1): 5–14.

Redón, J., Bartolin, V., Giner, V., Lurbe, E. (2001) Assessment of blood pressure: early morning rise. *Blood Pressure Monitoring* 6(4): 207–210.

Rees, J., Kanabar, D. (2000) *ABC of Asthma*, 4th edn. London: British Medical Journal Books.

Rehtmeyer, C. (2000) Seeing change as an opportunity. In F. Bower (ed.) *Nurses Taking the Lead*. Philadelphia: W.B. Saunders Co.

Reinke, L., Hoffman, L. (2000) Asthma education: creating a partnership. *Heart and Lung* 9(3): 225–236.

Renwick, D.S., Connolly, M.J. (1995) Prevalence and treatment of chronic airways obstruction in adults over the age of 45. *Thorax* 51(2): 164–168.

Resuscitation Council (2002) *The Emergency Medical Treatment of Anaphylactic Reactions*. London: Resuscitation Council.

Rich, A., Parker, D.L. (1995) Reflection and critical incident analysis: ethical and moral implications of their use within nursing and midwifery education. *Journal of Advanced Nursing* 22(6) 1050–1057.

Rich, K. (1999) In hospital cardiac arrest: pre-event variables and nursing response. *Clinical Nurse Specialist* 13(3): 147–153.

Riordan, S., Williams, R. (1997) Bioartificial liver support: developments in hepato-cyte culture and bioreactor design. *British Medical Bulletin* 53(4): 730–744.

Rithalia, S.V.S., Farrow, P., Doran, B.R.H. (1992) Comparison of transcutaneous oxygen and carbon dioxide monitors in normal adults and critically ill patients. *Intensive and Critical Care Nursing* 8(1): 40–46.

Roache, S. (1987) *The Human Act of Caring*. Ottowa: Canadian Hospital Association.

Robb, Y.A. (1998) Family nursing in intensive care part one: is family nursing appropriate in intensive care? *Intensive and Critical Care Nursing* 14(3): 117–123.

Roberts, B.L. (2001) Managing delirium in adult intensive care patients. *Critical Care Nurse* 21(1): 48–55.

Roberts, G.A. (1986) Burnout: Psychobabble or valuable concept? *British Journal of Hospital Medicine* 36(3): 194–197

Roberts, J. (2002) The management of poorly controlled asthma. *Nursing Standard* 16(21): 45–51.

Robinson, S.M., Mackenzie-Ross, S., Campbell, H., Egleston, C., Prevost, A.T. (1998) Psychological effects of witnessed resuscitation in bereaved relatives. *Lancet* 352: 614–617

Rodwell, C.M. (1996) An analysis of the concept of empowerment. *Journal of Advanced Nursing* 23(2), 305–313.

Rogers, E., Shoemaker, F. (1971) *Communication of Innovations*. New York: Free Press.

Rogers, J., Smith, M.B. (1998) Radial artery cannulation: a serious complication. *Clinical Intensive Care* 9(3): 134–135.

Rooke, G.A. (1995) Systolic pressure variation as an indicator of hypovolaemia. *Current Opinion in Anaesthesiology* 8(6): 511–515.

Roper, N., Logan, W., Tierney, A. (2000) *Elements of Nursing: A Model for Living*, 5th edn. Edinburgh: Churchill Livingstone.

Ropper, A.H., Rockoff, M.A. (1993) Physiology and clinical aspects of raised intracranial pressure. In A.H. Ropper (ed.) *Neurological and Neurosurgical Intensive Care*. New York: Raven Press, pp. 11–27.

Rossi, S., Zanier, E.R., Mauri, I., Columbo, A., Stocchetti, N. (2001) Brain temperature, body core temperature, and intracranial pressure in acute cerebral damage. *Journal of Neurology, Neurosurgery and Psychiatry* 71(4): 448–454.

Roumen, R.M.H., Hendriks, T., Van der Ven Jongekrijk, J. *et al.* (1993) Cytokine patterns in patients after major vascular surgery, haemorrhagic shock and severe blunt trauma. Relation with subsequent adult respiratory syndrome and multiple organ failure. *Annals of Surgery* 218(6): 769–776.

Royal College of Anaesthetists (2000) In J. Lack *et al.* (eds) *Royal College of Anaesthetists Raising the Standard*. London: Royal College of Anaesthetists.

Royal College of Surgeons/Royal College of Anaesthetists (1990) *Report of the Working Party on Pain after Surgery*. London: Royal College of Surgeons and College of Anaesthetists.

Rudat, K. (1994) *Black and Minority Ethnic Groups in England: Health and Lifestyles*. London: Health Education Authority.

Rudy, E.B., Turner, B.S., Baun, M., Stone, K., Brucia, J. (1993) Endotracheal suctioning in head-injured adults. *Heart and Lung* 20(6): 667–674.

Ruggenenti, P., Lutz, J., Remuzzi, G. (1997) Pathogenesis and treatment of thrombic microangiopathy. *Kidney International* 97(150): 101.

Runcimann, W.B., Ludbrook, G.L. (1996) The measurement of systemic arterial blood pressure. In C. Prys-Roberts, B.R. Brown, Jr. (eds) *International Practice of Anaesthesia*. Oxford: Butterworth-Heinemann, pp. 2/154/1-11.

Rushforth, H., Warner, J., Burge, D., Glasper, E. (1998) Nursing physical assessment skills: implications for UK practice. *British Journal of Nursing* 7(16): 965–970.

Rushton, C.H. (1991) Humanism in critical care: a blueprint for change. *Paediatric Nursing* 17(4): 399–402.

Russo-Magno, P., O.Brien, A., Panciera, T., Rounds, S. (2001) Compliance with CPAP therapy in older men with obstructive sleep apnea. *Journal of the American Geriatrics Society* 49(9): 1205–1211.

Ryder, S.D., Beckingham, I.J. (2001) Acute hepatitis. *British Medical Journal* 322(7279): 151–153.

Sakka, S.G., Klein, M., Reinhart, K., Meier-Hellmann, A. (2002) Prognostic value of extravascular lung water in critically ill patients. *Chest* 122(6): 2080–2086.

Salukhe, T.V., Wyncoll, D.L.A. (2002) Volumetric haemodynamic monitoring and continuous pulse contour analysis – an untapped resource for coronary and high dependency care units? *British Journal of Cardiology* 9(1 AIC): 20–25.

Santamaria, J.D. (1997) Acute pancreatitis. In T.E. Oh (ed.) *Intensive Care Manual*, 4th edn. Oxford: Butterworth-Heinemann, pp. 337–343.

Sauty, A., Uldry, C., Debétaz, L.-F., Leuenberger, P., Fitting, J.-W. (1996) Differences in PO_2 and PCO_2 between arterial and arterialized earlobe samples. *European Respiratory Journal* 9(2): 186–189.

Say, J. (1997) Nutritional assessment in clinical practice: a review. *Nursing in Critical Care* 2(1): 29–33.

Saylor, C. (1990) Reflection and professional education: art, science and competency. *Nurse Educator* 15(2): 8–11.

Scally, G., Donaldson, L.J. (1998) Clinical governance and the drive for quality improvement in the new NHS in England. *British Medical Journal* 317(7150): 61–65.

Scanlan, J.M., Chernomas, W.M. (1997) Developing the reflective teacher. *Journal of Advanced Nursing* 25(6): 1138–1143.

Schafheutle, E.I., Cantrill, J.A., Noyce, P.R. (2001) Why is pain management suboptimal on surgical wards? *Journal of Advanced Nursing* 33(6): 728–737.

Schierhout, G., Roberts, I. (1998) Fluid resuscitation with colloid or crystalloid solution in critically ill patients: a systematic review of randomised trials. *British Medical Journal* 316(7136): 961–964.

Schilling, R.J. (1994) Should relatives watch resuscitation? *British Medical Journal* 309(6951): 406.

Schiodt, F.V., Atillasoy, E., Shakil, A.O. *et al.* (1999) Etiology and outcome for 295 patients with acute liver failure in the United States. *Liver Transplantation and Surgery* 5(1): 29–34.

Schira, M. (2000) Renal assessment and diagnostic procedures. In L.D. Urden, K.M. Stacy (eds) *Priorities in Critical Care Nursing*, 3rd edn. St. Louis: Mosby.

Schofield, P. (2003) Pain assessment: how far have we come in listening to our patients? *Professional Nurse* 18(5) 276–279.

Schön, D.A. (1983) *The Reflective Practitioner*. New York: Basic Books.

Schön, D.A. (1991) *The Reflective Practitioner: How Professionals Think in Action*. Aldershot: Avebury.

Schön, D.A. (1995) The new scholarship requires a new epistemology. *Change* 27: 26–34.

Schulman, S.P., Fessler, H.E. (2001) Management of acute coronary syndromes. *American Journal of Respiratory and Critical Care Medicine* 164(6): 917–922.

Scott, A., Skerratt, S., Adam, S. (1998) *Nutrition for the Critically Ill*. London: Arnold.

Seaton, A.D., Leitch, A.G., Seaton, D. (2000) Clinical aspects. In *Crofton and Douglas's Respiratory Diseases*, 5th edn. London: Blackwell Science.

Seaton-Mills, D. (1999) Acute renal failure: causes and considerations in the critically ill patient. *Nursing in Critical Care* 4(6): 293–297.

Seers, K. (1987) Perceptions of pain. *Nursing Times* 83(48): 37–39.

Selye, H. (1956) *The Stress of Life*. New York: McGraw Hill Book Company.

Seneviratne, U. (2000) Guillain–Barré syndrome. *Postgraduate Medical Journal* 76(902): 774–782.

Serra, A. (2000) Tracheostomy care. *Nursing Standard* 14(42): 45–55.

Sevransky, J.E., Haponik, E.F (2003) Respiratory failure in elderly patients. *Clinical Geriatric Medicine* 19(1): 205–224.

Shah, S. (1999) Neurological assessment. *Nursing Standard* 13: 22, 49–56.

Shakil, A.O., Mazariegos, G.V., Kramer, D.J. (1999) Fulminant hepatic failure. *Surgical Clinics of North America* 79(1): 77–107.

Shapiro, C.M. (1993) *The ABC of Sleep Disorders*. London: British Medical Association.

Sharara, A.L. (2001) Gastroesophageal variceal hemorrhage. *New England Journal of Medicine* 345(9): 669–681.

Sharma, S. (2003) Respiratory failure, *Emedicine*, http: //www.emedicine.com/med/topic2011.htm accessed 20 May 2003.

Shaukat, N., Lear, J., Fletcher, S., de Bono, D., Woods, K.L. (1997) First myocardial infarction in patients of Indian subcontinent and European origin: comparison of risk factors, management and long term outcome. *British Medical Journal* 314(7125): 639–642.

Shaw, M. (1997) *Assessment Made Incredibly Easy*. Pennsylvania: Springhouse Corporation.

Shiotani, A., Graham, D.Y. (2002) Pathogenesis and therapy of gastric and duodenal ulcer disease. *Medical Clinics of North America* 86(6): 1447–1466.

Short, A., Cumming, A. (1999) Renal support. *British Medical Journal* 319(1): 41–44.

Shuldham, C. (1998) *Cardiorespiratory Nursing*. Cheltenham: Stanley Thornes.

Sikes, D.H., Ahrawal, N.M., Zhao, W.W., Kent, J.D., Recker, D.P., Verburg, K.M. (2002) Incidence of gastroduodenal ulcers associated with valecoxib compared with that of ibuprofen and diclofenac in patients with osteoathritis. *European Journal of Gastroenterology and Hepatology* 14(10): 1101–1111.

Sim, K.M. (2002) Respiratory emergencies. *Anaesthesia and Intensive Care Medicine* 3(11): 410–413.

Simmonds, P., Smith, D.B. (1999) Hepatitis C and G viruses – old or new? In A.G.

Dalgleish, R.A. Weiss (eds) *HIV and the New Viruses*, 2nd edn. San Diego: Academic Press, pp. 459–483.

Simpson, H. (2001) Diabetes and intensive care – medical management. *Care of the Critically Ill* 17(6): 194–197.

Simpson, T., Lee, E.R., Camaron, S. (1996) Relationships among sleep dimensions and factors that impair sleep after cardiac surgery. *Research in Nursing and Health* 19(3): 213–223.

Sin, D.D., Logan, A.G., Fitzgerald, F.S., Liu, P.P., Bradley, T.D. (2000) Effects of continuous positive airway pressure on cardiovascular outcomes in heart failure patients and without Cheyne-Stokes respiration. *Circulation* 102(1): 61–66.

Skowronski, G.A. (2003) Neuromuscular disease in intensive care. In A.D. Bersten, N. Soni (eds) *Intensive Care Manual*, 4th edn. Edinburgh: Butterworth-Heinemann, pp. 537–547.

Sleight, P. (1999) Acute myocardial infarction – diagnosis. In A.R. Webb, M. Shapiro, M. Singer, P.M. Suter (eds) *Oxford Textbook of Critical Care*. Oxford: Oxford University Press, pp. 201–203.

Smaha, D.A. (2001) Asthma emergency care: national guidelines summary. *Heart and Lung* 30(6): 472–474.

Smith, G. (2000) *ALERT: A Multiprofessional Course in Care of the Acutely Ill Patient*. University of Portsmouth.

Smith, P.M. (2000) Portal hypertension. *Surgery* 18(7): 153–156.

Smith, S.J (1993) Suctioning the airway. *Emergency* 25(3): 41–45.

Snell, C.C., Fothergill-Bourbonnais, F., Durocher-Henriks, S. (1997) Patient controlled analgesia and intramuscular injections: a comparison of patient pain experiences and postoperative outcomes. *Journal of Advanced Nursing* 25(4): 681–690.

Snowball, J. (1996) Asking nurses about advocating for patients: 'reactive' and 'proactive' accounts. *Journal of Advanced Nursing* 24(1): 67–75.

Somauroo, J.D., Wilkinson, M., White, V.J. *et al.* (2000) Effect of nasal bilevel positive airway pressure (BiPAP) and continuous positive airway pressure (CPAP) ventilation on cardiac haemodynamics in patients with congestive heart failure. *Heart* 83(suppl. II): A20.

Somerson, S., Craig, H., Somerson, S., Sicilia, M. (1996) Mastering emergency airway management: The skills you need to help your patient survive a code blue. *American Journal of Nursing* 96(5): 24–30.

Soni, N. (1995) Wonderful albumin? *British Medical Journal* 310(6984): 887–888.

Southwell, M.T., Wistow, G.S. (1995) Sleep in hospitals at night: are patient's needs being met? *Journal of Advanced Nursing* 21(6): 1101–1109.

Spencer, L. (1994) How do nurses deal with their own grief when a patient dies on an intensive care unit, and what help can be given to enable them to overcome their grief effectively? *Journal of Advanced Nursing* 19(6): 1141–1150.

Sprung, C.L. (1990) Changing attitudes and practices in foregoing life-sustaining treatments. *JAMA* 263(16): 2211–2215.

Stanley, A.J., Hayes, P.C. (1997) Portal hypertension and variceal haemorrhage. *Lancet* 350(9036): 1235–1239.

Stannard, C., Booth, S. (1998) *Churchill's Pocket Book of Pain*. London: Churchill Livingstone.

Steed, H.L., Capstick, V., Flood, C., Schepansky, A., Schultz, J., Mayes, D.C. (2002) A randomized controlled trial of early verses 'traditional' postoperative oral intake after major abdominal gynecologic surgery. *American Journal of Obstetrics and Gynecology* 186(5): 861–865.

Steinberg, W., Tenner, S. (1994) Acute pancreatitis. *New England Journal of Medicine* 330(17): 1198–1209.

Stenhouse, C., Coates, S., Tivey, M., Allsop, P., Parker, T. (2000) prospective evaluation of a modified early warning score to aid earlier detection of patients developing critical illness on a surgical ward. *British Journal of Anaesthesia* 84: 663.

Stocklmann, H.B.A.C., Hiemstra, C.A., Marquet, R.L., Jzermans, J.N.M. (2000) Extracorporeal perfusion for the treatment of acute liver failure. *Annals of Surgery* 231(4): 460–470.

Stone, K.S. (1991) The effect of lung hyperinflation and endotrachael suctioning on cardiopulmonary haemodynamics. *Nursing Research* 40: 315.

Storer, J. (1996) The liver. In S.M. Hinchliff, S.E. Montague, R. Watson (eds) *Physiology for Nursing Practice*, 2nd edn. London: Baillière Tindall, pp. 504–529.

Storey, N. (2001) What is clinical governance? *Bulletin* 1(12): 1–9.

Strickland, W.J., Strickland, D.L. (1996) Partnership building with special populations. *Family Community Health* 19(3): 21–34.

Strunin, L., Rowbotham, D., Miles, A. (1999) *The Effective Management of Post-Operative Nausea and Vomiting*. London: Aesculapius Medical Press.

Subbe, C.P., Kruger, M., Rutherford, P., Gemmel, L. (2001) Validation of a modified Early Warning Score in medical admissions. *Quarterly Journal of Medicine* 94(10): 521–526.

Suerbaum, S., Michetti, P. (2002) *Helicobacter Pylori* infection. *New England Journal of Medicine* 347(15): 1175–1186.

Sung, J. (1997) Acute gastrointestinal bleeding. In T.E. Oh (ed.) *Intensive Care Manual*, 4th edn. Oxford: Butterworth-Heinemann, pp. 329–336.

Sutcliffe, J. (1997) Assessment of cerebral function. In D.R. Goldhill, P.S. Withington (eds) *Textbook of Intensive Care*. London: Chapman and Hall, pp. 631–637.

Swartz, M. (2002) *Textbook of Physical Diagnosis – History and Examination*. Philadelphia: W.B. Saunders.

Swearingen, P., Keen, J. (2001) *Manual of Critical Care Nursing*, 4th edn. St. Louis: Mosby.

Tang, A., Hooper, T., Ragheb, H. (1999) A regional survey of chest drains: evidence-based practice? *Postgraduate Medical Journal* 75(886): 471–474.

Tannahill, A. (1985) What is health promotion? *Health Education Journal* 44(4): 167–168.

Taylor, B. (1994) *Being Human: Ordinariness in Nursing*. Melbourne: Churchill Livingstone.

Teasdale, G., Jennett, B. (1974) Assessment of coma and impaired consciousness. *Lancet* ii(7872) 81–83.

Teasdale, K. (1998) *Advocacy in Health Care*. Oxford: Blackwell Science.

Teekman, B. (2000) Exploring reflective thinking in nursing. *Journal of Advanced Nursing* 31(5): 1125–1135.

Terman, M., Lewy, A.J., Dijk, D., Boulous, Z., Eastman, C.L., Campbell, S.S. (1995)

Light treatment for sleep disorders: Consensus report. *Journal of Biological Rhythms* 10(2): 135–147.

Thabut, G., Thabut, D., Myers, R.P. *et al.* (2002) Thrombolytic therapy of pulmonary embolism. *Journal of the American College of Cardiology* 40(9): 1660–1667.

Tham, T.C.K., Collins, J.S.A. (2000) *Gastrointestinal Emergencies*. London: British Medical Journal Books.

Thangathurai, D., Charbonnet, C., Roessler, P., Wo, C.C., Yorhida, R., Shoemaker, W.C. (1997) Continuous intraoperative noninvasive cardiac output monitoring using a new thoracic bioimpedance device. *Journal of Cardiothoracic and Vascular Anaesthesia* 11(4): 440–444.

Therapondos, G., Hayes, O.C. (2002) Management of gastro-oesophageal varices. *Clinical Medicine* 2(4): 297–302.

Thomas, H.C. (1999) Hepatitis B and D. *Surgery* 27(1): 34–36.

Thomas, V., Wilson-Barnett, J., Goodhart, F. (1998) The role of cognitive-behavioural therapy in the management of pain in patients with sickle cell disease. *Journal of Advanced Nursing* 27(5): 1002–1009.

Thompson, C.S., Ashley, J., Smith, D.L. (1999) Arterialised earlobe blood gases: use for LTOT prescription. *Thorax* 55(Suppl. 3): A77.

Thompson, L. (2000) *Suctioning Adults with an Artificial Airway*. The Josanna Briggs Institute for Evidence Based Nursing and Midwifery, Systemic Review, No. 9.

Thomson, C. (2002) The value of research in clinical decision-making. *Nursing Times* 98(42): 30–34.

Tigner, R. (1998) Handling a sickle cell crisis. *Registered Nurse* July 61(7): 32–35.

Tingle, J. (2002a) Clinical negligence and the need to keep professionally updated. *British Journal of Nursing* 11(20): 1304–1306.

Tingle, J. (2002b) The professional standard of care in clinical negligence. *British Journal of Nursing* 11(19): 1267–9.

Tingle, J., Cribb, A. (1995) *Nursing, Law and Ethics*, 2nd edn. Oxford: Blackwell Science.

Todd, N. (1997) The physiological knowledge required by nurses caring for patients with unstable angina. *Nursing in Critical Care* 2(4): 17–24.

Tones, K. (1991) Health promotion, empowerment and the psychology of control. *Journal of the Institute of Health Education* 29(1): 17–26.

Topf, M., Thompson, S. (2001) Interactive relationships between hospital patients' noise-induced stress and other stress with sleep. *Heart and Lung* 30(4): 237–243.

Treadwell, L., Mendelow, D., Head Injury Audit Team (1994) Audit of head injury management in the northern region. *British Journal of Nursing* 3(3): 136–140.

Turk, D., Melzack, R. (2001) *Handbook of Pain Assessment*. London: The Guildford Press.

Turner, S. (2001) NT practice solutions. *Nursing Times* 97(40): 41.

Uhl, W., Isenmann, R., Buchler, M.W. (1998) Infections complicating pancreatitis: diagnosing, treating, preventing. *New Horizons* 6(Suppl. 2): S72–S79.

Uhl, W., Buchler, M.W., Malfertheiner, P., Begar, H.G., Adler, G., Gaus, W. (1999) A randomised, double-blind, multicentre trial of octreotide in moderate to severe acute pancreatitis. *Gut* 45(1): 97–104.

Upton, D. (1999) How can we achieve evidence-based practice if we have a theory–practice gap in nursing today? *Journal of Advanced Nursing* 29(3): 549–555.

Urden, L.D., Stacy, K.M. (eds) (1999) *Priorities in Critical Care Nursing*, 3rd edn. St. Louis: Mosby.

van den Berghe, G. (2000) Euthyroid sick syndrome. *Current Opinion in Anaesthesiology* 13(2): 89–92.

van den Berghe, G., Wouters, P., Weekers, F. *et al.* (2001) Intensive insulin therapy in critically ill patients. *New England Journal of Medicine* 345(19): 1359–1367.

van Welzen, M., Carey, T. (2002) Autonomic dysreflexia: guidelines for practice. *Connect* 2(1): 13–21.

Vargas, H.E., Gerber, D., Abu-Elmagd, K. (1999) Management of portal hypertension-related bleeding. *Surgical Clinics of North America* 79(1): 1–22.

Vespa, P. (1998) Neurological complications of critical medical illness and transplantation. *Current Opinion in Critical Care* 4(2): 69–75.

Vianello, A., Bevilacqua, M., Arcaro, G., Gallan, F., Serra, E. (2000) Non-invasive ventilatory approach to treatment of acute respiratory failure in neuromuscular disorders. A comparison with endotracheal intubation. *Intensive Care Medicine* 26(4): 384–390.

Wahr, J.A., Tremper, K.K. (1996) Oxygen measurement and monitoring techniques. In C. Prys-Roberts, B.R. Brown (eds) *International Practice of Anaesthesia*. Oxford: Butterworth-Heinemann.

Wainright, S.P., Gould, D. (1996) Endotracheal suctioning: an example of the problems of relevance and rigor in clinical research. *Journal of Clinical Nursing* 5(6): 389–398.

Waldmann, C., Thyveetil, D. (1998) Management of head injury in a district general hospital. *Care of the Critically Ill* 14(2): 65–69.

Wall, P.D., Melzack, R.W. (1999) *Textbook of Pain*, 4th edn. Edinburgh: Churchill Livingstone.

Wallace, D. (1996) Using reflective diaries to assess students. *Nursing Standard* 10(36): 44–47.

Walsh, M. (1997) Accountability and intuition: justifying nursing practice. *Nursing Standard* 11(23): 39–41.

Walsh, M. (2000) *Nursing Frontiers: Accountability and the Boundaries of Care*. Oxford: Butterworth-Heinemann.

Walsh, M. (2002) Caring for the patient with a disorder of the renal system. In M. Walsh (ed.) *Watson's Clinical Nursing and Related Sciences*, 6th edn. London: Baillière Tindall.

Walsh, M., Ford, P. (1989) *Nursing Rituals*. Oxford: Butterworth-Heinemann.

Walters, A.J. (1995) The life world of relatives of critically ill patients: a phenomenological hermeneutic study. *International Journal of Nursing Practice* 1: 18–25.

Ward V., Wilson, J., Taylor, L., Cookson, B., Glynn, A. (1997) *Hospital-Acquired Infection; Surveillance, Policies and Practice. Preventing Hospital Acquired Infection, Clinical Guidelines*. London: Public Health Laboratory Service.

Waterworth, S., Luker, K.A. (1990) Reluctant collaborators: do patients want to be involved in decisions concerning care? *Journal of Advanced Nursing* 15(8): 971–976.

Watson, J. (1999) *Post Modern Nursing and Beyond*. New York: Churchill Livingstone.

Watson, R. (2000a) Assessing pulmonary function in older people. *Nursing Older People* 12(8): 27–28.

Watson, R. (2000b) *Anatomy and Physiology for Nurses*, 11th edn. Edinburgh: Baillière Tindall.

Waugh, A., Grant, A. (2001) *Anatomy and Physiology in Health and Illness*, 9th edn. Edinburgh: Churchill Livingstone.

Weatherall, D. (1999) Genetic disorders of haemoglobin. In A. Hoffbrand, S. Lewis, E. Tuddenham (eds) *Post Graduate Haematology*, 4th edn. Oxford: Butterworth-Heinemann.

Weeks, S.K., O'Connor, P.C. (1994) Concept analysis of family and health: a new definition of family health. *Rehabilitation Nursing* 19(4): 207–210

Weiskittle, P.D. (2001) Renal urinary dysfunctions. In P.L. Swearingen, J.H. Keen (eds) *Manual of Critical Care Nursing*, 4th edn. St. Louis: Mosby.

Welch, J. (2000) Using assessment to identify and prevent critical illness. *Nursing Times* 96(20): 3–4.

Welie, J., Welie, S. (2001) Patient decision-making competence: Outlines of a conceptual analysis. *Medicine, Health Care and Philosophy* 4(2): 127–138.

Welsh, F.K.S., Farmery, S.M., MacLennan, K. *et al.* (1998) Gut barrier function in malnourished patients. *Gut* 42(3): 396–401.

Weston, C. (1996) Current status of thrombolytic therapy. Part 1: Acute myocardial infarction and unstable angina. *Care of the Critically Ill* 12(3): 106–108.

White, R.D. (1996) Enhanced neonatal intensive care design: A physiological approach. *Journal of Perinatology* 16: 381–384.

Whitehead, D. (2000) Health promoting clinical practice and its related educational issues: towards a common consensus. *Advancing Clinical Nursing* 3(4): 156–161.

Whittaker, J., Ball, C. (2000) Discharge from intensive care: a view from the ward. *Intensive and Critical Care Nursing* 16(3): 135–143.

WHO (1986) *Ottawa Charter for Health Promotion*. Geneva: World Health Organisation.

WHO (1996) *Cancer Pain Relief*, 2nd edn. Geneva: World Health Organisation.

Wiessner, W., Casey, I., Zhilut, J. (1995) Treatment of sepsis and septic shock: A review. *Heart and Lung* 24(5): 380–392.

Wigfull, J., Welchew, E. (2001) Survey of 1057 patients receiving postoperative patient-controlled epidural analgesia. *Anaesthesia* 56(1): 70–75.

Wilkes, M.M., Navickis, R.J. (2001) Patient survival after human albumin administration. A meta-analysis of randomized, controlled trials. *Annals of Internal Medicine* 135(3): 205–208.

Wilkinson, J. (1999) Implementing reflective practice. *Nursing Standard* 13, 36–40.

Wilkinson, P. (1995) A qualitative study to establish the self-perceived needs of family members of patients in a general intensive care unit. *Intensive and Critical Care Nursing* 11(2): 77–86.

Wilson, C., Imrie, C.W. (1991) Systemic effects of acute pancreatitis. In C.D. Johnson, C.W. Imrie (eds) *Pancreatic Disease: Progress and Prospects*. Berlin: Springer-Verlag, pp. 287–297.

Wilson, J., Tingle, J. (1999) *Clinical Risk Modification: A Route to Clinical Governance*. Oxford: Butterworth-Heinemann.

Windsor, A.C., Kanwar, S., Li, A.G.K. *et al.* (1998) Compared with parenteral nutrition, enteral feeding attenuates the acute phase response and improves disease severity in acute pancreatitis. *Gut* 42(3): 431–435.

Winer, J.B. (1994) Diagnosis and treatment of Guillain–Barré syndrome. *Care of the Critically Ill* 10(1): 23–25.

Wirtz, K.M., La Favor, K.M., Ang, R. (1996) Managing chronic spinal cord injury: issues in critical care. *Critical Care Nurse* 16(4): 24–37.

Withington, P.S. (1997) Acute severe head injury. In D.R. Goldhill, P.S. Withington (eds) *Textbook of Intensive Care*. London: Chapman and Hall Medical, pp. 621–629.

Wood, C. (1998) Endotracheal suctioning: a literature review. *Intensive and Critical Care Nursing* 14(3): 124–136.

Woodrow, P. (1997) Ethical and Legal. Nurse advocacy: is it in the patient's best interests? *British Journal of Nursing* 6(4): 225–229.

Woodrow, P. (1999) Pulse oximetry. *Nursing Standard* 13(42): 42–46.

Woodrow, P. (2000) *Intensive Care Nursing: A Framework for Practice*. London: Routledge.

Wright, B. (1991) *Sudden Death. Intervention Skills for the Caring Professionals*. Edinburgh: Churchill Livingstone.

Wright, B. (1996) *Sudden Death. A Research Base for Practice*, 2nd edn. Edinburgh: Churchill Livingstone.

Wright, I.O. (1998) Esophageal varices: implications and treatment. *Gastroenterology Nursing* 21(1): 2–5.

Wright, L.M., Leahey, M. (1994) *Nurses and Families*. Philadelphia: F.A. Davies Company.

Wyncoll, D.L. (1999) The management of severe acute necrotizing pancreatitis: an evidence-based review of the literature. *Intensive Care Medicine* 25(2): 146–156.

Wyncoll, D.L.A. (2003) Management of acute poisoning. In A.D. Bersten, N. Soni (eds) *Intensive Care Manual*, 5th edn. Edinburgh: Butterworth-Heinemann, pp. 823–832.

Yates, D.W., Elison, G., McGuiness, S. (1990) Care of the suddenly bereaved. *British Medical Journal* 301(6742): 29–31.

Yin, A.T., Bradley, T.D., Liu, P.P. (2001) The role of continuous positive airway pressure in the treatment of congestive heart failure. *Chest* 120(5): 1675–1685.

Young, K.K., Oh, T.E. (1997) Diabetic emergencies. In T.E. Oh (1997) *Intensive Care Manual*, 4th edn. Butterworth-Heinemann, pp. 443–450.

Yu, N., Nardella, A., Pechet, L. (2000) Screening tests for disseminated intravascular coagulation: guidelines for rapid and specific laboratory diagnosis. *Critical Care Medicine* 28(6): 1777–1780.

Zacharisen, M.C. (2002) Occupational asthma. *Medical Clinics of North America* 86(5): 951–972.

Zarzaur, B.L., Fukatsu, K., Kudsk, K.A. (2000) The influence of nutrition on mucosal immunology and endothelial cell adhesion molecules. In J.-L. Vincent (ed.) *Yearbook of Intensive Care and Emergency Medicine*. Berlin: Springer, pp. 63–71.

Zwarenstein, M., Atkins, J., Barr, H., Hammich, M., Koppel, I., Reeves, S. (1999) A systematic review of interprofessional education. *Journal of Interprofessional Care* 13(4): 417–424.

Index

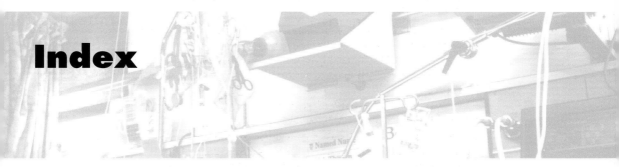

Page numbers in *italic* refer to figures and tables: **emboldened** numbers to 'boxed' text